The New Medicine

CARDIOLOGY

The New Medicine

An Integrated System of Study

The New Medicine

An Integrated System of Study

Series Editors R. Harden and A. Marcus

Volume 3

CARDIOLOGY

Edited by Hamish Watson

The New Medicine Series has been produced in collaboration with Update Publications Limited

SPRINGER-SCIENCE+BUSINESS MEDIA, B.V.

Published by
MTP Press Limited
Falcon House
Lancaster, England

British Library Cataloguing in Publication Data

Watson, Hamish
    Cardiology.—(The New medicine)
    1. Cardiology
    I. Title II. Series
    616.1′2   RC681

ISBN 978-0-85200-403-6   ISBN 978-94-011-7251-6 (eBook)
DOI 10.1007/978-94-011-7251-6

Typeset by Servis Filmsetting Ltd., Manchester

CONTENTS

LIST OF CONTRIBUTORS

EDITOR

Hamish Watson, TD, MD, FRCP, FRCPE
Chairman, Section of Cardiology, Department of
Medicine; Postgraduate Dean and Director of
Postgraduate Medical Education, University of
Dundee: Consultant Cardiologist, Tayside Area,
Scotland

CONTRIBUTORS

J.S. Davidson, BSC, PHD
Lately Senior Lecturer, Department of Physiology,
University of Dundee, Scotland (now at University of
Calgary, Canada)

D. Emslie-Smith, MD, FRCP, FRCPE
Reader in Medicine, University of Dundee; Honorary
Consultant Physician, Ninewells Hospital, Dundee,
Scotland

Mary Fulton, MB, CHB, DPH, FRCPE, FFCM
Senior Lecturer, Department of Community Medicine,
University of Edinburgh, Scotland

R.J. Kellet, MA, MB, BCH, FRCP
Consultant Physician, Eastern General Hospital,
Edinburgh, Scotland

A.R. Lorimer, MD, FRCP, FRCPG
Consultant Cardiologist, Royal Infirmary, Glasgow,
Scotland

K.G. Lowe, CVO, MD, FRCP, FRCPE, FRCPG
Honorary Professor of Medicine, University of Dundee;
Consultant Physician, Ninewells Hospital, Dundee,
Scotland

J.B. McGuinness, MD, FRCP, FRCPG
Consultant Physician, Victoria Infirmary, Glasgow,
Scotland

D. Maclean, PH.D, MB, CHB, FRCPE
Senior Lecturer in Pharmacology and Therapeutics,
University of Dundee; Honorary Consultant Physician,
Ninewells Hospital, Dundee, Scotland

G.P. McNeill, PHD, MB, CHB, MRCPE
Consultant Physician, Ninewells Hospital, Dundee,
Scotland

H.C. Miller, BSC, MB, CHB, FRCPE
Consultant Cardiologist, Royal Infirmary, Edinburgh,
Scotland

D.N. Ross, BSC, MB, CHB, FRCS
Director, Department of Surgery, Institute of
Cardiology; Consultant Surgeon, National Heart
Hospital, London, England

G.B. Shaw, CBE, BSC, MB, CHB, FRCP, FRCPE, FRCPG
Consultant Physician and Cardiologist, Southern
General Hospital, Glasgow, Scotland

M.G. Walker, CHM, FRCSE
Senior Lecturer in Surgery, University of Dundee;
Honorary Consultant Surgeon, Ninewells Hospital,
Dundee, Scotland

W.F. Walker, DSC, CHM, FRCS, FRCSE
Honorary Reader in Surgery, University of Dundee;
Consultant Surgeon, Ninewells Hospital, Dundee,
Scotland

Hamish Watson, TD, MD, FRCP, FRCPE
Consultant Cardiologist, Ninewells Hospital, Dundee,
Scotland

SERIES EDITORS

Professor R. McG. Harden, MD, FRCP(GLAS)
Centre for Medical Education
Ninewells Hospital and Medical School
University of Dundee
Scotland

Dr A. Marcus, MB, BCH
Chairman
Update Publications Ltd
London
England

CO-ORDINATING EDITOR

Dr R. Cairncross
Centre for Medical Education
Ninewells Hospital and Medical School
University of Dundee
Scotland

INTRODUCTION

The need for a new approach to textbooks

Many books have been written for students of medicine. The conventional textbook, however, imposes many constraints upon the reader and the author. While a considerable effort has been put into developing newer, more sophisticated methods of learning such as television, audio-tape and slides, and computers, few attempts have been made to improve the more traditional approach – the book. The aim of this series of textbooks is to minimize the limitations of the standard text and to maximize the usefulness of the book as an aid to learning.

We believe that in a number of ways this series is unique. It is the first textbook to be produced as a collaborative project between a publisher and a University Department of Medical Education. The intenton has been to produce a series of textbooks which take into account three significant trends in medical education: a move towards a more integrated approach to teaching, an increased emphasis on student-centred learning, and greater use of problem-based learning.

A more integrated text

Firstly, there is a general move to a more integrated approach to learning, a trend reflected in the curricula of many schools. This involves a shift from subject- or discipline-based teaching where the emphasis is on the individual subjects or disciplines such as medicine, surgery and therapeutics, to a multi-disciplinary or integrated approach where the student is encouraged to take a more holistic view of medicine and to learn the appropriate medicine, surgery or therapeutics in relation to each system such as the cardiovascular system, respiratory system, etc. Unfortunately, textbooks, in general, have not kept pace with these developments and many textbooks still look at medicine from the point of view of each separate discipline. Patients, however, present to the doctor with symp-toms such as abdominal pain, or swellings in the neck, and don't come neatly labelled as a surgical case or a medical case. The examination of the patient, and his further investigation and management, must take into account both 'medical' and 'surgical' pathologies. The advantages and indications for medical treatment must be reviewed alongside those of surgical intervention. This series of medical textbooks presents such an integrated view of medicine and has been written by a multi-disciplinary team.

One approach to the production of an integrated textbook is to ask a series of specialists from different backgrounds each to prepare a chapter or section looking at the subject from his own view point. Unfortunately, such a strategy frequently results in a disjointed look at the subject and the juxtaposition of sections written by a surgeon, a physician and a general practitioner is a poor substitute for a truly integrated book.

In this book the contributors have worked together as a team, planning and writing the book under the direction of an editor. As a group they have taken overall responsibility for its contents. It is hoped that the result will be a more meaningful integration of the subjects.

A useful aid to the student

A second trend in medical education is the move towards more student-centred learning where the emphasis is on the student and what he learns rather than what he is taught. This is a move away from a more teacher-centred approach when the emphasis is on the teacher and what he teaches.

A student-centred approach results in more effective learning and prepares the student better for his continuing education or life-long learning. This series of books has been designed to provide the teacher and the student with an effective resource for learning. It can be used as a basis for a course where the emphasis is on independent learning, as a resource to provide background information for small group work and as a text for use in relation to a lecture course.

Each volume contains questions relating to the content of the volume. The reader can use these to assess his knowledge of the subject. They can be used either before or after he reads the relevant sections of the book. The reader by trying to answer the questions can obtain an indication as to the extent to which he has mastered the subject and to which further reading is necessary.

A more problem-based approach to medicine

A third trend in medical education is the move towards a more problem-based approach to learning. In the past the emphasis in medical education has been placed on the teaching of facts about patients and their diseases rather than on the application of the facts and the use of the information to solve problems relating to patients. To take account of this trend, each volume in the series contains a section which looks at how patients present with problems relating to the system under consideration. It is hoped that this will encourage a more problem-based approach to medicine and provide a resource which can be used in more problem-based curricula.

Format of books

The volumes in the series have a standard format. Each volume has five sections and each section tackles the subject from a different direction. Section one presents appropriate background information and briefly reviews the relevant general anatomy, physiology, biochemistry, pathology and epidemiology. Section two considers how to take a history from a patient and conduct a physical examination in relation to the system under consideration. Section three discusses the investigation and management of the common clinical presentations and leads to a series of differential diagnoses. Section four considers the diseases relating to the system and discusses their management. Section five covers in more detail some aspects of the pharmacology and therapeutics.

For whom is the text intended?

Undergraduate students can use the books in this series as they work their way through the curriculum. The series will be of value not only in schools with integrated curricula but in more traditional schools. The texts will provide the necessary information on each subject while at the same time encouraging the student to relate the various subjects he is studying one to another. While the books will be of particular value in the later years of the cirriculum, they can also serve to introduce students to medicine in the earlier years. Many teachers have attempted in recent years to introduce a more clinical approach in the early phases of the medical school curriculum and to relate the basic and paramedical sciences to clinical medicine. This series has been designed to encourage the student to relate the medical sciences to the practice of medicine.

The series also has a place in postgraduate and continuing education. For postgraduate students the series can serve as introductory texts in each area. For doctors who have completed their vocational training, it can provide a useful and up-to-date review of medicine. While participation in courses, attendance at meetings, reading of journals and interaction with colleagues are all useful in continuing medical education, a readily available reference source is also necessary. This series of books can be used for this purpose.

SECTION I

Background to Cardiovascular Disease

MORTALITY AND MORBIDITY

Cardiovascular diseases are common causes of death, illness and disability particularly in the middle-aged and elderly. This section looks at the magnitude of the problem and points to some of the implications.

Mortality

Diseases of the cardiovascular system are the main cause of death in adults in the developed countries of the world. In most Western countries they account for about 49% of deaths (LD-1).

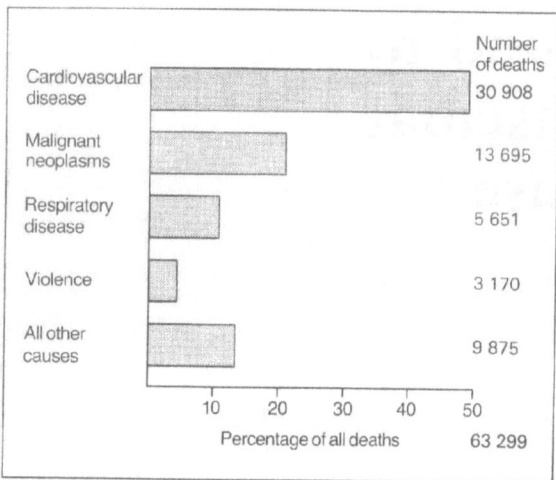

LD-1. *Relative frequency of cause of death – typical Western country, 1980*

They are made up of a number of conditions, but the major contributors are coronary heart disease and cerebrovascular disease with chronic rheumatic heart disease, hypertensive and other forms of heart disease, (e.g. congenital, pericardial, myocardial and pulmonary) as smaller contributors. The exact proportions vary in different countries and typical data are shown in LD-2. In Japan, the contribution of cerebrovascular disease (57%) is much larger.

Mortality from cardiovascular conditions increases with age and this increase is particularly steep in coronary heart disease and cerebrovascular disease (LD-3). The various components contribute different proportions at different ages (Table 1).

In cardiovascular disease, as in other diseases, women have lower mortality rates than men and, in middle age, their rates are less than half those of men (Table 2).

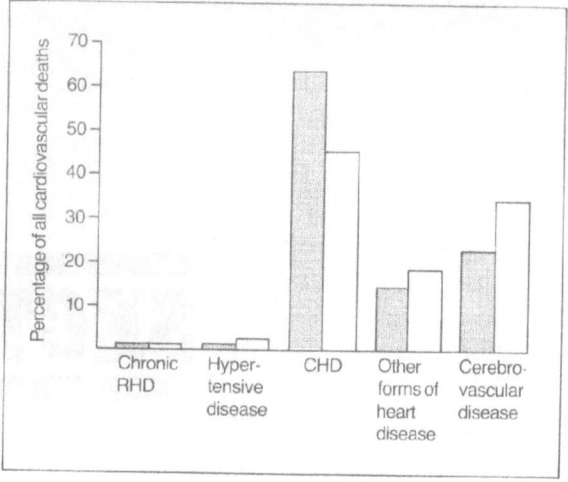

LD-2. *Relative frequency of death from different forms of cardiovascular disease – typical Western country, 1980. Key:* ▨ *= males;* ▢ *= females; RHD, rheumatic heart disease; CHD, coronary heart disease*

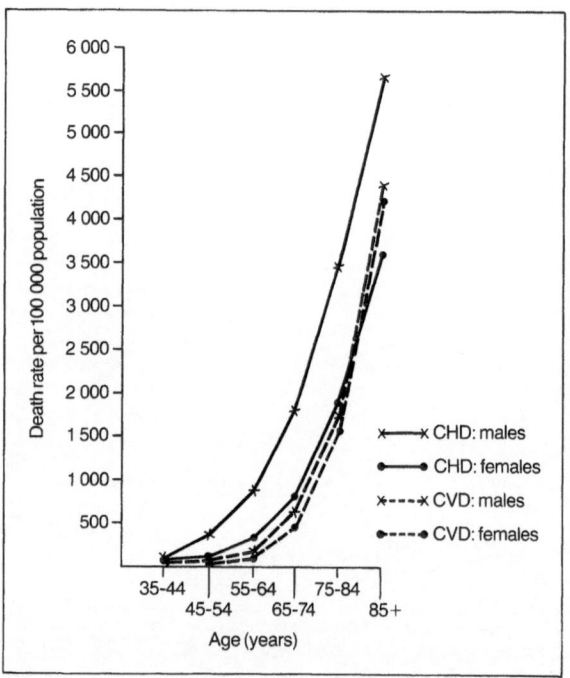

LD-3. *Coronary heart disease (CHD) and cerebrovascular disease (CVD) age and sex specific death rates – typical Western country, 1980*

Time trends

Myocardial infarction was first described in 1911 and first diagnosed clinically in Edinburgh in 1927. Death rates from coronary heart disease subsequently increased steadily until the late 1960s. Since then, there has been some slowing down and the rates in some countries have now flattened out. In some countries there has been a fall which, in the USA, has been of the order of 20%.

Death rates from cerebrovascular disease have fallen steadily since 1950 as have those associated with hypertensive disease. These changes started before the widespread introduction of antihypertensive drugs. Mortality from rheumatic heart disease has also declined markedly since 1945.

TABLE 1 The components of cardiovascular disease and the percentage they contribute to total cardiovascular mortality at different ages in males and females, typical Western country, 1980

Disease	Sex	Age/Percentage				
		25–34	35–44	45–54	55–64	65–74
Coronary heart	M	44	74	80	77	65
disease	F	16	38	51	60	58
Cerebrovascular	M	29	11	11	15	22
disease	F	48	40	28	24	27
Chronic	M	2	2	1	1	1
rheumatic heart	F	3	3	5	5	2
disease						
Hypertensive	M	2	1	1	1	2
disease*	F	3	1	2	2	2
Other forms of	M	23	12	7	6	10
heart disease	F	30	18	14	9	11
Total		100	100	100	100	100

* Also contributes to coronary and cerebrovascular disease.

International comparisons

International comparisons of cardiovascular disease show considerable differences between countries, mainly due to the coronary heart disease (CHD) component. Table 3 shows that CHD mortality varies by a factor of up to 10 between countries: in Finland and Scotland men and women have mortality rates from CHD that are amongst the highest in the world. The extent of the variation in different parts of the world, combined with the rapid increase in death rates in this century, strongly suggests the importance of environmental factors in the aetiology of this disease.

Variations occur not only between countries but also within them. The best documented are those in Britain (LD-4) and Finland. In Britain, the lowest rates are in south-east England and the highest in south and west Scotland.

Considerable emphasis has been given to death data because they provide the most complete information at present available. Although they are often criticized, mortality rates are quite adequate for making broad comparisons and following trends.

The natural history of the different cardiovascular diseases varies considerably. Many of those who develop coronary heart disease die soon after the illness begins whereas hypertension, rheumatic heart disease and many kinds of congenital cardiac malformations are compatible with a long life. This can be seen when mortality is compared with morbidity and population data.

Morbidity

Hospital admissions

Typically, in the West, 10% of all admissions to hospital are for cardiovascular disease, and 46% of

TABLE 2 Death rates per 100 000 from cardiovascular disease by age and sex, typical Western country, 1980

Disease	All ages		Under 25		25–34		35–44		45–54		55–64		65–74		75–84		85+	
	M	F	M	F	M	F	M	F	M	F	M	F	M	F	M	F	M	F
Chronic RHD	4	9	—	—	0	0	2	1	5	8	11	24	16	27	31	31	30	35
Hypertensive disease	9	11	—	—	0	0	1	0	5	3	14	9	46	26	84	75	129	224
CHD	405	293	—	—	6	2	69	14	337	84	885	312	1842	898	3512	1970	5733	3728
Other heart disease	47	70	1	2	2	2	6	4	17	12	46	31	142	105	608	458	2570	2148
Cerebrovascular disease	143	210	1	1	4	5	10	15	44	46	168	124	623	424	1793	1612	4478	4322
Congenital heart disease	3	3	5	6	1	1	2	1	1	2	1	1	0	0	0	1	0	0
Total	611	595	8	9	14	10	91	36	410	156	1125	500	2670	1464	5978	4120	12833	10484

TABLE 3 Death rates from coronary heart disease in
different countries at age 55–64 (rates per 100 000)

Year	Country	Males	Females
1975	Finland	997	214
1978	Scotland	900	294
1977	Northern Ireland	888	311
1971	USA	756	246
1977	Australia	731	231
1971	England and Wales	711	197
1981	Sweden	564	129
1977	West Germany	463	107
1981	Switzerland	321	70
1976	France	212	49
1977	Japan	95	36

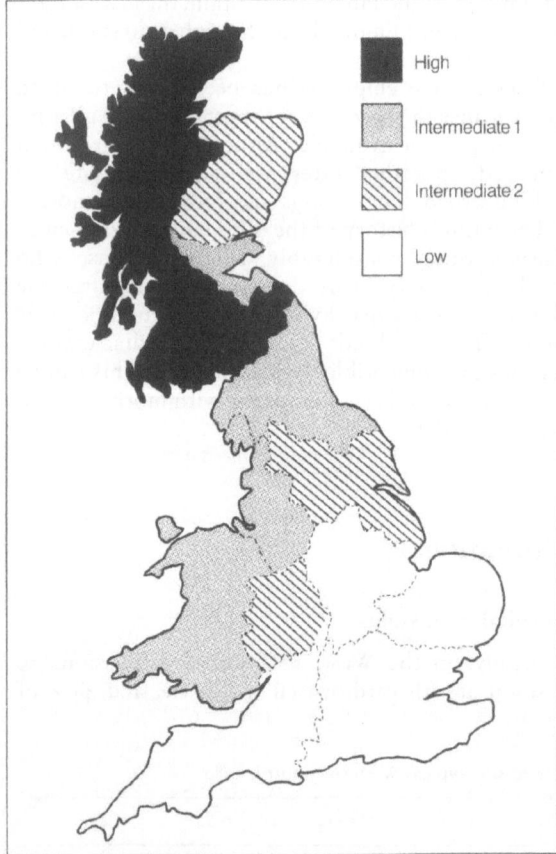

LD-4. *Mortality rates from coronary heart disease in men aged 45–54 in England, Wales and Scotland. Based on death rates per 100 000*

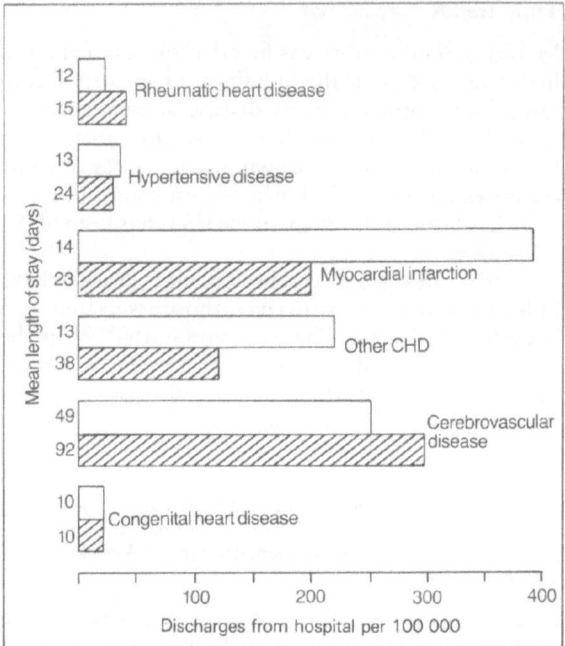

LD-5. *Discharges from hospital rates per 100 000 – typical Western country, 1980. ☐ = males; ▨ = females*

these are under the age of 65. The highest admission rates are found in men admitted with acute myocardial infarction and next come women admitted with cerebrovascular disease (LD-5). Though rates are lower for rheumatic heart disease, hypertensive disease and congenital heart disease, these conditions are responsible for a substantial proportion of admissions. As expected, congenital heart disease makes a particular contribution in the under-15 age group.

LD-5 also shows the mean length of stay in hospital. It tends to be longer in women than in men and reaches the very high figure of 92 days in women with cerebrovascular disease. The burden on the hospital service and on the community services after they have been discharged from hospital needs no underlining.

Data on hospital outpatient attendances are not available.

Consultations in general practice

Cardiovascular disease accounts for 9% of all consultations in general practice. The highest rates are found in hypertension (Table 4). This is in keeping with the long survival and continuing care required by these patients. Next in rank are the different manifestations of coronary heart disease.

Cardiovascular disease as a cause of disability

Estimates suggest that 3.3 million men and women of all ages in Britain are physically handicapped or

TABLE 4 Consultations in general practice by age and sex
(rates per 1000 population)

| | All ages | | 45–64 | |
	Males	Females	Males	Females
Hypertension	60	157	151	183
Angina and other CHD	37	32	82	40
Acute myocardial infarction	24	7	59	11
Cerebrovascular disease	20	19	28	12
Rheumatic heart disease	3	6	6	15
Congenital heart disease	1	1	0	0
All cardiovascular disease (including those not listed)	234	273	472	377

disabled. In 15% of these the cause is cardiovascular, but no further details are available.

Special studies in the population as a whole

Morbidity data are restricted in their range and completeness and are also limited in the sense that they only provide information on patients who seek medical help and reach a hospital or general practitioner.

A more complete picture of the frequency of cardiovascular disease can only be obtained by carrying out specially designed studies in the population as a whole. These studies may take the form of an examination of a representative sample of men or women in a specified age group and then following them up in subsequent years. The initial examination reveals those who have disease at the time and the follow-up provides information about new cases. The natural history of disease can also be studied in this way, risk factors can be identified and the need for medical and social services can be estimated.

For example, if a sample of 1000 British men aged 50–59 (including those with a past history of myocardial infarction) were examined for coronary heart disease by asking them standard questions about chest pain and recording an electrocardiogram (ECG), the following results could be expected:

55 would answer positively to the questions on angina of effort

75 would answer positively to the questions on possible myocardial infarction

74 would have ischaemic changes (mostly minor) on the resting ECG.

The total number affected would come to 169 because some would fall into more than one group. Out of the 1000 men, 40 would be under the care of their general practitioner for 'heart or blood pressure'.

If the same 1000 men were followed for 5 years, 25 would die from coronary heart disease during that period. Of these deaths:

18 would occur outside hospital, mostly at home

15 would occur before medical help arrived

13 would occur within 1 hour of the onset of symptoms

12 would occur among those who had had chest pain or ischaemic changes on their ECG.

Another 39 would develop non-fatal myocardial infarcts. Of these:

19 would be first infarcts

20 would be second or subsequent infarcts

35 would be sent to hospital

4 would be looked after at home.

A further example can be drawn from experience in measuring blood pressure. Several studies have now shown the benefit of lowering blood pressure in the control of stroke, congestive cardiac failure and hypertensive renal disease. Samples of the adult population have had their blood pressure measured and have answered questions about previous recordings and the use of antihypertensive drugs. Raised levels are quite common and prevalence figures are shown in Table 5. Analysis of the answers reveals that in only half the patients found to have a raised blood pressure is this known to their doctors. Of those who are known, only half are on treatment with antihypertensive drugs and of these only half have a blood pressure that might reasonably be considered to be well controlled (a diastolic blood pressure below 100 mmHg). It is therefore apparent that only one in eight patients with raised blood pressure is on effective treatment – hardly a satisfactory state of affairs, but one that has now been confirmed in several parts of the developed world. Studying only those hypertensive patients attending a hospital or general practice clinic may thus give a false impression of the true nature and extent of the problem.

Epidemiological studies provide information that cannot be gained in any other way and more of them are needed. However, they are difficult to carry out, bristle with pitfalls and require careful appraisal. For example, the ECG is widely used in the assessment of

TABLE 5 Prevalence of hypertension per 1000 adults at different ages

Age	Diastolic BP ⩾ 115 mmHg	Diastolic BP ⩾ 95 mmHg
Males		
35–44	5	53
45–54	12	127
55–64	71	330
65–74	68	302
Females		
35–44	17	124
45–54	49	208
55–64	77	364
65–74	97	660

cardiovascular disease, but its interpretation is not always straightforward. LD-6 shows the extent of observer variation among 14 experienced cardiologists in the interpretation of a series of records taken after exercise. Special precautions have to be taken to minimize this sort of problem in epidemiological work.

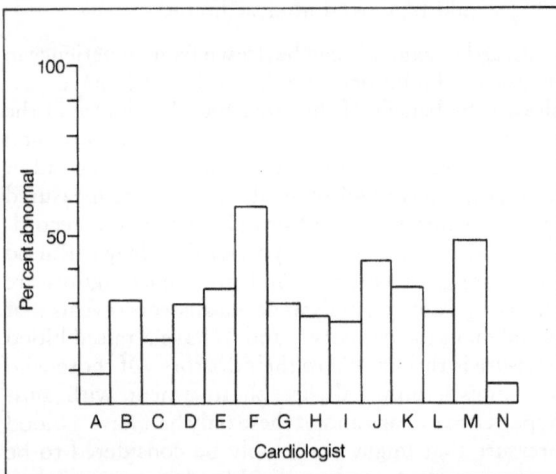

LD-6. *Opinions of 14 cardiologists on the abnormality of 38 postexercise ECGs*

Conclusion

The aim of this section has been to provide an overall picture of the prevalence of cardiovascular disease. More detailed discussion of individual diseases will be found in other chapters.

Descriptive data of this sort are extremely valuable. They define the magnitude of the problem of cardiovascular disease, provide a record of what is being achieved in its control and give guidance on the allocation of resources. The variations between age, sex, ethnic and social groups, between different regions and countries and the alterations that take place over time provide starting points for further investigation and a framework against which to test new theories.

EMBRYOLOGY

A basic knowledge of embryology is helpful when studying the cardiovascular system. A detailed knowledge is essential for those who wish to understand congenital cardiac malformations.

The development of the heart

A cardiovascular system is required by the growing embryo. It is established at a very early stage of development and is the first system in the body to function.

To begin with, the heart is a simple tube. During the fourth week of intra-uterine life, when the embryo is about 5 mm long, three constrictions appear and divide the tube into four primitive chambers: the sinus venosus, the atrium, the ventricle and the bulbus cordis. The bulbus cordis is continuous with the truncus arteriosus, the main blood vessel leaving the heart.

As a result of differential growth, the tube becomes U-shaped (LD-7) and during the next 4 weeks a remarkable series of developments turns the primitive heart with four common chambers into one not much different from that found after birth.

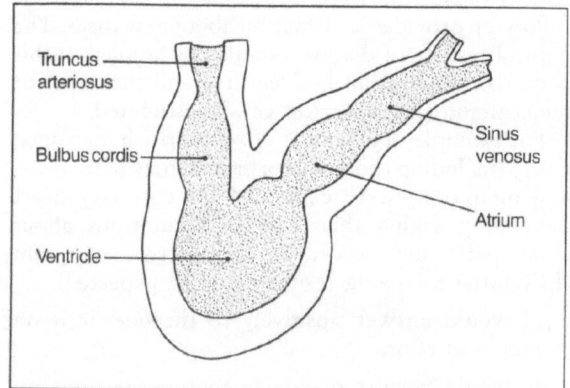

LD-7.

The atria and ventricles

The common atrium is divided into a right atrium and a left atrium by the atrial septum. The atrial septum has a thin lower part, the septum primum, and a thicker upper part, the septum secundum. The septum secundum overlaps the right side of the septum primum and allows blood to flow between them through the foramen ovale from the right atrium into the left atrium during fetal life (LD-8).

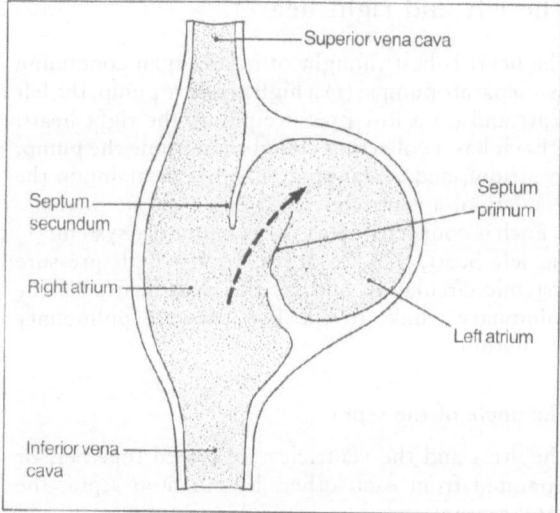

LD-8.

The common ventricle is divided into a right ventricle and a left ventricle by the ventricular septum. The ventricular septum is mostly muscular, but has a membranous component in its upper part below the root of the aorta.

Two proliferations of subendothelial tissue, the endocardial cushions, divide the common atrio-ventricular (AV) canal into separate right and left AV orifices, each with its own AV valve, the mitral valve and the tricuspid valve.

The endocardial cushions meet in the midline with the lower part of the atrial septum above and the upper part of the ventricular septum below, thus dividing the heart into four chambers (LD-9).

If either the atrial septum or the ventricular septum is incompletely formed or the common AV canal incompletely septated, the chambers and valves may communicate with each other. Such holes in the heart account for almost half of all congenital cardiac malformations.

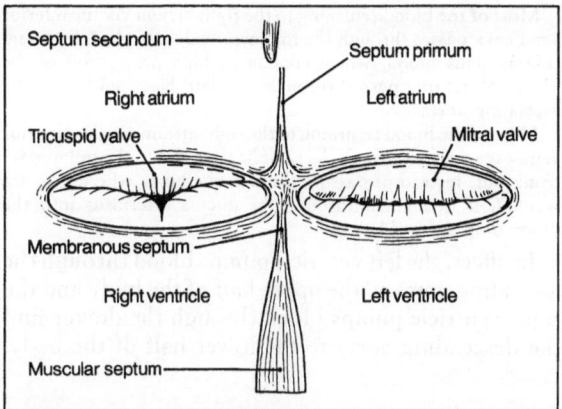

LD-9.

The great arterial trunks

The proximal part of the bulbus cordis is incorporated into the outflow tracts of the ventricles, particularly into the infundibular portion of the right ventricle. The distal part of the bulbus merges with the truncus arteriosus, which, by a process of septation and rotation, forms the aorta and pulmonary trunk.

During the course of development six pairs of aortic arches are formed, but they are never all present at the same time and only parts of some of them persist in the cardiovascular system; the remainder atrophy and disappear. For practical purposes the 4th and the 6th arches are the most important.

Both 4th arches persist; the left as the definitive arch of the aorta, the right as part of the right subclavian artery. The ventral parts of both 6th arches persist to form the right and left pulmonary arteries. The dorsal part of the 6th left arch becomes the ductus arteriosus.

The fetal circulation

Before birth, the lungs have no function and, like all other organs, receive only what blood is required for their development. As a consequence, the pulmonary circulation in the fetus is small and very little blood is returned through the pulmonary veins to the left atrium.

The right atrium, on the other hand, receives not only the whole of the systemic venous return but also all the blood that returns to the heart from the placenta. Two large right to left shunts compensate for the small pulmonary blood flow, as follows.

Most of the blood returning to the right atrium via the inferior vena cava passes through the foramen ovale into the left atrium (LD-9). This blood, which contains a high proportion of the placental return, passes through the left heart and into the ascending aorta.

Most of the blood returning to the right atrium via the superior vena cava passes through the right heart and into the pulmonary trunk but, instead of passing through the lungs where it is not wanted, it is shunted through the ductus arteriosus into the descending aorta (LD-10).

In effect, the left ventricle pumps blood through the ascending aorta to the upper half of the body and the right ventricle pumps blood through the ductus and the descending aorta to the lower half of the body.

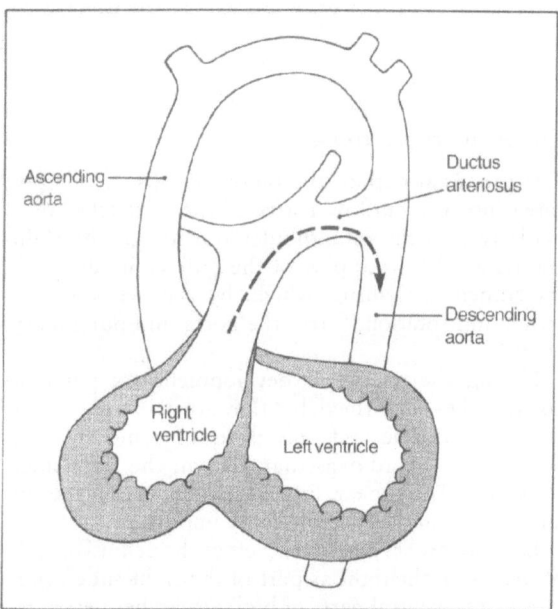

LD-10.

Until birth, and for a short time afterwards, both ventricles maintain the same systemic pressure and it is only after expansion of the lungs and the establishment of the pulmonary circulation with its low vascular resistance that pressures in the right heart fall to normal levels.

During the first few days of life the shunting mechanisms used by the fetus may persist and cause intermittent cyanosis.

Congenital cardiac malformations interfere, to a greater or lesser degree, with the normal pressure/flow relationships that exist between the left heart with its high pressure systemic arterial circulation and the right heart with its low pressure pulmonary arterial circulation.

ANATOMY

A good working knowledge of the correct orientation of the heart and great vessels, and of the relationships of their component parts to one another, is of fundamental importance when examining the cardiovascular system and eliciting the physical signs that are produced in health and disease.

The left and right hearts

The heart is best thought of as an organ containing two separate pumps: (1) a high pressure pump, the left heart and (2) a low pressure pump, the right heart.

Each has a collecting chamber to prime the pump, an atrium, and a pumping chamber to maintain the circulation, a ventricle.

Each is connected to its own circulatory system: (1) the left heart, via the aorta, to the high pressure systemic circulation and (2) the right heart, via the pulmonary trunk, to the low pressure pulmonary circulation.

The angle of the septa

The atria and the ventricles are joined together, or separated from each other, by common septa, the atrial septum and the ventricular septum.

These septa are in line with each other and lie at an angle of 45° to the median plan (LD-11). Because of this obliquity of the septa, when viewed from the front, the right heart lies anterior and to the right of the left heart so that the right heart chambers make up most of the anterior surface of the heart.

The atria lie to the right of, behind and to a lesser extent above their respective ventricles and, again because of the obliquity of the septa, blood flows forwards and to the left as it passes from the atria into the ventricles.

The left heart chambers are at a slightly higher level in the thorax than their right-sided counterparts with the result that the atrial and ventricular septa also lie at an oblique angle when viewed in the vertical plane (LD-12).

The heart and great vessels in the mediastinum

Forward projection of the vertebral column into the thoracic cavity considerably reduces the anteropost-

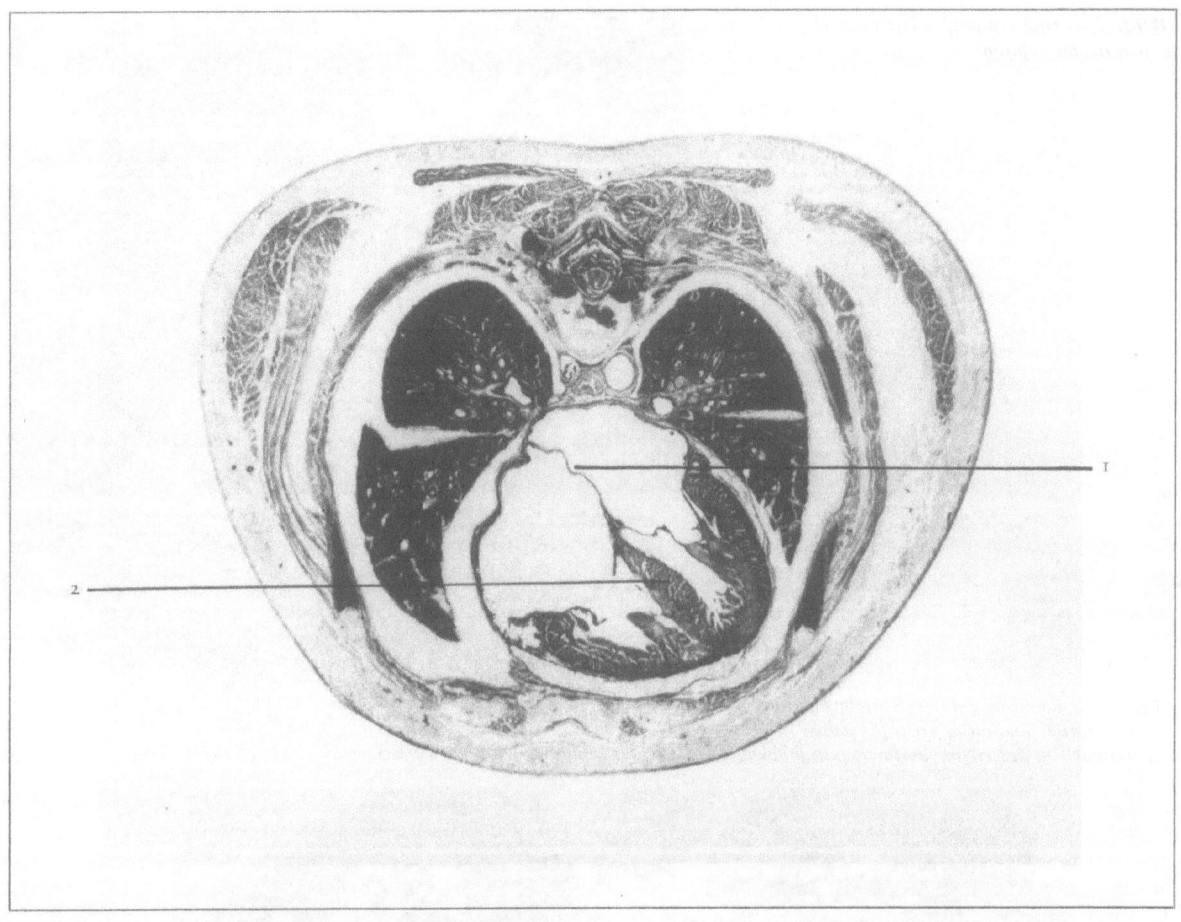

LD-11. *1, Atrial septum; 2, ventricular septum*

erior diameter of the mediastinum in the median plane. The heart and great vessels occupy virtually all of the available space between the posterior surface of the sternum and the anterior surface of the vertebrae (LD-13 and 14).

In childhood the heart is relatively mobile, but in adult life it becomes fairly firmly anchored within the mediastinum and maintains its central position unless subjected to inordinate unilateral pressures or traction.

With so little room for expansion or contraction, any enlargement of the heart or contraction of the thoracic cage affects the relationships of the thoracic contents and consequently their apparent size and shape.

The fibrous skeleton of the heart

The cardiac skeleton is the strong central framework that prevents the heart and great arteries from tearing themselves apart during several thousand million contractions in an average lifespan. The chambers, valves and great arteries are bound together in a way that provides great strength while at the same time permitting a considerable amount of movement during systole and diastole.

The skeleton is mainly fibrous. Fibrocartilage and fibroelastic tissue have been described, but do not make a major contribution to it. True cartilage and bone, found in some domestic animal hearts, are not found in man, although calcification may occur with age.

The atrioventricular annuli

In the human heart, the skeleton is formed largely by the fibrous annuli that surround the heart valves and extensions arising from them (LD-15). Three of these annuli, the aortic, mitral and tricuspid valve rings, are

LD-12. *1, Atrial septum; 2, left ventricle;*
3, ventricular septum

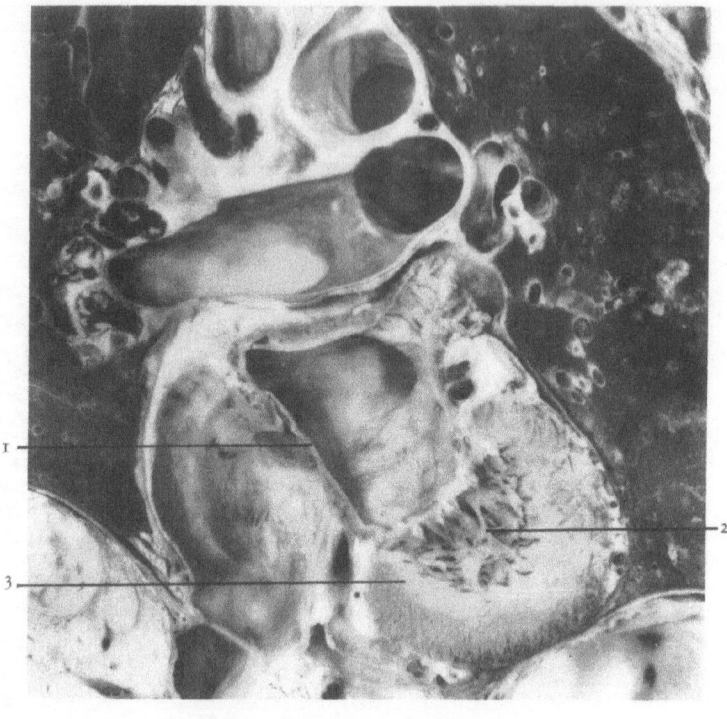

LD-13. *1, Vertebral column; 2, right pulmonary*
vein; 3, atrial septum; 4, tricuspid valve;
5, sternum; 6, descending aorta; 7, mitral valve; 8, ventricular septum

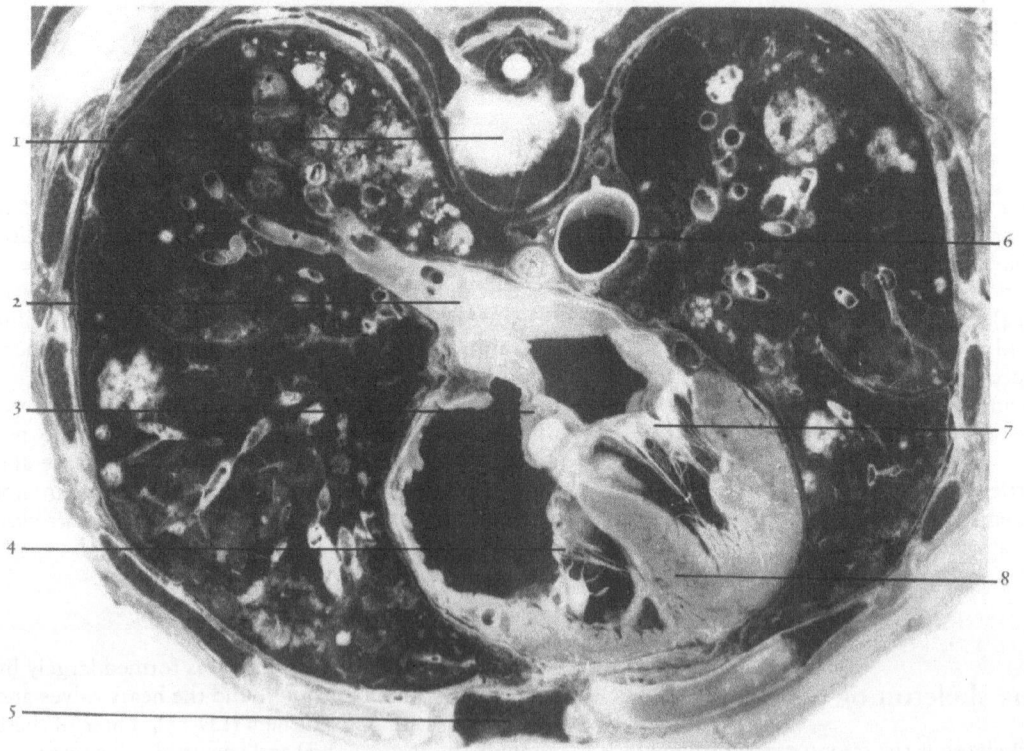

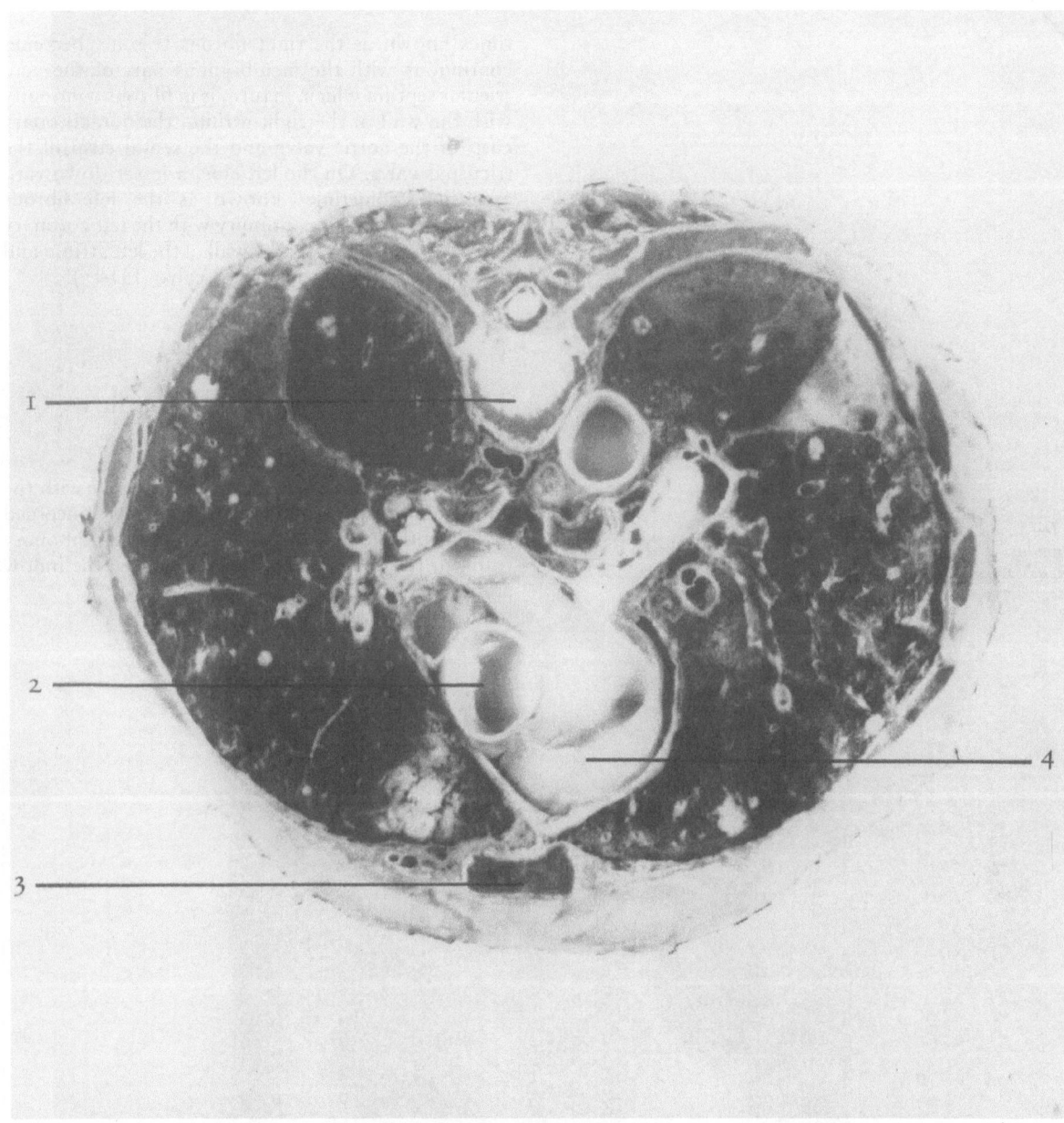

LD-14. *1, Vertebral column; 2, ascending aorta; 3, sternum; 4, pulmonary trunk*

intimately related to one another (LD-16). The fourth, the annulus of the pulmonary valve, lies at a higher level and has little fibrous continuity with the rest of the heart.

The atrioventricular annuli separate the atrial myocardium from that of the ventricles and give attachment to the muscle fibres of these chambers. They also give attachment to the cusps of the valves.

The central fibrous body

A strong band of fibrous tissue known as the central fibrous body lies between the posterior wall of the aortic root and the upper parts of the mitral and tricuspid valves. It thickens and extends downwards between the adjacent mitral and tricuspid annuli. The atrial septum is attached to its central part.

On the right side, a downward extension, some-

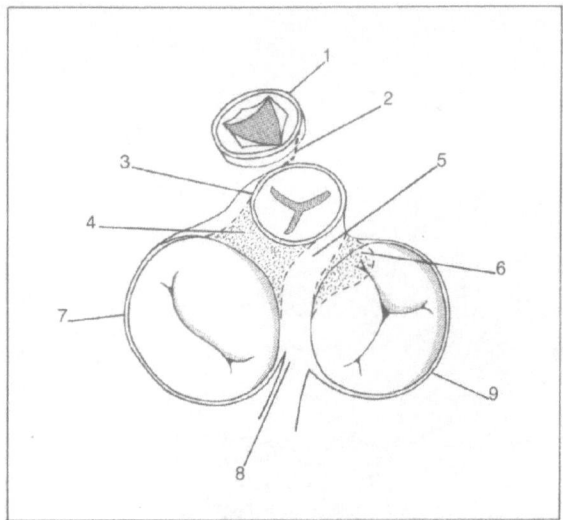

times known as the right fibrous trigone, becomes continuous with the membranous part of the ventricular septum which, in turn, is in fibrous continuity with the wall of the right atrium, the non-coronary cusp of the aortic valve and the septal cusp of the tricuspid valve. On the left side, a lesser downward extension, sometimes known as the left fibrous trigone, is in fibrous continuity with the left coronary cusp of the aortic valve, the wall of the left atrium and the anterior cusp of the mitral valve (LD-17).

LD-15. 1, *Pulmonary annulus;* 2, *conus ligament;* 3, *aortic annulus;* 4, *intervalvar septum;* 5, *central fibrous body;* 6, *membranous part of ventricular septum;* 7, *mitral annulus;* 8, *atrial septum;* 9, *tricuspid annulus*

The ventricular inflow and outflow tracts

Each ventricle has a part concerned mainly with the inflow of blood from the atrium and a part concerned mainly with the outflow of blood into the pulmonary trunk or the aorta. These parts are called the inflow and outflow tracts.

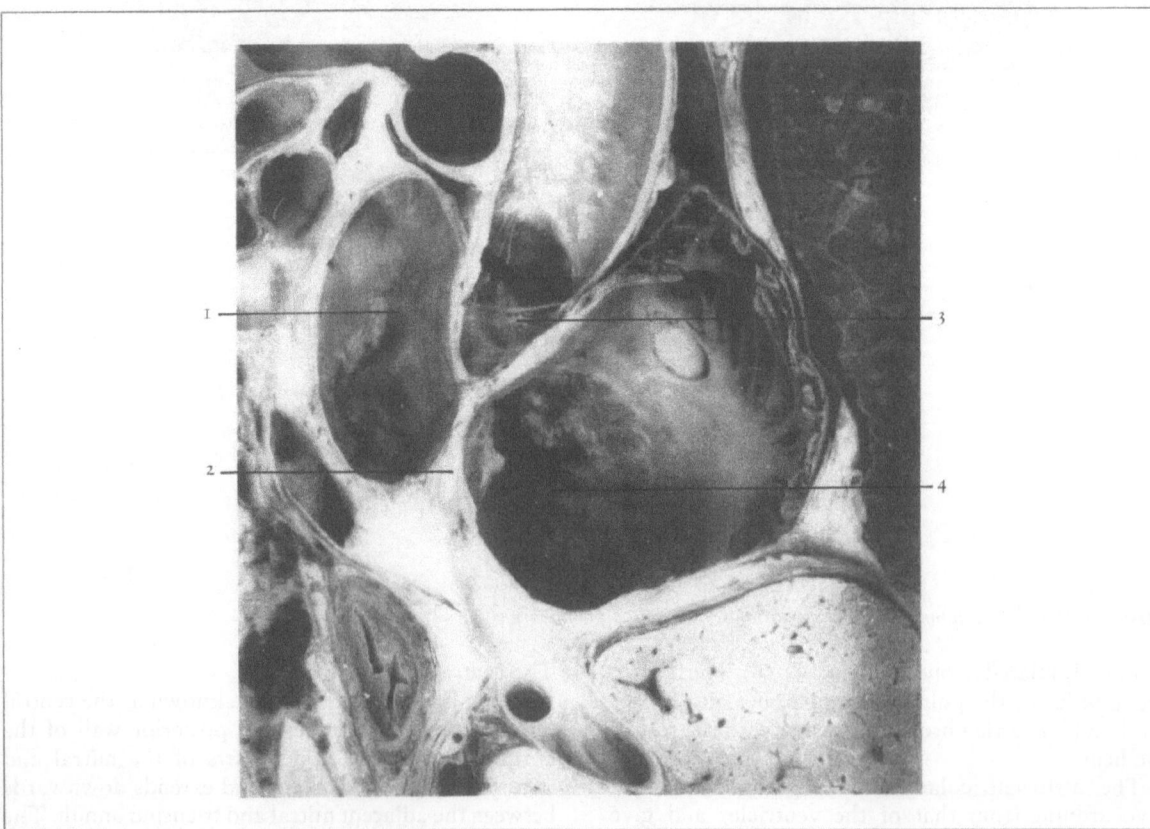

LD-16. 1, *Mitral valve;* 2, *atrial septum;* 3, *aortic valve;* 4, *tricuspid valve*

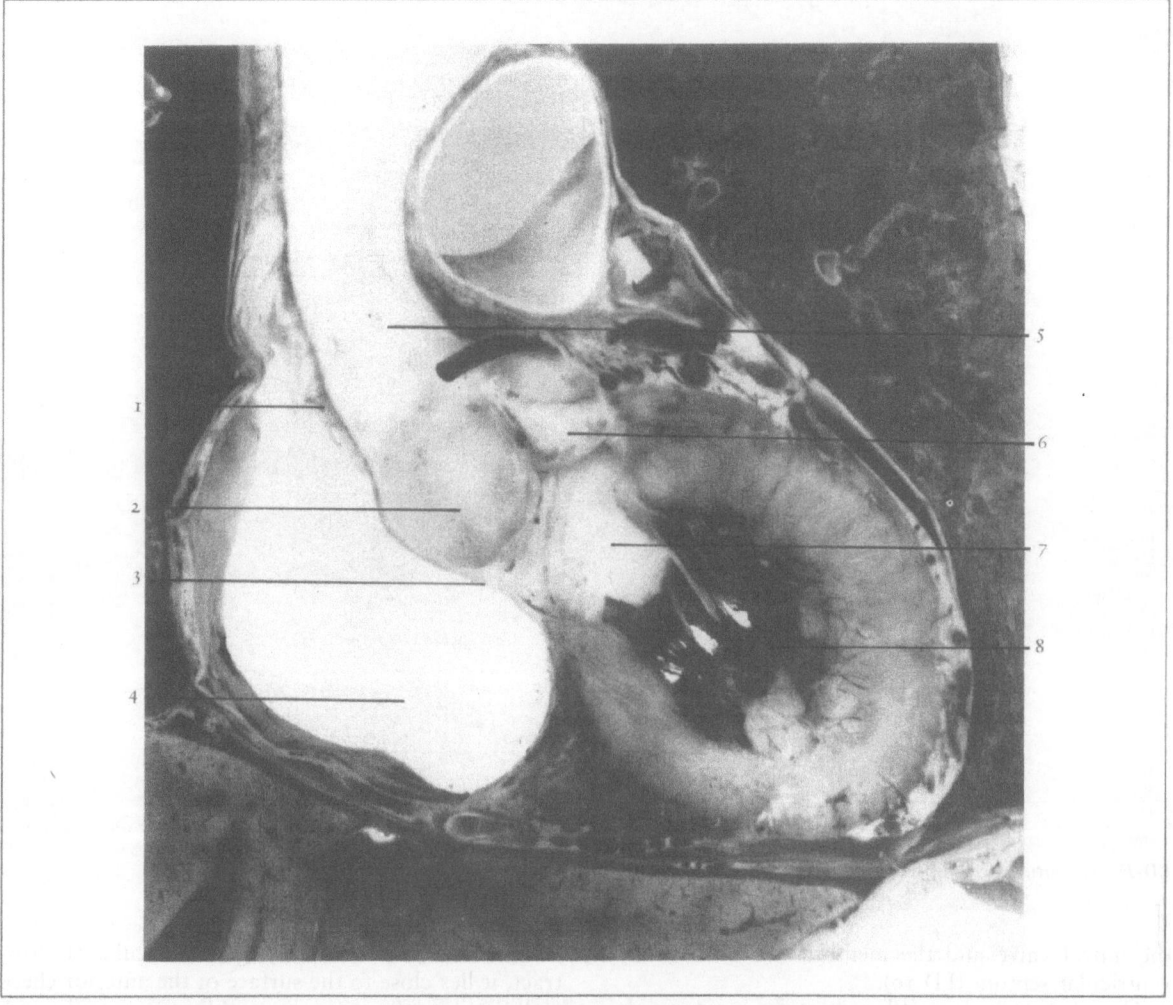

LD-17. *1, Medial wall, right atrium; 2, non-coronary aortic sinus; 3, membranous part, ventricular septum; 4, right atrium; 5, ascending aorta; 6, left coronary cusp, aortic valve; 7, anterior cusp, mitral valve; 8, left ventricle*

The *inflow tracts* extend from the atrioventricular valves to the apices of the ventricles and their walls are trabeculated, the right much more so than the left.

The *outflow tracts* extend from the apices of the ventricles to the semilunar valves and their walls are smooth.

It is thought that the trabeculae slow the blood as it flows into the ventricles during diastole and that the smooth walls accelerate its passage out of them during systole.

The outflow tracts lie above and to some extent in front of their ventricular chambers and are therefore nearer to the anterior chest wall – a fact that has relevance in auscultation.

The right ventricular outflow tract

This, although embryologically complex, is functionally a simple muscular tube (LD-18). It is longer than the left ventricular outflow tract, starting at a lower level, because all the right heart chambers are at a lower level than the left heart chambers, and finishing at higher level, because the pulmonary valve lies at a higher level than the aortic valve.

The left ventricular outflow tract

This is a complex fibromuscular canal. Its anterior wall is formed by the muscular part of the ventricular septum and its posterior wall by the anterior cusp of

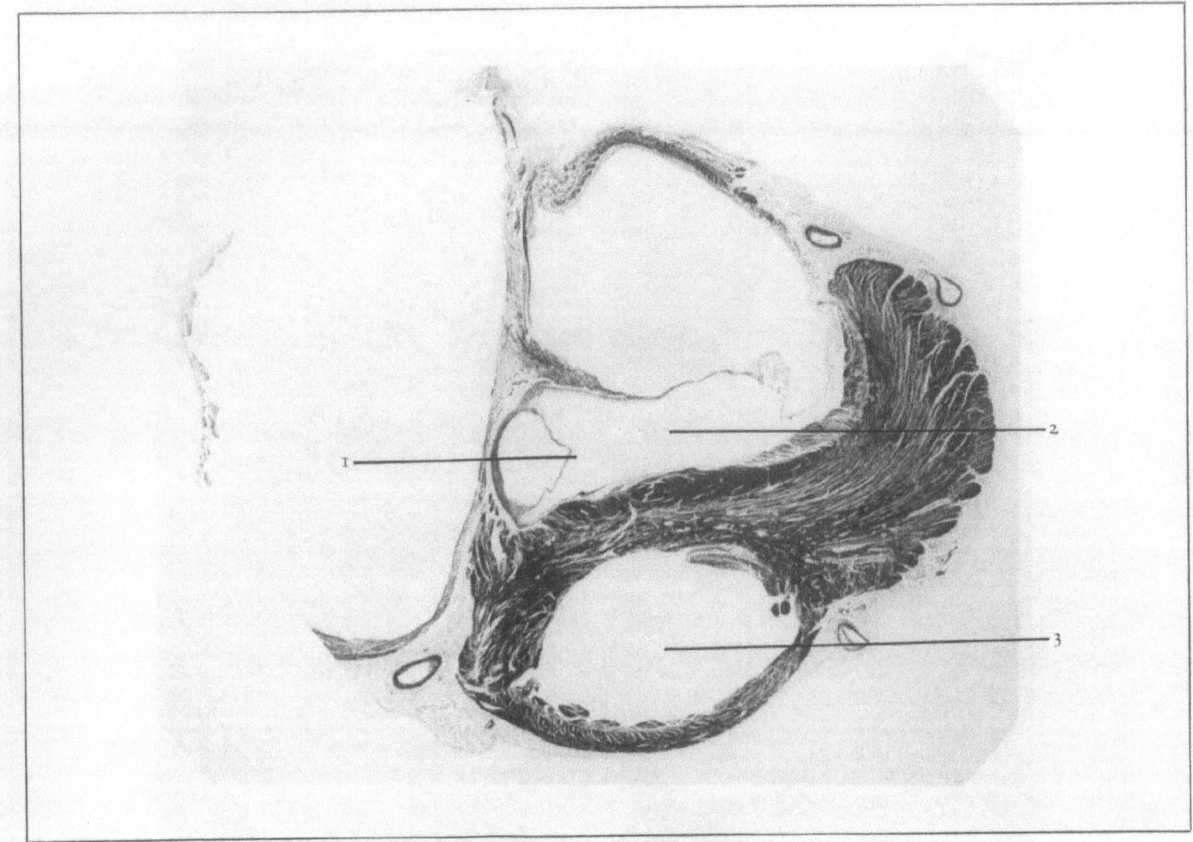

LD-18. *1, Aortic valve cusps; 2, left ventricular outflow tract; 3, right ventricular outflow tract*

the mitral valve and the membranous part of the ventricular septum (LD-19).

The left ventricular outflow tract crosses upwards from left to right behind the right ventricular outflow tract so that the outflow tracts resemble a Saint Andrew's cross (✗). In this way the ventricular mass becomes increasingly compact during systole as the myocardial fibres contract and shorten.

The sites of the valves

Many of the sounds heard during auscultation of the heart are produced at or by the valves. Their position within the heart and their relationships within the thorax are therefore of considerable importance.

The pulmonary valve

The pulmonary valve is higher than the aortic valve

and anterior to it. With the right ventricular outflow tract, it lies close to the surface of the anterior chest wall in the left precordium (LD-20). Sounds and murmurs produced there are best heard along the left upper sternal edge. This is known as the pulmonary area. Systolic murmurs are propagated upwards towards the inner third of the left clavicle. Diastolic murmurs are propagated downwards along the left sternal border.

The aortic valve

The aortic valve lies deep within the thorax in the centre of the heart. Sounds and systolic murmurs are propagated through the aorta and are best heard where the ascending aorta comes towards the surface in the right upper precordium (LD-21). This is known as the aortic area, though it is far from the aortic valve. Diastolic murmurs, like those associated with the pulmonary valve, are propagated downwards along the left sternal edge.

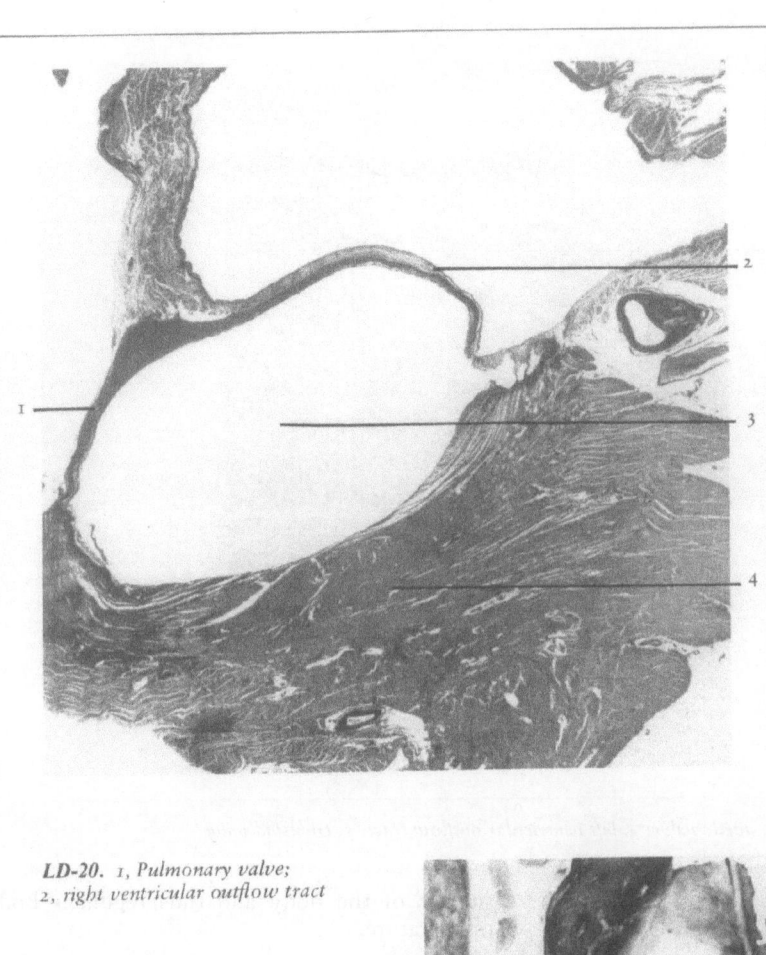

LD-19. 1, Membranous part, ventricular septum; 2, anterior cusp, mitral valve; 3, left ventricular outflow tract; 4, muscular part, ventricular septum

LD-20. 1, Pulmonary valve; 2, right ventricular outflow tract

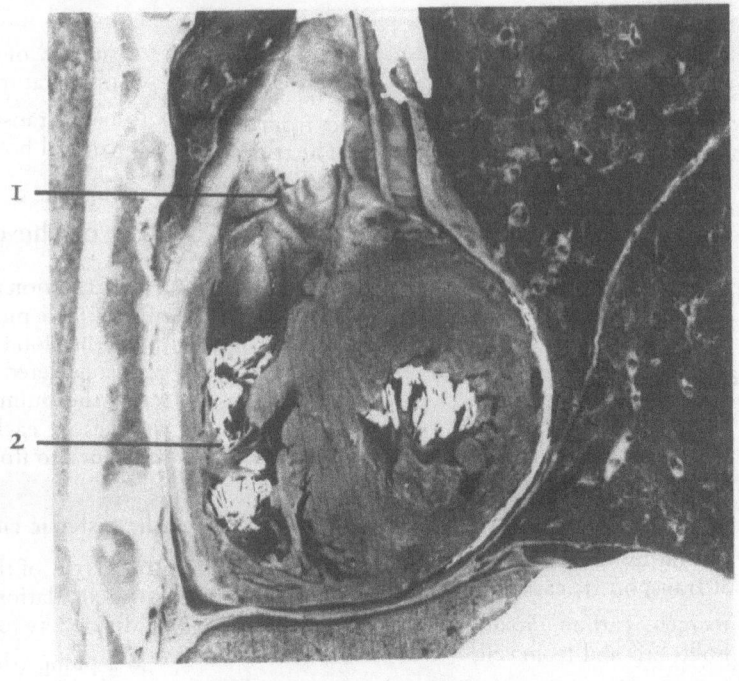

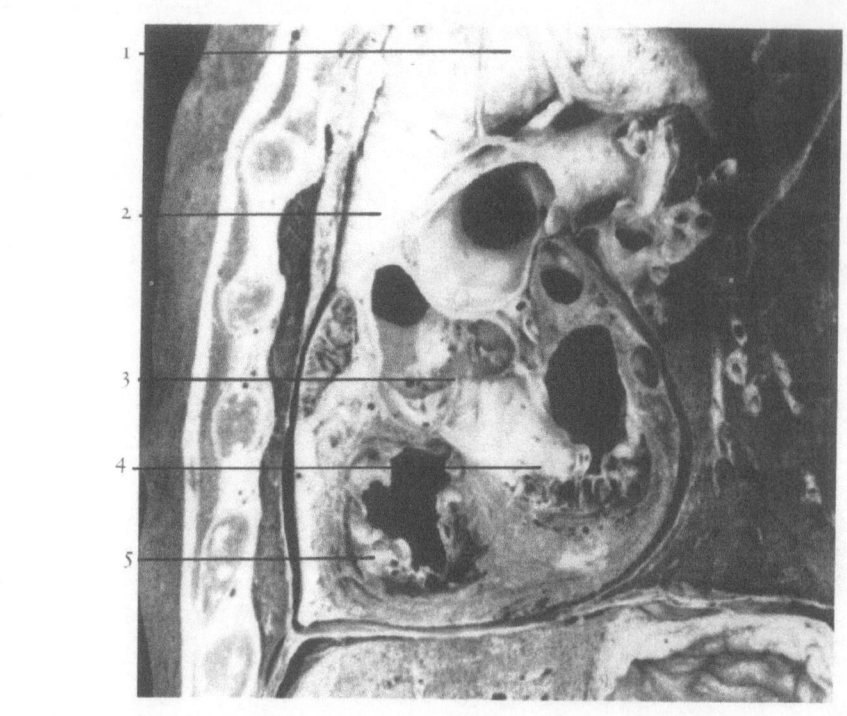

LD-21. *1, Aortic arch; 2, ascending aorta; 3, aortic valve; 4, left ventricular outflow tract; 5, tricuspid valve*

The tricuspid and mitral valves

Because of the plane of the septa, blood flows obliquely through the atrioventricular valves from the atria towards the apices of the ventricles. The tricuspid valve lies much closer to the surface than the mitral valve which, like the aortic valve, lies deep within the thorax in the centre of the heart (LD-11 and 13). For this reason, tricuspid sounds and murmurs are loudest over the lower sternum. Mitral sounds and murmurs are best heard where they are propagated, in this case towards the apex of the heart in the midclavicular line.

PHYSIOLOGY

The central function of the cardiovascular system is one of transport. It carries:

- oxygen, carbon dioxide, nutrients and metabolites to and from cells
- heat produced by metabolic activity, to the

surface of the body and thus regulates body temperature.

- neurotransmitter substances and hormones that control body functions.

Plan of the circulation

The circulation is a closed hydraulic system consisting of a variable pump, the heart, and a series of flexible tubes, the blood vessels. After the neonatal period, it is best considered as two connected but separate systems, the pulmonary circulation and the systemic circulation, each with its own pump, capacity and resistance to flow.

The systemic circulation

About 85% of the blood is contained within this part of the circulation. It is a high resistance circuit and can be divided as follows:

- a pump (the left ventricle) containing 4–5% of the blood

- a distributing system of elastic vessels (the aorta and arteries) containing about 12% of the blood. The terminal portion (the arterioles) functions as a variable resistance

- an exchange system (the capillaries) which, with the arterioles, contains about 8% of the systemic circulation

- a collecting and reservoir system (venules, veins, venae cavae and right atrium) containing about 60% of the blood. The capacity of the veins can be altered, thereby bringing about a redistribution of blood.

The pulmonary circulation

This contains about 15% of the blood. It begins with the right ventricle emptying into the pulmonary arteries and ends with the pulmonary veins draining into the left atrium. The resistance to flow in the pulmonary circuit is low, about one fifth of that in the systemic circuit, and the pressures are correspondingly lower. The effects of gravity are also less pronounced.

The volumes shown above are approximate. As will be seen later, considerable shifts in the distribution of blood throughout the two systems can occur in response to certain conditions.

Consequences of the basic plan

A careful consideration of the organization of this closed-system, double circulation should make it apparent that certain conditions must be maintained for the continuous circulation of blood. Over even a short space of time, the output from each side of the heart and the venous return to it must be matched: see 'Cardiac output and venous return' (p. 20).

The heart

Central to the working of the circulatory system are the mechanisms that regulate the heart. It is a muscular organ providing the motive power for the circulation by its inherent rhythmic contractile activity. This subsection describes the mechanism of cardiac muscle contraction, the sequence of events within the heart during the rhythmic sequence of contraction and relaxation, and the intrinsic and extrinsic mechanisms that regulate its function.

Contraction of heart muscle

The contraction of the heart is achieved by the filaments of actin and myosin that make up the contractile elements sliding between one another. The electrical activity that precedes contraction is described in the section on Electrocardiography (p. 34). The action potential passes over the myocardium and spreads to the T-tubules. During the plateau phase of the action potential, Ca^{2+} enters the cell and triggers the release of stored Ca^{2+} from the lateral cisternae of the sarcoplasmic reticulum (LD-22). Calcium binds to the regulator protein, troponin, altering the configuration of the troponin–tropomyosin complex and thus exposing the active sites on the actin filaments. The rise in intracellular calcium also activates the myosin filaments by the splitting of adenosine 5′-triphosphate (ATP). The myosin heads attach to the active sites on the actin filaments forming crossbridges that cause the overlap between actin and myosin filaments to increase. The muscle contracts. The Ca^{2+} is then returned to the sarcoplasmic reticulum by ATP dependent pumps, the process reverses and the muscle relaxes. During this relaxation phase, the Ca^{2+} that entered the cell during the action potential plateau is pumped out by an active process. The Ca^{2+} in the sarcoplasmic reticulum tubules is translocated to the cisternae where it is stored until released by the next action potential. As heart rate increases, the period of relaxation is shortened, and Ca^{2+} levels might not be fully restored. The resulting elevation of intracellular Ca^{2+} leads to enhanced contractility (Bowditch staircase effect).

The cardiac cycle

The cardiac cycle is an orderly sequence of contraction (systole) and relaxation (diastole). The duration of the cycle and its components varies with the heart rate (LD-23). Note how, as the heart rate increases, the duration of diastole is reduced to a greater extent than the duration of systole. This sequence of contraction followed by relaxation generates the rhythmic pressure fluctuations that determine the opening and closing of the heart valves and the filling of the ventricles that pump blood into the pulmonary and systemic circulations.

Electrical events of cardiac cycle

The initiation and synchronization of contractions of individual myocardial fibres is caused by a wave of electrical excitation that travels through the myocardium. This wave of excitation (depolarization) can be recorded on the surface of the body as the ECG. The activity originates in the sinoatrial(SA) node (pacemaker) and is conducted through the atrium (P wave)

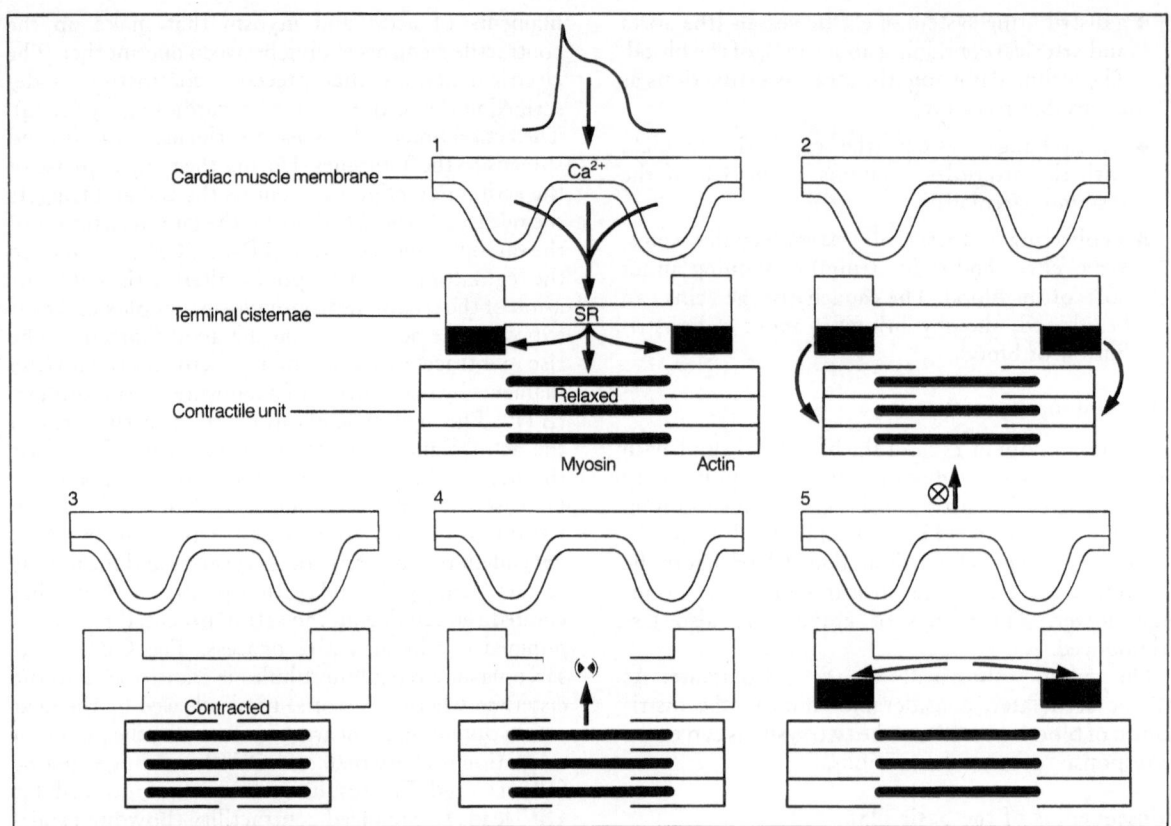

LD-22. (*1*) *As the action potential passes over the muscle membrane and through the T-tubule system, calcium passes into the cell from the interstitial fluid (during the plateau phase) and is also released from membrane bound sites. (2) This raises the free ionic cytoplasmic calcium, which can then activate the contractile machinery, thus initiating contraction. The calcium can also act on the terminal cisternae of the sarcoplasmic reticulum (SR), causing the release of calcium stored there, further increasing the free cytoplasmic calcium. (3) Contraction is now complete. (4) During diastole, calcium is pumped back into the sarcoplasmic reticulum and ultimately returned to the stores in the terminal cisternae (5). At the same time (5), pumps in the external membrane eliminate the excess Ca^{2+} that entered from the interstitial fluid during the action potential*

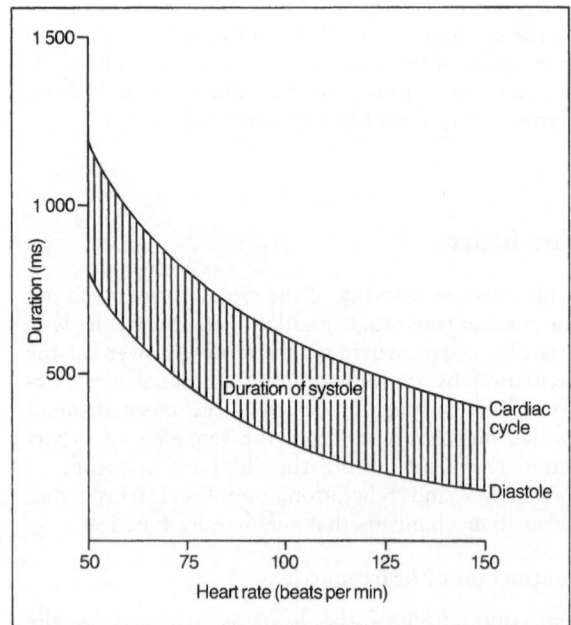

LD-23. *As the heart rate increases, the duration of each cardiac cycle falls (upper curve). This is due largely to a fall in the duration of the diastolic interval (lower curve). The duration of systole (i.e. the difference between corresponding points on the upper and lower curves) changes by a relatively small amount*

initiating atrial contraction. The impulse then passes to the AV node where it is delayed by the slow rate of conduction through this tissue. The delay allows time for the atria to expel their contents into the ventricles before the ventricles contract. From the AV node, the impulse passes via the bundle of His and its left and right branches to the ventricular myocardium. The PR interval represents the time taken for the impulse to pass through the AV junctional tissues (LD-24). The wave of excitation subsequently spreads through the ventricular muscle (QRS complex), initiating a contraction that begins at the apex of the heart and moves towards the base. As the ventricles repolarize (T wave), relaxation spreads from the apex towards the base.

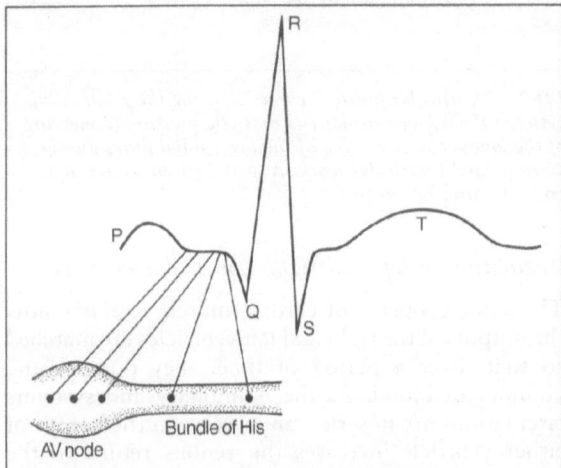

LD-24. *Time taken for electrical excitation to pass through conducting system. Note how much of the PR interval is caused by delay in the AV node*

Mechanical events of cardiac cycle

The mechanical events of the cardiac cycle can be monitored as intracardiac pressure or volume changes and as heart sounds. This general description of the cycle applies to the right and left hearts, the differences between them being largely quantitative (LD-25). During atrial diastole, which begins while the ventricles are still contracting, blood flows into the collecting chambers from the great veins. This causes the atrial pressure to rise and when, during ventricular diastole, it exceeds the pressure in the ventricles, the AV valves open. During this period of total diastole, up to 80% of ventricular filling occurs without the help of the atrial pump. The rate of filling depends upon the pressure gradient between the great veins and the ventricles. As this is fairly constant, the

degree of filling depends upon the duration of diastole. If this is shortened by an increase in heart rate (LD-23), filling is less complete.

During atrial systole, the atria contract, the atrial pressures rise and the flow through the atrioventricular valves increases. This, the 'atrial transport function', contributes about 20% to ventricular filling. Some blood is also regurgitated into the great veins during this phase of the cycle, but the amount is limited by narrowing of their orifices when the surrounding atrial muscle contracts.

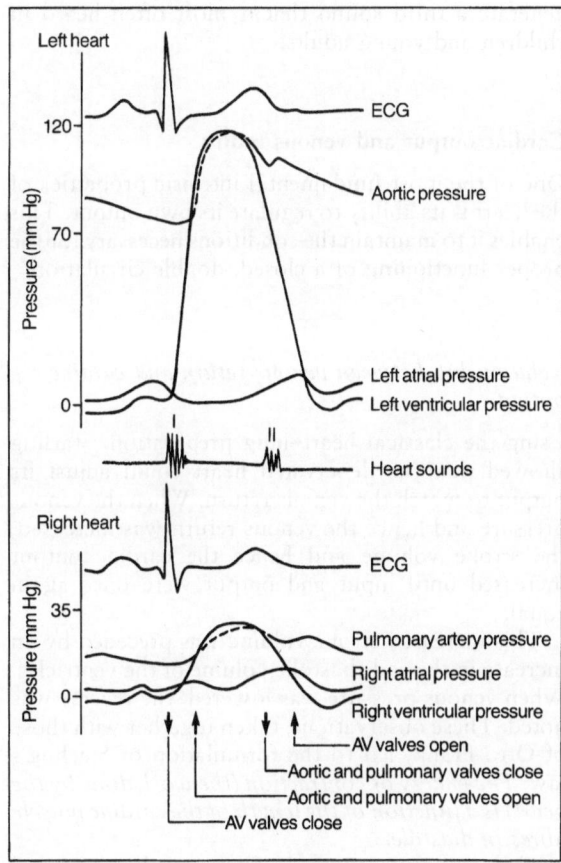

LD-25. *Electrical and mechanical events of the cardiac cycle*

The ventricles now contract so that ventricular pressure rises. When it exceeds the atrial pressure, the atrioventricular valves close, generating the first heart sound (LD-25). As both the inflow (mitral and tricuspid) and outflow (aortic and pulmonary) valves are now closed, the ventricular contraction is isovolumetric, i.e. there is no change in volume. Consequently, the intraventricular pressures rise steeply until they exceed the pressures in the aorta and pulmonary artery. At this point, the aortic and pulmonary valves open and the ventricles empty, at first rapidly and then more slowly as the contraction begins to weaken.

As the ventricular myocardium relaxes, the pressure in the ventricles falls again and, when it is less than the pressures in the aorta and pulmonary artery, the aortic and pulmonary valves close, causing the second heart sound. When the pressure in the ventricles falls below the pressure in the atria, the AV valves open and the cycle repeats itself. Towards the end of the phase of rapid ventricular filling, vibrations generate a third sound that is most often heard in children and young adults.

Cardiac output and venous return

One of the most fundamental intrinsic properties of the heart is its ability to regulate its own output. This enables it to maintain the conditions necessary for the proper functioning of a closed, double circulation.

Relationship between venous return and cardiac output

Using the classical heart–lung preparation, Starling showed that the denervated heart could adjust its output to match the venous return. When the venous pressure and hence the venous return was increased, the stroke volume and hence the cardiac output increased until input and output were once again equal.

This increased stroke volume was preceded by an increase in the end-diastolic volume of the ventricles. When venous pressure was lowered, the reverse was noted. These observations, taken together with those of Otto Frank, led to the formulation of Starling's law: *The energy of contraction (the work done by the heart) is a function of the length of the cardiac muscle fibres in diastole.*

This property of muscle fibres can be expressed graphically (LD-26). As will be seen, the force of contraction is dependent upon the initial length of the cardiac muscle fibre. As the fibre is stretched, it generates more tension over a wide range of fibre lengths. However, at greater lengths, the mechanism fails and the tension falls off. This inherent property of the cardiac muscle can be demonstrated in the intact heart and it has been found that when cardiac nerves are stimulated, although the curve shifts, the basic relationship between initial fibre length and work done persists (LD-26).

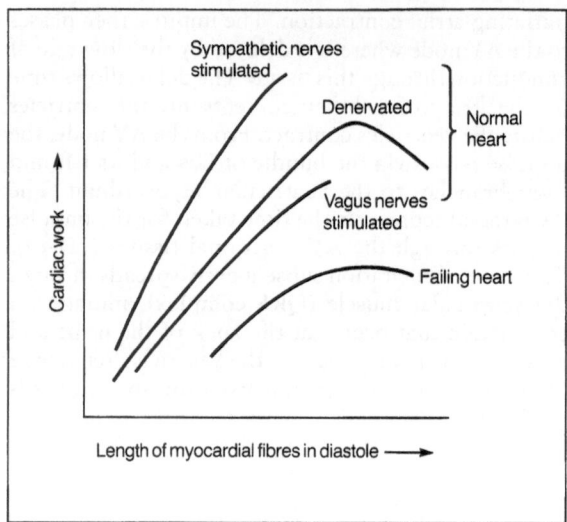

LD-26. Ventricular function curves showing the relationship between the left ventricular end diastolic pressure (a measure of the amount of stretching of the myocardial fibres during diastole) and ventricular work. At very high pressures, note how the curve begins to fall

Regulation of left and right ventricular outputs

The same property of cardiac muscle explains how the outputs of the right and left ventricles are matched so that, over a period of time, they pump equal volumes of blood. As the pulmonary and systemic circulations are in series, an increase in the output of either ventricle increases the venous return to the other, which then increases its own end-diastolic volume and hence its stroke volume. Thus, within the space of a few cycles, the outputs of the two ventricles are once again equal. Inequalities between the output of the ventricles are therefore transient and rapidly corrected.

Heart rate and cardiac output

Cardiac output is the product of heart rate and stroke volume. An increase in heart rate might therefore be expected to produce a proportional increase in cardiac output. However, it is important to realize that heart rate and stroke volume are not independent of one another, so that the above prediction does not necessarily hold true in all circumstances. As an increase in heart rate is achieved largely at the expense of diastole, the time available for ventricular filling is reduced. This leads to a reduction in the end-diastolic volume and, in consequence, the stroke volume is reduced. So, unless the increase in heart rate is accompanied by other changes, such as an increase in central venous pressure or increased contractility, the cardiac output changes little if at all and may actually fall with very rapid rates, because the increase cannot compensate for the greatly reduced diastolic filling time.

It is worth noting, however, that many of the extrinsic cardiac control mechanisms do ensure that an increased rate is accompanied by an increased filling pressure so that stroke volume is not reduced and cardiac output is increased. (See also Bowditch staircase effect, p. 17.)

Extrinsic control of the heart

Although the heart has the remarkable inherent ability to regulate its output in response to haemo-dynamic changes in the circulation, its ability to respond to the demands of other organs requires an extrinsic control system. This extrinsic control is mediated by the autonomic nervous system via the parasympathetic (vagus) and cardiac sympathetic nerves, and through the release of adrenaline from the adrenal medulla (LD-27).

LD-27. *The autonomic innervation of the heart in schematic form. The parasympathetic supply originates in the brainstem and reaches the heart via branches of the vagus nerve. Fibres supply the SA and AV nodes and the atria but not the ventricular myocardium. The sympathetic preganglionic fibres originate mainly in the upper thoracic region and pass mainly to the cervical ganglia of the sympathetic chain where they synapse with the postganglionic neurons. These supply the SA node, the atria and the ventricles. They also form a plexus around the aorta and its main branches where they mingle with the vagal preganglionic fibres. The adrenal medulla can be regarded as an extension of the sympathetic system*

The parasympathetic system (vagus)

The parasympathetic nervous system is largely concerned with regulating heart rate and has little or no direct effect on ventricular contractility or on the peripheral vasculature. All parts of the heart are able to initiate impulses at different inherent rates. The SA node has the highest inherent rate (LD-28) and normally functions as the cardiac pacemaker. The vagus affects heart rate by direct action on the SA node.

Stimulation of the vagus causes slowing of the heart rate (negative chronotropic effect) and, if sufficiently intense, can cause cardiac arrest. Usually, when this happens, the ventricles start beating at their own intrinsic rate despite continued vagal stimulation. This is known as ventricular escape.

In the moment-to-moment regulation of heart rate at rest, the vagal influence is dominant and, particularly in athletes with low resting heart rates, this 'vagal tone' can be considerable. Changes in heart rate under resting conditions tend to result from changes in vagal 'tone' rather than changes in sympathetic drive.

The effects of the vagus on the heart are mediated by acetylcholine (ACh), which activates only one kind of receptor – the 'muscarinic' receptor. Activation of this muscarinic receptor leads to an increase in potassium conductance. This decreases the slope of the pacemaker prepotential which therefore takes longer to trigger the action potential (LD-29). In this way, the heart rate is slowed. It is necessary for the vagus to influence the atria and the AV node at the same time as the SA node, because their inherent rates are also fast and they would otherwise take over the

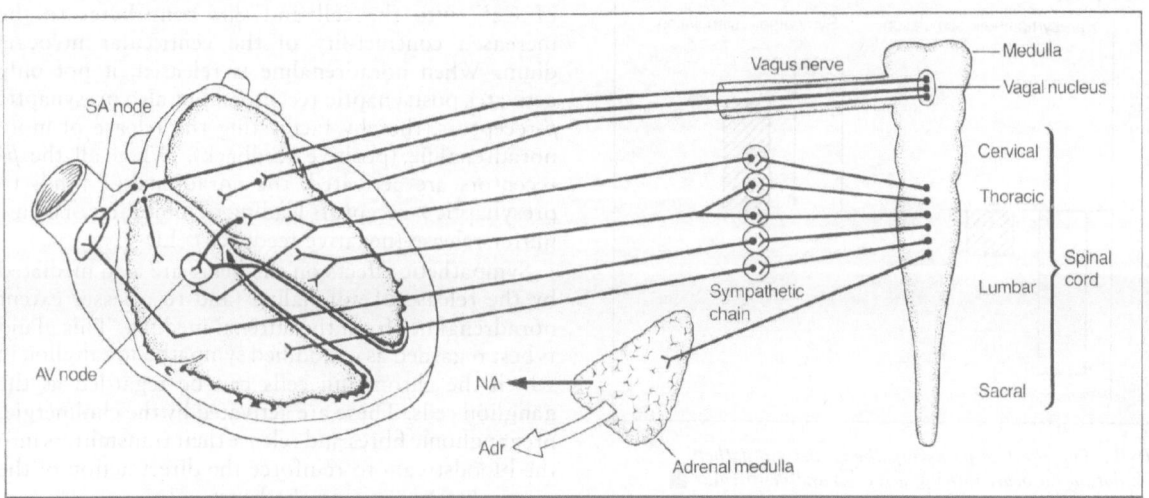

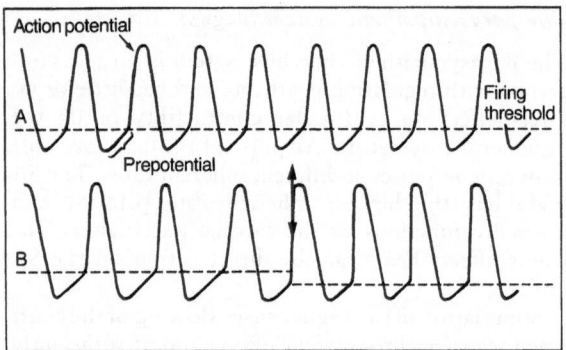

LD-28. *Pacemaker potentials showing prepotential and firing threshold. Cell B has a lower intrinsic discharge rate than cell A. When they are coupled (↕) as in the intact heart, cell A drives cell B. There is no change in prepotential slope. Effectively, the firing threshold of B has been lowered*

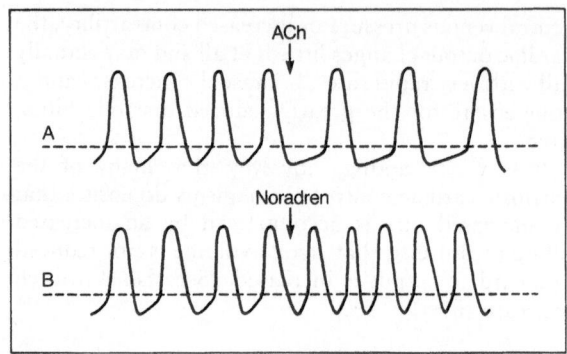

LD-29. *Pacemaker potentials showing how acetylcholine (ACh) reduces the slope of the prepotential and hence slows the heart rate (A). Noradrenaline increases the slope of the prepotential, thereby increasing the heart rate (B)*

pacemaker activity as soon as the rate of the SA node had been reduced below their own inherent rate.

The vagus has no direct effect on ventricular contractility (LD-30) as it does not innervate the ventricular myocardium to any significant extent. However, because it slows the heart rate, it would cause indirectly an increase in stroke volume (page 20), thereby offsetting the effect of a slower heart rate on cardiac output. On the other hand, because the vagus innervates the atrium, it can reduce ventricular filling by decreasing atrial contractility (negative inotropic effect) and in this way would cause a modest fall in cardiac output.

The sympathetic system and the adrenals

Sympathetic nerve fibres are widely distributed

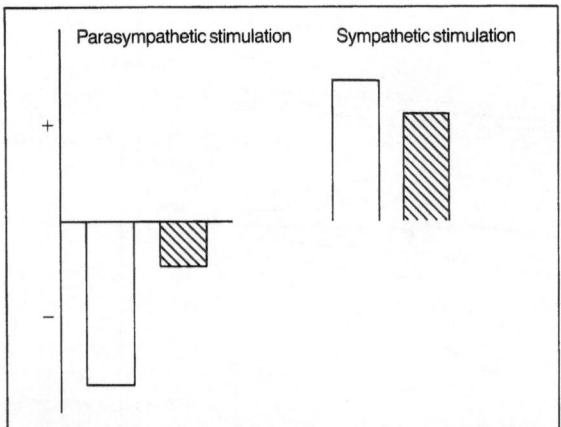

LD-30. *The effect of parasympathetic and sympathetic stimulation on heart rate* □*, atrial* ◩ *and ventricular* ■ *contractility*

throughout the heart. An increase in sympathetic discharge increases heart rate (positive chronotropic effect) by acting on the SA node and increases contractility (positive inotropic effect) by acting on the ventricular myocardium (LD-30). Although, at rest, the sympathetic fibres have less influence than the vagus, they play an important role in the response of the heart to stress and exercise.

The transmitter that mediates the effect of the sympathetic nerves on the heart is noradrenaline. This activates receptors that, in the heart, are predominantly of the β type. Activation of these receptors in the SA node leads to an increased K^+ influx and increased Na^+ efflux. This increases the slope of the pacemaker prepotential, thereby reducing the time taken to trigger the action potential and hence increasing the heart rate (LD-29).

Sympathetic stimulation also accelerates the influx of Ca^{2+} into the cell and this contributes to the increased contractility of the ventricular myocardium. When noradrenaline is released, it not only activates postsynaptic receptors, but also presynaptic β-receptors, thereby facilitating the release of more noradrenaline (positive feedback). When all the β-receptors are activated, the noradrenaline binds to presynaptic α-receptors leading to inhibition of transmitter release (negative feedback) (LD-31).

Sympathetic effects on the heart are also mediated by the release of adrenaline (and to a lesser extent noradrenaline) from the adrenal medulla. This gland is best regarded as a modified sympathetic ganglion in which the chromaffin cells can be regarded as the ganglion cells. These are activated by the cholinergic, preganglionic fibres and release their transmitters into the bloodstream to reinforce the direct action of the sympathetic nerves on the heart.

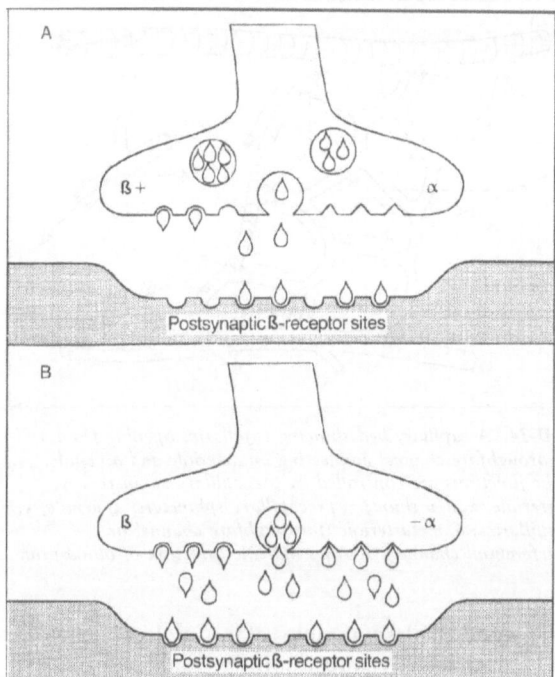

LD-31. *Autoregulation of transmitter release. When first released (A), noradrenaline stimulates presynaptic β-receptors, stimulating further release of transmitter (+). As the concentration in the synaptic cleft increases (B), presynaptic receptors are activated leading to inhibition (−) of transmitter release*

The vascular system

The blood is pumped from the heart to the tissues through the vascular system. The blood vessels constituting the vascular system, far from being passive conduits, are, like the heart itself, subject to various control mechanisms that affect cardiac output and its distribution. This section will describe the subdivisions of the vasculature and explain their characteristics.

General plan

The blood vessels can be divided into four systems:

- the arteries
- the arterioles
- the capillaries
- the veins

Each has different characteristics that determine its special role in regulating the circulation.

The arteries

The walls of the arteries possess a well developed tunica media containing considerable quantities of elastic tissue. The elastic properties, particularly of the aorta and large arteries, are important in smoothing out flow. During systole, the walls of the aorta distend; during diastole, they recoil and help to maintain the pressure and therefore the flow between contractions. By the time blood reaches the small arterioles, the flow is steady rather than pulsatile and this is due in large measure to the elasticity of the arterial system acting against a peripheral resistance (LD-32). A loss of elasticity in old age leads to a higher pulse pressure.

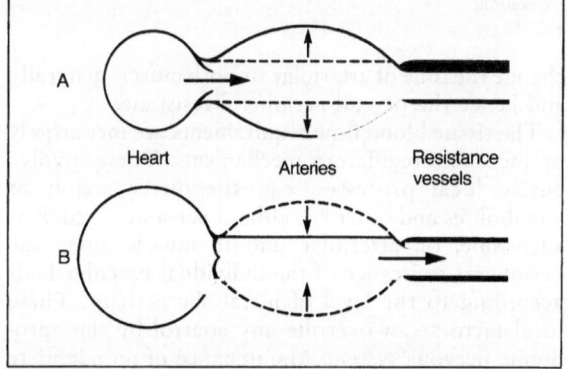

LD-32. *In systole (A) the heart expels blood against the resistance of the arterioles. The elastic arteries therefore distend to accommodate this volume. During diastole (B) the elastic vessels recoil against the peripheral resistance, thus maintaining pressure and flow*

The arterioles

These are the small terminal parts of the arterial tree. Their media consists of richly innervated smooth muscle. By contracting the smooth muscle in their walls, they vary the size of their lumens and thus the resistance to flow through them. The distribution of blood throughout the body therefore depends upon the degree of constriction of the arterioles in the different tissues. As the resistance to flow through a vessel varies inversely with the fourth power of its radius, a small change in diameter will produce a large effect on resistance and hence flow (LD-33). Control of peripheral resistance serves two distinct purposes:

- the regulation of arterial blood pressure
- the regulation of flow through individual organs

The arterial blood pressure is regulated by the autonomic nerves (mainly sympathetic), which

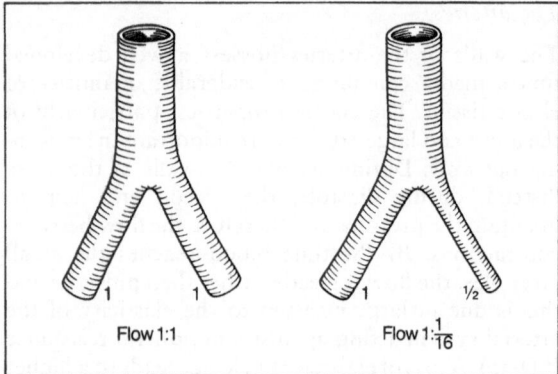

LD-33. *According to Poiseuille's law, halving the radius of a blood vessel increases resistance and hence decreases flow sixteenfold*

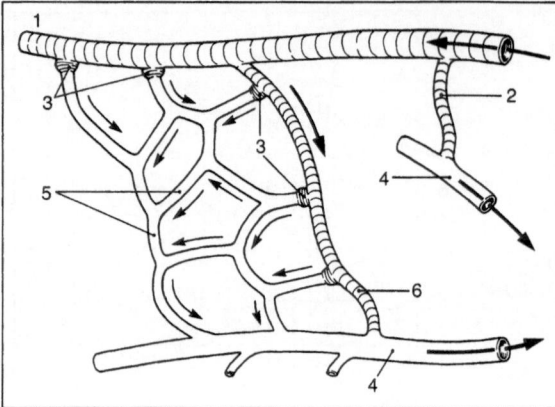

LD-34. *A capillary bed showing capillaries opening from a thoroughfare channel connecting an arteriole and a venule. The junctions are controlled by precapillary sphincters. 1, arteriole; 2, a–v shunt; 3, precapillary sphincters; 4, venule; 5, capillaries; 6, metarteriole (thoroughfare channel or preferential channel). Arrows indicate direction of blood flow*

change the tone of arteriolar smooth muscle generally and hence the overall peripheral resistance.

The tissue blood flow requirements are met largely by local autoregulatory mechanisms. These involve purely local processes, e.g. the direct action of metabolites and other vasodilator substances, such as adenosine, on arteriolar smooth muscle alters the peripheral resistance of the individual vascular beds according to the level of metabolic activity. These local factors can override any control by the autonomic nervous system. Maintenance of an adequate blood pressure is essential for the perfusion of all organs, particularly to ensure adequate perfusion of the brain.

Capillaries

Capillaries are the smallest blood vessels. The exchange of gases, nutrients and metabolites between the blood and the cells takes place through their walls. The general organization of a capillary bed is shown in LD-34.

The resistance of individual capillaries is high, but their combined resistance is less than that of arterioles because of their vast number and parallel arrangement. Flow through the capillaries is slow, to allow adequate time for exchange processes. The perfusion of individual sections of the capillary network is controlled by the precapillary sphincters that can be seen to open and close at intervals of 0.5–3 min.

Exchange across capillaries is the result of two processes:

- diffusion
- bulk flow

Because the capillary endothelium is permeable to water and all plasma solutes of low molecular weight, these move freely into the interstitial fluid. O_2 and nutrients move out of the capillary because the cells that constantly metabolize them create a concentration gradient between the plasma and the interstitial fluid. Conversely, CO_2 and metabolites, constantly produced by tissue cells, are in higher concentration in the interstitial fluid and diffuse into the capillaries.

Fluid flows across the capillary wall because osmotic pressure inside the capillary is higher than it is in the interstitial fluid. The pressure gradient results from (1) the hydrostatic pressure within the capillary and (2) the colloid osmotic pressure of the plasma proteins, which remain in the capillaries and do not pass into the interstitial fluid (LD-35).

Veins

Veins carry blood from the tissues back to the heart. They tend to be elliptical in cross-section and this allows them to increase their capacity without increasing the venous pressure. Collectively, they constitute the main reservoir of blood in the body. By varying the state of contraction of the smooth muscle in their walls, they can vary their capacity and through this mechanism the central venous pressure is controlled.

The control is exerted by the sympathetic nerves that innervate the smooth muscle. The consequence of venoconstriction, however, is quite different from that of arteriolar constriction (vasoconstriction). In

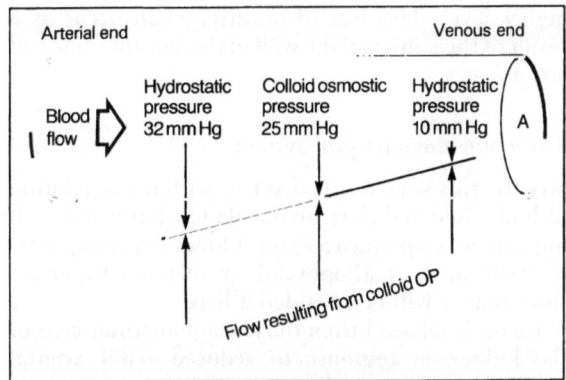

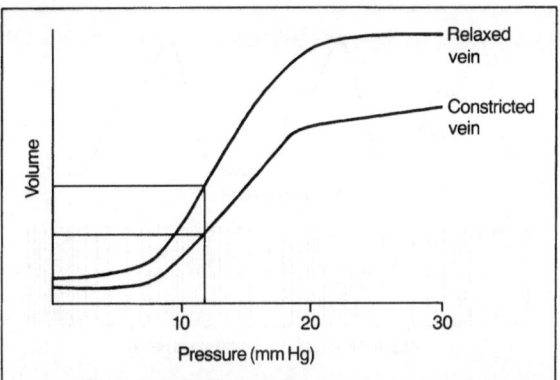

LD-35. *Fluid flow across capillaries. At the arterial end, hydrostatic pressure exceeds colloid osmotic pressure (OP), so there is a net flow of fluid into the interstitial space. At the venous end, the osmotic pressure exceeds hydrostatic pressure, and net flow is reversed. If hydrostatic pressure falls, as in haemorrhage, more fluid enters the capillaries than leaves them, so helping restore blood volume and pressure. If there is a sustained rise in blood pressure, a fall in plasma protein concentration or a leak of protein into the interstitial fluid, flow into the interstitial fluid will be increased and cause oedema*

LD-36. *Volume contained by a vein at different distending pressures. In the constricted state, at any given pressure the volume contained is less. If volume is held constant, then it follows that constriction must lead to a rise in pressure*

arterioles, a small change in radius leads to a great increase in resistance, but arterioles contain so little blood that this has little influence on its overall distribution. Veins, in contrast, contain such a large volume of blood that even small changes in their radius cause large changes in venous capacity and a redistribution of blood. As venous resistance is already low, a change in radius has little effect on overall peripheral resistance.

The compliance of veins is shown graphically in LD-36. Because of their distensibility, veins can accommodate a large volume of blood with little or no rise in pressure. Thereafter, pressure and volume are linearly related. Eventually, compliance is so reduced that quite high distending pressures produce little change in volume or, conversely, small volume changes lead to a rapid rise in pressure. When a vein is constricted by venomotor activity, the pressure/volume curve remains the same shape but shifts to the right; i.e. at any given distension pressure, the volume is less. In other words, compliance is reduced. If compliance of a small group of veins is reduced, the excess capacity in other veins readily accommodates the displaced blood. When a large number of veins contract simultaneously, venous pressure increases causing an increased venous return and hence an increased cardiac output. In this way, the capacity of the venous reservoir is reduced and blood is redistributed to the arterial side of the circulation.

Regulation of arterial blood pressure

As the arterial pressure provides the main force for the perfusion of tissues, particularly of the brain, its regulation is of paramount importance. The motor pathway for this regulation is provided mainly by the sympathetic nerves that innervate the smooth muscle in the walls of the arterioles. These are mainly noradrenergic and constrictor acting through α-adrenoceptors, though some cholinergic dilator fibres are found in some vascular beds.

The regulation of pressure also requires a sensory system to detect disturbances and trigger the appropriate reflex compensatory response.

Baroreceptor reflexes

Nerve endings, sensitive to pressure changes in the arterial system, are found in the carotid sinus and aortic arch. They are called 'baroreceptors', though the effective stimulus is stretching of the vessel wall rather than pressure *per se*.

These receptors discharge continuously during the cardiac cycle, their discharge being modulated by the pulse pressure (LD-37). When blood pressure rises, baroreceptor activity also rises, inhibits the vasomotor centre and causes a reduction in sympathetic constrictor tone. The baroreceptors also slow the heart, largely by stimulating the cardio-inhibitory centre but also by inhibiting the cardio-acceleratory centre. These pathways are shown schematically in LD-38. When blood pressure falls, these processes are reversed.

There is evidence that, in hypertension, the sensitivity of the baroreceptors is reduced so that, although they continue to regulate pressure, they do so at a

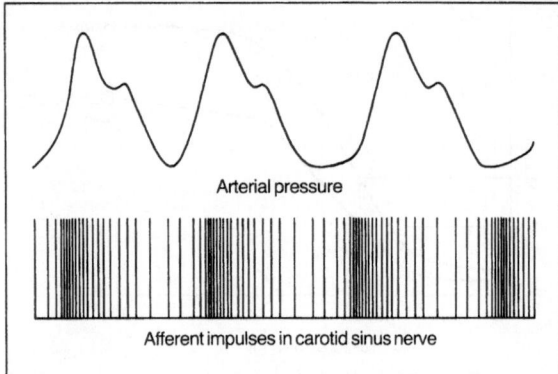

LD-37. Impulses in baroreceptor during cardiac cycle. Although they can discharge during diastole, baroreceptors are particularly sensitive to the rate of rise in pressure during systole

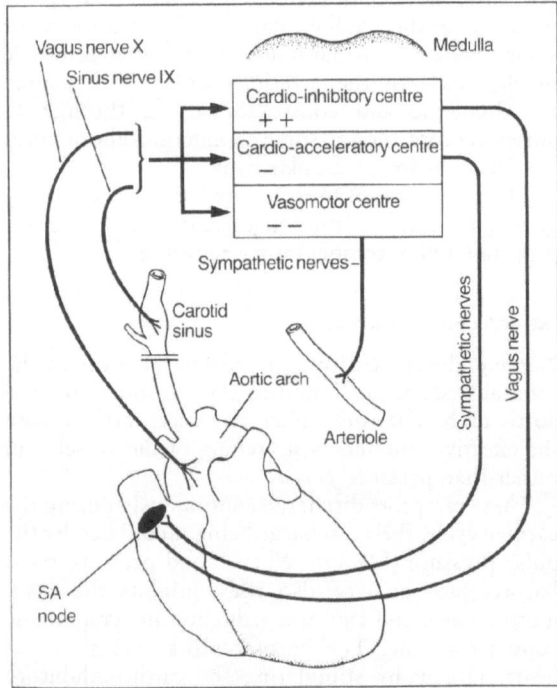

LD-38. Pathways of the baroreceptor reflexes showing the site of action of baroreceptor afferents in the medulla. A rise in pressure leads to a rise in baroreceptor discharge. This leads to excitation (+) of the cardio-inhibitory centre and, to a lesser extent, inhibition (−) of the cardio-acceleratory centre. Thus heart rate slows. More importantly, they also inhibit the vasomotor centre, thereby reducing vasoconstrictor tone

higher level. This loss of sensitivity can occur as a result of thickening of the wall of the carotid sinus and aorta.

The renin–angiotension system

Strictly, this system is concerned with the regulation of body fluid and electrolyte balance, but it has such important consequences on blood pressure, particularly in the pathophysiology of renal hypertension, that it will be considered here.

Renin is released from the juxtaglomerular cells of the kidney in response to reduced renal arterial pressure or increased sympathetic nerve activity acting on β-adrenoceptors in the cells, and also from the adjacent macula densa in response to a fall in sodium load (LD-39).

The renin acts on a substrate produced in the liver and normally present in the plasma, to produce angiotension I. This is further acted on by a converting enzyme from lung and kidney to yield angiotension II, a powerful constrictor of arteriolar smooth muscle and therefore strongly hypertensive.

In addition, it releases aldosterone and antidiuretic hormone (ADH) which influence circulating volume and indirectly influence blood pressure.

Regulation of central venous pressure

As described above, central venous pressure can be controlled by altering the compliance of the veins through changes in venomotor tone. To illustrate the consequences of this process, LD-40 shows, in a somewhat simplified way, the compensatory responses that take place following a fall in central venous pressure caused by haemorrhage.

The pulmonary circulation

Peripheral resistance in the lungs is much lower than in the systemic circulation and the mean arterial pressure is correspondingly lower (12–15 mmHg). The pressure gradient across the pulmonary capillary bed is only about 5–10 mmHg.

The low pressure in the pulmonary capillaries is exceeded by the osmotic pressure of the plasma proteins. This would prevent fluid movement out of the capillaries were it not for the presence of protein in the pulmonary interstitial fluid. Bulk flow of water does occur, though it is considerably restricted and so prevents water entering the alveoli and interfering with gas exchange. The pulmonary lymphatics are also important in removing excess fluid. A rise in pulmonary capillary pressure in diseases leads to the

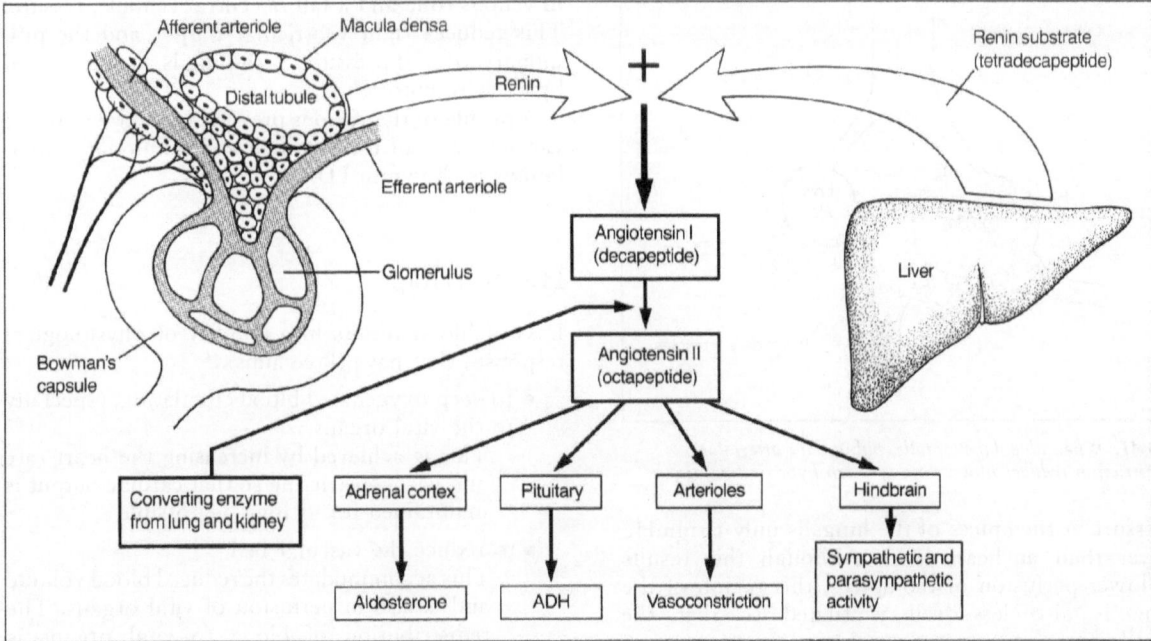

LD-39. *The sites of release of renin and a summary of the renin–angiotensin system*

production of excessive fluid and hence dyspnoea, particularly when in the supine position.

The low resistance of the pulmonary arterioles and their elasticity ensures that they distend when right ventricular output increases, thereby further decreasing their resistance. This automatic adjustment ensures that the increased output has little net effect on pulmonary arterial pressure. However, pulmonary arteriolar resistance, and hence pulmonary pressure, can be affected by hormonal influences, pulmonary gas tensions and, in some pathological conditions, by nervous influences. The most important of these factors is the constriction of the pulmonary arterioles in response to low alveolar PO_2, the converse of the systemic arteriolar response. This assures that the better ventilated parts of the lung are better perfused with blood (LD-41).

The pulmonary circulation can operate at low pressures because it is not exposed to large hydrostatic forces. In the upright position, the mean arterial

LD-40. *Effect of a fall in central venous pressure on cardiac output and reflex compensatory mechanisms. The increased sympathetic discharge will compensate for the fall in arterial pressure by causing arteriolar constriction. While this will restore systemic arterial pressure, it will also tend to reduce central venous pressure further, unless accompanied by the venoconstriction shown above*

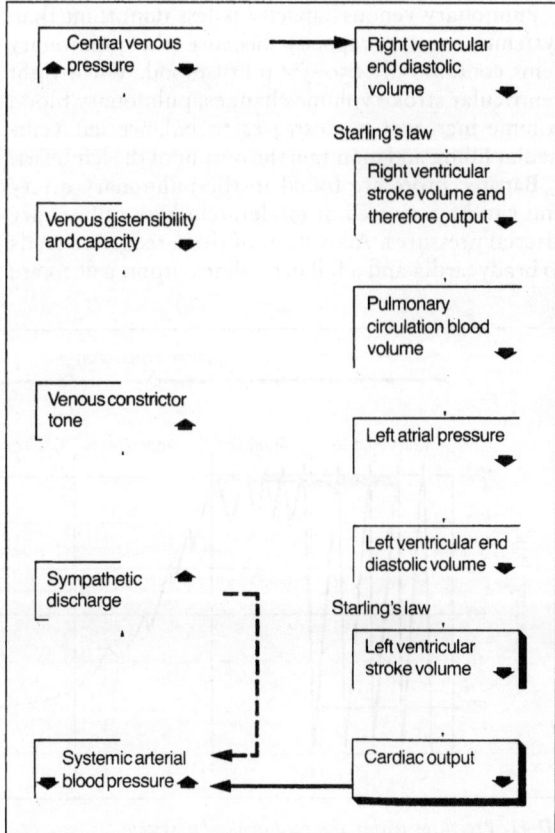

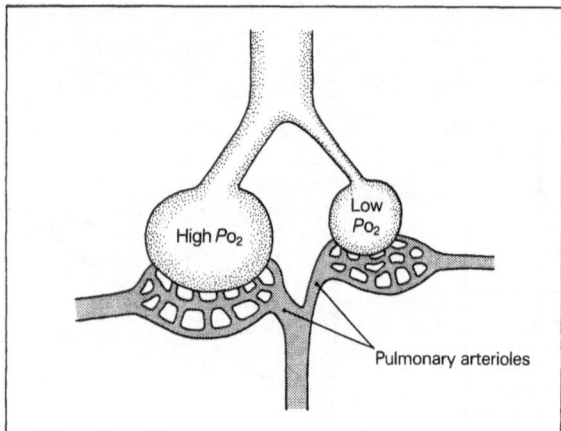

LD-41. *When alveolar* Po$_2$ *falls, pulmonary arteriolar constriction reduces blood flow through hypoxic lung tissue*

pressure at the apices of the lungs is only 10 mmHg lower than at heart level. Although this results in lower perfusion of the apices, this region of the lung is also less well ventilated so that the ventilation/perfusion ratio remains fairly constant throughout the lungs.

Pulmonary venous capacity is less important than systemic venous capacity because the pulmonary veins contain only 250–300 ml of blood. When right ventricular stroke volume changes, pulmonary blood volume increases or decreases to balance left ventricular filling and maintain the output of the left heart.

Baroreceptors are found in the pulmonary artery and can be activated at moderately high pulmonary arterial pressures. Activation of these receptors leads to bradycardia and a fall in cardiac output, a decrease

in venous tone and a fall in central venous pressure. This reduces right ventricular output and the pulmonary arterial pressure. Breathing is also depressed by these receptors.

A profile of the various pressures found within the various parts of the systemic and pulmonary circulations is shown in LD-42.

Haemorrhage

Loss of blood results in a number of physiological responses that have three aims:

- to keep oxygenated blood circulating, especially to the vital organs
  This is achieved by increasing the heart rate and vasoconstricting so that cardiac output is maintained for as long as possible

- to reduce the vascular bed
  This accommodates the reduced blood volume and assists in perfusion of vital organs. The redistribution of blood to vital organs is assured by changes in vascular tone. The vessels to the skin and gut are constricted whereas those to the heart and brain dilate. The total vascular bed is thus reduced and the perfusion pressure in the tissues is maintained

- to restore blood volume
  This starts immediately blood is lost and is related to capillary exchange. Because of the lowered capillary pressure, more fluid passes into the venules from the interstitial tissues (plasma refill).

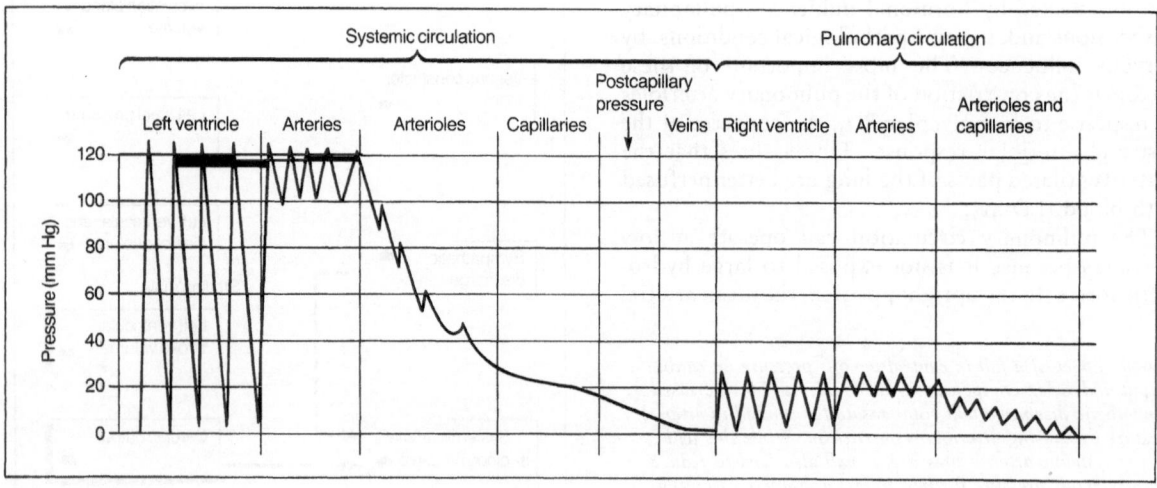

LD-42. *Pressures within the cardiovascular system*

Physiological changes

The first two aims are accomplished by neurogenic and hormonal actions.

Neurogenic control

À fall in blood pressure stimulates the baroreceptors:
- the low pressure venous baroreceptors
- the high pressure arterial baroreceptors

The low pressure baroreceptors in the atria and great veins of the thorax respond to a fall in central venous pressure. The high pressure arterial baroreceptors in the aortic arch and carotid sinus respond to a fall in arterial pressure. The baroreceptors relax their inhibitory action on the vasomotor centres which then stimulate the sympathetic nervous system to produce peripheral vasoconstriction. This raises the peripheral resistance and arterial blood pressure.

Hormonal control

Various hormones are released into the circulation to raise blood pressure and blood flow through the tissues. These act on specific receptor sites in the smooth muscle of arteries and include the adrenal medullary hormones, adrenaline and noradrenaline. Noradrenaline acts on the receptors in the vessel wall to produce vasoconstriction. Adrenaline acts on both the α- and β-receptors, the proportion of these receptors in the blood vessel wall determining the response to the hormones. For example, in the skin, β-receptors predominate so that vasoconstriction occurs; in the coronary arteries β-receptors predominate so that vasodilatation occurs.

A fall in pressure in the renal arteries causes release of renin. This changes angiotensinogen to angiotensin I, which is changed into angiotensin II, a potent vasoconstrictor. Vasopressin, a vasoconstricting hormone, comes from the posterior lobe of the pituitary. Locally produced kinins, such as bradykinin, have a vasodilator action on the arterioles and are produced in response to ischaemia.

Capillary exchange

When the arteriolar pressure falls, fluid passes into the capillaries from the interstitial tissues to aid in restoring blood volume. The speed of refill is governed by the degree of drop in arteriolar pressure. This fluid dilutes the blood and not only helps to restore blood volume and pressure, but aids blood flow by allowing the blood cells to pass more quickly through the capillaries.

Restoration of plasma proteins is slower and takes some days. It depends on the breakdown of muscle proteins and the synthesis of amino acids to form albumin in the liver. Red cells also take longer to return to normal as they are manufactured in the bone marrow in response to erythropoietin from the kidney.

Shock

There are many definitions of shock. It may simply be regarded as a state where, because of diminished blood flow, the tissues suffer from lack of oxygen.

Shock, therefore, exists when the body is unable to contain a change in the:
- blood volume
- circulatory bed
- pumping action of the heart

Under each of these headings there are many causes of shock. Common examples are:
- hypovolaemic shock due to blood loss
- septic shock due to expansion of the circulatory bed
- cardiogenic shock due to pump failure

The effects of shock are many but all lead to deficient oxygen supply to cells.

Shock due to change in capillary bed

In septic shock the problem is more complex. It is due mainly to release of endotoxins from bacteria and is sometimes referred to as endotoxic shock. These toxins come mainly from Gram-negative organisms but septic shock may be associated with any organisms.

Blood volume is lost into dilated veins and capillaries throughout the body. Capillary leakage also occurs, so that plasma escapes into the interstitial tissues. If this occurs in areas such as the lungs, it is difficult for oxygen to pass from the alveoli into the blood stream and the respiratory distress syndrome (RDS) becomes evident. There is a low blood PO_2 that will not respond to oxygen therapy. The toxins may also affect the heart to cause cardiac failure and the kidneys to cause renal failure.

Shock due to change in pump action of heart

Cardiogenic shock follows massive myocardial infarction. The exact mechanism of its production is still uncertain but it is a consequence of acute left heart failure and results in progressive hypotension, sweating, cold extremities and mental torpor.

Massive pulmonary embolism results in acute right-sided heart failure. Shock is caused by a sudden reduction of cardiac output with a severe fall in systemic blood pressure.

PATHOLOGY

Congenital heart disease

Most congenital cardiac malformations occur at a very early stage of fetal development. As with other congenital malformations, the cause is seldom apparent. Usually, it is multifactorial and the result of a complex interplay between hereditary and environmental influences.

Some are associated with chromosomal abnormalities, some occur as part of a genetic disorder and some are caused by viral infections.

The total number with identifiable causes is still less than 10% and much remains to be learned about this aspect of heart disease.

Rheumatic heart disease

The heart is commonly affected in the generalized connective tissue or 'collagen' disorders, and acute rheumatic fever is much the most important of these.

The occurrence of a latent period between the episode of acute streptococcal infection and the characteristic symptoms of rheumatic fever suggests an abnormal immune response to the common Group A β-haemolytic streptococcal infection. A genetic influence is also probable in those so affected. Acute rheumatic fever lasts some weeks or months and recurrences are common. Although arthritis is the most common clinical feature, carditis is the most sinister. It is more commonly present in first attacks in children than in adults. Acute carditis often leads to chronic rheumatic heart disease. Many cases of chronic disease are seen without any clear history of acute rheumatism.

Pathological findings

Fibrinous pericarditis, cardiac enlargement and acute

endocarditis are characteristic postmortem findings in fatal cases of acute rheumatic fever.

The specific histological lesion is the Aschoff body. These lesions may be widespread throughout the myocardium. They are granulomata in which degenerate collagen and multinucleated cells are prominent.

Valvulitis in non-fatal cases is responsible for permanent and progressive valve damage (either predominant stenosis or incompetence). The order of frequency of valve involvement may be related to the pressure at which the valve leaflets close as suggested in Table 6.

TABLE 6

Order	Valve	Valve closing pressure
1	Mitral	left ventricular systolic
2	Aortic	aortic diastolic
3	Tricuspid	right ventricular systolic
4	Pulmonary	pulmonary diastolic

In the stage of acute endocarditis, the leaflets are oedematous with erosions and small sterile vegetations consisting of fibrin and platelets. Subsequent scarring and distortion of the valves with fusion or retraction of cusps accounts for a wide variety of lesions from almost pure stenosis to gross incompetence.

Inflammatory heart disease

The following may be present, singly, or in combination:

- pericarditis
- myocarditis
- endocarditis

Pericarditis

This may be of several types:

- fibrinous
- serofibrinous
- purulent
- adhesive
- constrictive

There are a variety of causes:

- bacteria

- viruses
- acute rheumatism
- trauma
- neoplasm
- uraemia
- myocardial infarction
- collagen disease
- arteritis
- idiopathic

Myocarditis

In severe cases of acute myocarditis, the heart is dilated and flabby, with an acute inflammatory exudate (polymorphonuclear or mononuclear) that may be diffuse or focal.

Bacterial infections

The heart may be involved in septicaemia or when infection is localized elsewhere in the body, either by the invading organisms or their toxins. The cardiac involvement may be trivial and not clinically evident, perhaps only being shown by electrocardiographic changes. On the other hand, it may be severe or fatal, a classical example being diphtheritic myocarditis.

Viral infections

The best known examples are infection with Coxsackie B, poliomyelitis and influenza. Here again, there may be a wide spectrum in the severity of cardiac involvement.

Other myocarditides

These include:

- rheumatic heart disease
- Chagas disease
- toxoplasmosis

The myocardium may also be involved in:

- many generalized diseases, e.g. syphilis, sarcoidosis
- poisonings, e.g. carbon monoxide, tricyclic antidepressants
- physical injury, e.g. irradiation, car accidents

Endocarditis

Infective endocarditis

This usually occurs in patients with acquired or congenital cardiac lesions. It is most commonly blood borne, but is increasingly seen following cardiac surgery or investigative procedures. Bacteria, Rickettsia or fungi may be the causative agents.

Endocardial vegetations may be large or small and are usually friable. Destruction of valves or other structures may be considerable. Emboli, being infective, can give rise to mycotic aneurysms. The myocardium may contain frank abscesses or merely non-specific foci of mononuclear cells. One of the most serious complications is glomerulonephritis, which may be diffuse or focal.

Rheumatic endocarditis

This is the most important of the non-infective endocarditides.

New growths

Primary

These are very rare and include:

- myxoma – the commonest
- sarcoma
- simple tumours – fibroma, haemangioma

Cardiac myxomata are usually found in the atria, particularly the left, closely related to the fossa ovalis. They are round or lobulated, smooth or irregular, and there may be overlying thrombus. They give rise to symptoms by blocking the orifices of valves or by arterial embolism.

Secondary

Metastatic deposits in the myocardium or pericardium are common. Practically any primary tumour may spread to the heart; carcinoma of the bronchus and reticuloses are the commonest. Such metastases cause surprisingly little in the way of symptoms, but may give rise to dysrhythmias or cause heart block from involvement of the conduction system. Occasionally, cardiac tamponade results from pericarditis or extensive pericardial deposits.

Coronary heart disease

The clinical patterns include:

- angina

- sudden death
- cardiac infarction
- cardiac failure

Atheroma of the coronary arteries is far and away the commonest cause of cardiac ischaemia.

Other causes are:

- coronary embolism – as in infective endorcarditis
- arteritis – polyarteritis nodosa and giant-celled arteritis
- impaired coronary blood flow – due to severe disease of the aortic valve or first part of the aorta

Atheroma

This consists of raised patchy intimal lesions. A core of lipid-rich material is covered by connective tissue. The elements vary in different lesions. Calcification, ulceration, overlying thrombus and intramural haemorrhage further diversify the form of the patches of atheroma.

Cardiac implications

Impaired coronary blood flow can lead to myocardial infarction with either necrosis in the distribution of a diseased coronary artery or a more diffuse subendocardial distribution.

Papillary muscle necrosis or rupture can result in mitral valve incompetence. Ventricular aneurysm, rupture of the ventricular septum (acquired ventricular septal defect) and rupture into the pericardium are other severe or fatal complications.

Fibrinous pericarditis is common and may become haemorrhagic in patients receiving anticoagulant therapy.

The infarcted area consists of a central yellowish area of necrotic material surrounded by ischaemic tissue. Healing occurs by organization and fibrosis of the dead tissue.

In cases of sudden unexpected death or in those dying during the first few hours, less than half show the histological features seen in patients who die on the second or subsequent days. In some, this is because there has been insufficient time for evidence of infarction to appear; in others, it is because no infarction has occurred.

Cardiac hypertrophy

Hypertrophy of a cardiac chamber is a compensatory mechanism required to overcome:

- increased pressure loads caused by such things as arterial hypertension or stenosed valves
- increased volume loads caused by such things as arteriovenous shunts or valves that allow regurgitation

Increase in size of individual fibres is followed, when necessary, by an increase in the number of fibres and a proportional increase in capillaries.

The heart is smaller in females than in males and there is a rough relationship with both height and weight. There is, however, a wide range of individual chamber weights and volumes, and it is difficult to be sure of slight hypertrophy.

Moderate or severe degrees of hypertrophy and enlargement are usually evident on inspection, by measurement of wall thickness or by weighing.

Cardiomyopathy

This is a term that was used originally for myocardial disease of unknown aetiology. Most of the pathological changes are fairly non-specific with varying amounts of round-cell infiltration and fibrosis in chambers that show varying degrees of enlargement and hypertrophy.

Over the years, a number of aetiological agents have been detected (alcohol, collagen diseases etc.) and the number qualifying under this heading has been slowly diminishing. The term has been retained, however, with the prefix Primary used for those whose aetiology remains a mystery and the prefix Secondary used for those where the cause is thought to have been discovered.

Primary cardiomyopathies

Hypertrophic cardiomyopathy

This often disproportionately affects the ventricular septum, predominantly on the left side. It is characterized by abnormally arranged myocardial fibres and excessive connective tissue, and can interfere not only with the function of the left ventricle but also with that of the aortic and mitral valves.

Congestive cardiomyopathy

This is characterized by a flabby myocardium with dilated cardiac chambers and is associated with unexplained heart failure.

Obliterative cardiomyopathy (endomyocardial fibrosis)

Here there is unexplained endocardial thickening and reduction in the size of cardiac chambers that interferes with function in much the same way as constrictive pericarditis.

Secondary cardiomyopathy

These are diseases of the myocardium of known aetiology, some of which have a characteristic histological pattern. Examples include:

- cardiac haemosiderosis
- glycogen storage disease
- cardiac disease associated with skeletal myopathy

Other causes include:

- nutritional disorders – beriberi
- electrolyte disorders – potassium deficiency
- poisoning – severe chronic alcoholism

Pathology of the specialized conducting tissue

The commonest congenital abnormalities are accessory atrioventricular pathways. These account for ventricular pre-excitation and the circus rhythms that are frequently associated with it, e.g. the Wolff–Parkinson–White syndrome.

Progressive idiopathic fibrosis of the conducting pathways in elderly patients with otherwise healthy hearts is much the commonest cause of heart block. Less common causes are:

- coronary heart disease
- calcific aortic valve disease
- cardiomyopathy
- trauma

Heart failure

Here there is likely to be evidence of intrinsic heart disease – myocardial infarction, valvular disease or cardiac hypertrophy in response to a pressure load. It is right ventricular in patients with such conditions as chronic diffuse lung disease or pulmonary thromboembolic disease and left ventricular in those with systemic arterial hypertension or mitral regurgitation.

The heart fails when compensatory mechanisms become inadequate to maintain the forward flow of blood. The cardiac chambers usually dilate because of lengthening of myocardial sarcomeres and fail to empty properly. The venous inflow is impeded and as a result the venous pressure rises, the veins become distended and congestion results. In left heart failure, there is congestion in the lung vessels with interstitial and intra-alveolar oedema. In right heart failure, there is systemic venous congestion with dependent peripheral oedema and fluid collection in serous cavities. The abdominal viscera are engorged with blood. The liver, especially, becomes enlarged and also fibrotic when heart failure has been long-standing.

Poor forward blood flow, especially in the presence of widespread arterial atheroma, may be associated with infarction of the brain or other organs. Systemic venous distension and stasis may give rise to venous thrombosis and the risk of pulmonary embolism.

The lungs and the pulmonary vascular bed

Chronic respiratory disease imposes an increased load on the right ventricle by making it work harder to pump blood through the lungs. In severe cases, this may eventually lead to right heart failure. Cor pulmonale is the term by which this type of secondary heart disease is commonly known.

The lungs are also involved in diseases affecting the left heart. In obstructive lesions such as mitral stenosis, for example, there is chronic pulmonary arterial hypertension because of increased tone in the pulmonary arterioles. Under such circumstances, irreversible obliterative changes occur in the pulmonary vascular bed that increase the work of the right heart in much the same way as in chronic cor pulmonale.

Pulmonary hypertension, an obligatory response in certain conditions, is less predictable in others. Some patients with mitral stenosis develop a considerable increase in their pulmonary artery pressures while others, with seemingly identical lesions, do not.

The ageing heart

The heart changes little with age except for an increase in the pigment lipofuscin. This increase in pigment, together with cardiac atrophy, constitutes brown atrophy. It is seen in generalized wasting diseases, which are more frequent in the elderly, particularly when associated with neoplasia.

Calcification of the aortic and mitral valves is increasingly common with advancing age, as is mucoid or myxomatous degeneration of the mitral valve. These are by no means innocent conditions and carry a significant morbidity and mortality.

Amyloid degeneration confined to the heart is common in those over 70. In the great majority, it causes no symptoms although it occasionally accounts for otherwise unexplained cardiac failure.

ELECTROCARDIOGRAPHY

The electrocardiogram (ECG) registers the electrical activity of the heart, which is generated by individual cardiac cells. It is easily recorded and often provides essential diagnostic information. Interpretation of the electrocardiogram is therefore an integral part of any cardiological assessment.

Cellular electrophysiology

Electrical events within cardiac cells have been extensively studied in animal preparations and to a considerable extent in humans.

Microelectrode recordings from within cardiac cells demonstrate that a resting potential of approximately -90 mV is present across the cell membrane. This resting membrane potential is generated by distribution of ions between intracellular and extracellular fluids. There is active (i.e. energy requiring) outward transport of Na^+ ions and inward transport of K^+ ions. This results in a negative potential within the cell and a relatively positive potential on the surface of the cell. The cell membrane is therefore polarized. At rest, permeability to potassium is high, so the resting membrane potential is largely dependent upon extracellular potassium concentration.

Pacemaker cells

Most cardiac cells maintain a stable resting membrane potential, but at several sites pacemaker cells are present. These are characterized by a spontaneous fall in their resting membrane potential or diastolic depolarization (LD-43a). Diastolic depolarization is due to a gradual inward leakage of Na^+ ions and a

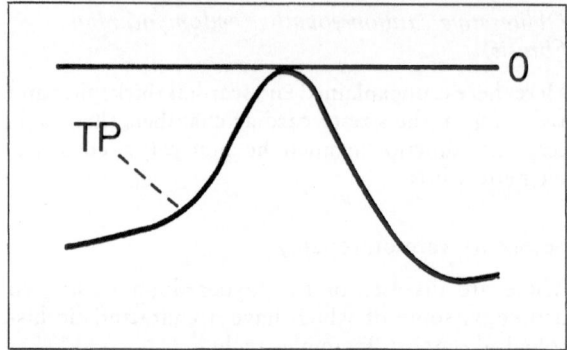

LD-43a. *Cardiac action potential. The action potential from a pacemaker cell is shown. Instead of the normal stable resting membrane potential (phase 4), there is gradual spontaneous depolarization until a threshold potential (TP) is reached when depolarization is self-perpetuating*

reduced outward flux of K^+ ions. When a threshold level of about -60 mV is reached, the process becomes self-perpetuating and more rapid depolarization occurs. These events can be recorded by an intracellular microelectrode as an action potential. Rapid depolarization spreads from the pacemaker cells to adjacent cells (LD-43b). These, in turn, are depolarized to threshold level, thus generating further depolarization and sequential activation of cardiac tissue.

Pacemaker activity is detectable in the

- sinus node
- lower part of the AV node
- His Bundle (the AV junction)
- Purkinje system

It is usually most rapid in sinus node cells and slowest in distal Purkinje cells. It is generally absent from normal atrial and ventricular muscle but may be present in these tissues when they are unduly excitable or ischaemic. As the most rapid pacemaker rhythm is usually in the sinus node, sinus rhythm dominates and suppresses pacemaker activity at other sites. If the sinus rate should slow, subsidiary rhythms may emerge from other sites and are termed 'escape' rhythms.

The cardiac action potential

Depolarization in non-pacemaker cells occurs when a cell is excited by an external electrical stimulus or is activated by spread of electrical activity from adjacent tissue. The action potential that results has several characteristics (LD-44). Rapid depolarization (phase 0) is followed by short-lived relatively rapid repolariz-

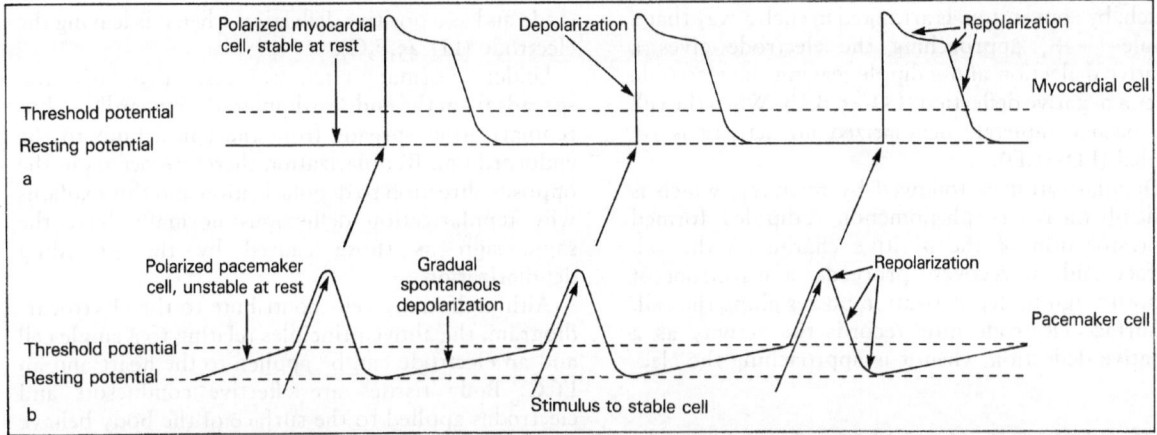

LD-43b. *Cardiac action potential. Gradual spontaneous depolarization of pacemaker cells provides constant stimuli to myocardial cells that are stable at rest*

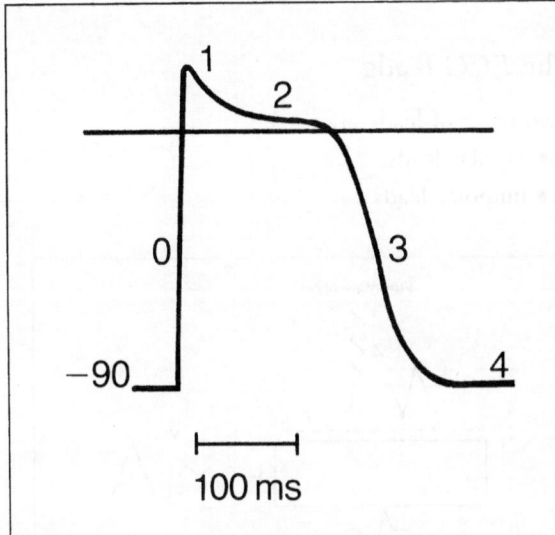

LD-44. *Cardiac action potential. The typical cardiac action potential has five phases numbered 0–4. Conduction velocity of the action potential is dependent on the rate of rise of phase 0. The duration of the action potential determines the refractory period and varies for different cardiac tissues*

the ECG and repolarization corresponds to the T wave.

Each phase of the action potential is due to different ionic fluxes.

Phase 0
Rapid depolarization, is due to a sudden increase in permeability of the cell membrane to Na^+ ions and is largely complete in a few milliseconds.

Phase 1
Repolarization, is due to an inward current of Cl^- ions.

Phase 2
The plateau phase, is due to a slow inward Na^+ current and in some cells an inward Ca^{2+} current contributes.

Phase 3
Repolarization, is due to an outward K^+ current.

Some antidysrhythmic drugs affect these different ionic fluxes.

ation (phase 1), a plateau phase (phase 2), a repolarization phase with restoration of the resting potential (phase 3) and finally the resting phase (phase 4).

The cell is inexcitable or 'refractory' during the action potential and normal excitability only returns with return of the membrane potential to resting values. The cell is 'relatively refractory' during phase 3 as the membrane potential returns to normal. Depolarization corresponds to the QRS complex of

The genesis of the ECG

The genesis of the ECG can best be appreciated by considering a single cell. When a cell is depolarized, the surface of the cell becomes relatively negative. Adjacent cell surfaces remain positively charged so that positively and negatively charged areas become contiguous, forming a dipole (LD-45,A). Current flows from positive to negative areas so that activation and the dipole spread along the cell (LD-45,C). This activity can be recorded by a surface electrode, which, by convention, is arranged in such a way that a dipole (− +) approaching the electrode gives a positive deflection and a dipole leaving the electrode gives a negative deflection (LD-45,B,C). When the cell has been completely depolarized no activity is recorded (LD-45,D).

Depolarization is followed by recovery, which is basically the reverse phenomenon. A dipole is formed by restoration of the positive charge on the cell surface and, as recovery proceeds, a wavefront of opposite sign to depolarization passes along the cell. A surface electrode now records the activity as a negative deflection when it is approaching the elec-

trode and as a positive deflection when it is leaving the electrode (LD-45,F,G).

Under normal circumstances, depolarization spreads from the endocardium to the epicardium, but repolarization spreads from the epicardium to the endocardium. Repolarization therefore occurs in the opposite direction to depolarization and this explains why repolarization deflections normally have the same sign as those caused by the preceding depolarization.

Although many cells contribute to the electrocardiogram, the above principles relating to a single cell and an electrode can be applied to the heart and an ECG. Body tissues are effective conductors and electrodes applied to the surface of the body behave similarly to those applied to the surface of the heart.

LD-45. Depolarization and repolarization. A, The resting cell surface is positively charged. B, depolarization results in a dipole (− +) that moves along the cell surface (B→D). Activation leaving electrode X is recorded as a negative potential but the same activation approaching electrode Y is recorded as a positive potential. Recordings from Z are biphasic. When depolarization is complete (D,E), repolarization follows and results in the formation of a dipole (+ −) (F). This has the opposite configuration to the dipole of depolarization, i.e. it leads with a negative charge. It also moves in the opposite direction resulting in a repolarization wave (T) with the same sign as depolarization. The configuration of the T wave varies in the electrodes X, Y and Z

The ECG leads

Two types of leads are used:

* bipolar leads
* unipolar leads

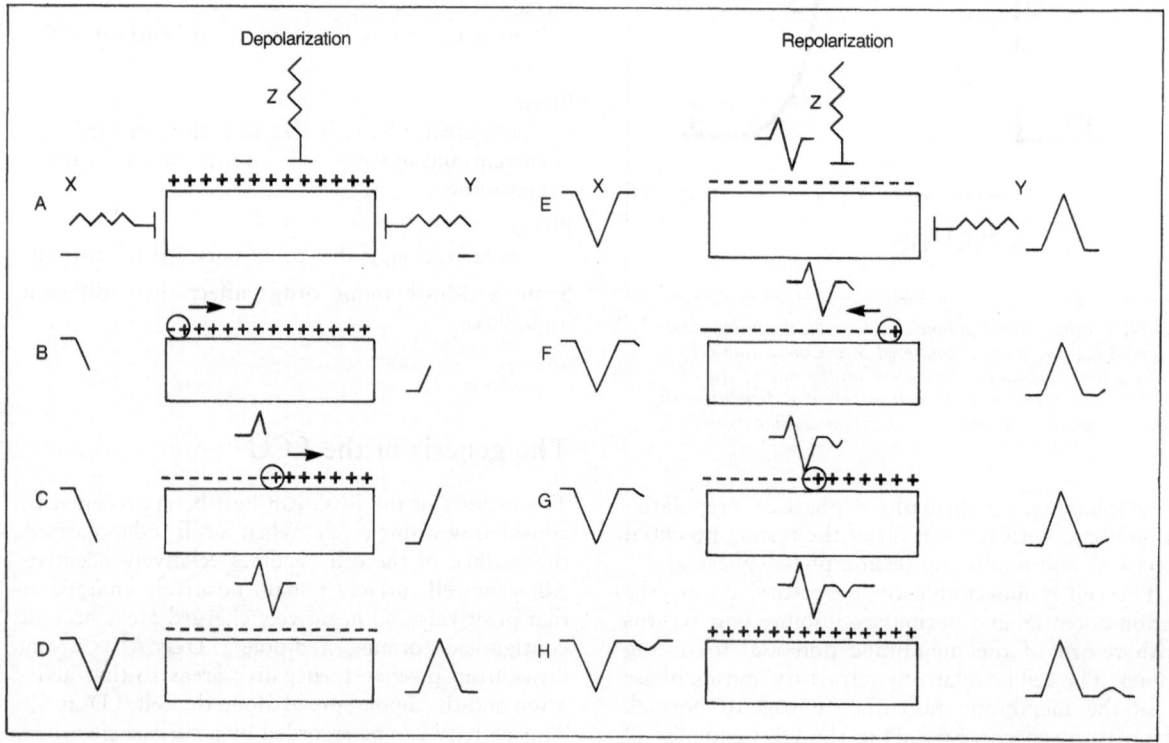

Bipolar leads

Two of three limb electrodes are used and electrical activity is recorded between them. (Table 7). A fourth electrode on the right leg acts as an earth lead.

TABLE 7

	Negative electrode	Positive electrode
Lead I	Right arm	Left arm
Lead II	Right arm	Left leg
Lead III	Left arm	Left leg

Events affecting the anterior surface of the heart are best seen in Lead 1 and those affecting the inferior surface in Leads 2 and 3 (LD-46).

Local events are more readily recorded by unipolar leads.

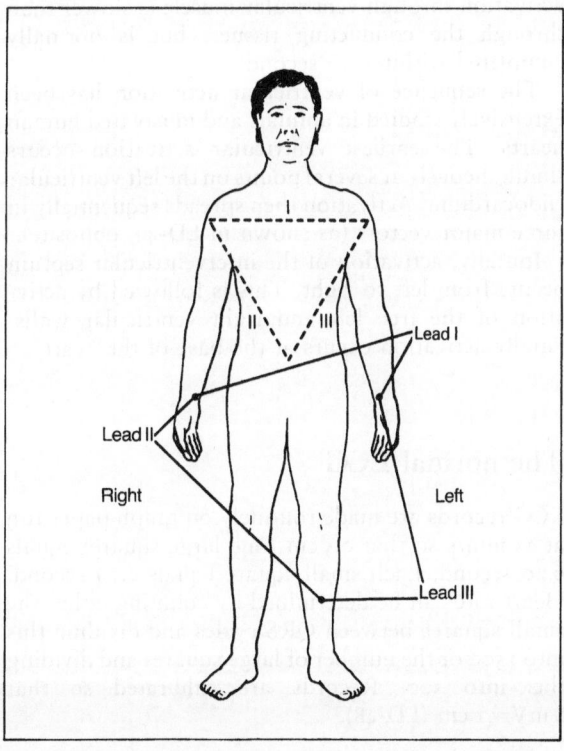

LD-46. The standard limb leads are shown. Conventionally the electrodes are placed distally on the limbs. The body tissues act as conductors giving the same effect as having the electrodes much more proximally. Lead I records activity from the anterior surface of the heart, leads II and III record activity from the inferior surface

Unipolar leads

These use a single exploring electrode to record cardiac activity. The second electrode is an indifferent electrode and is maintained at zero potential. In practice, zero potential is achieved by connecting all the limb leads together at a central common terminal where electrical activity is cancelled out. Unipolar leads record local electrical activity and, conventionally, recordings are taken from six chest positions, V_1–V_6, as shown in LD-47.

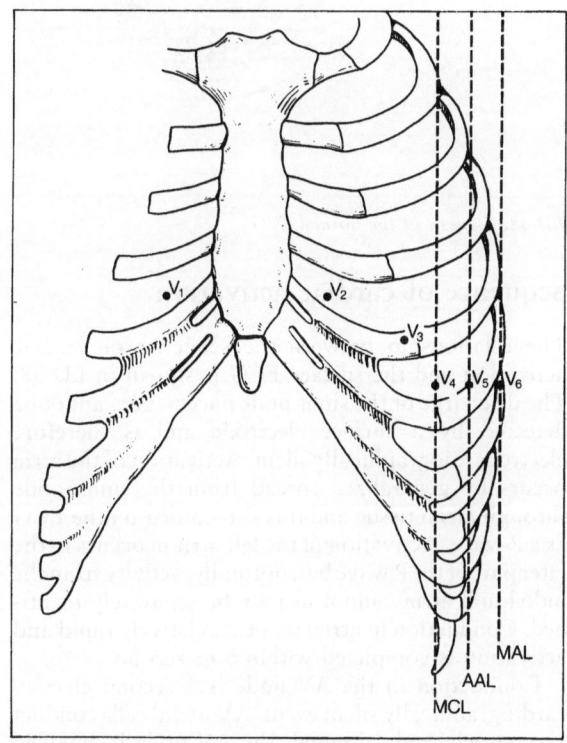

LD-47. The position of the unipolar chest leads is shown. V_1 is in the fourth right intercostal space just to the right of the sternum. V_2 is in the fourth left intercostal space just to the left of the sternum. V_4 is in the fifth intercostal space in the midclavicular line (MCL). V_3 is midway between V_2 and V_4. V_5 and V_6 are in the anterior axillary line (AAL) and the midaxillary line (MAL) at the same horizontal level as V_4

Unipolar recordings are also taken from electrodes on the right arm, left arm and left leg. The indifferent electrode is again taken from the central common terminal but the lead from the limb concerned is detached in order to augment the electrical activity recorded. Hence these are properly termed augmented unipolar leads (aVR, aVL and aVF).

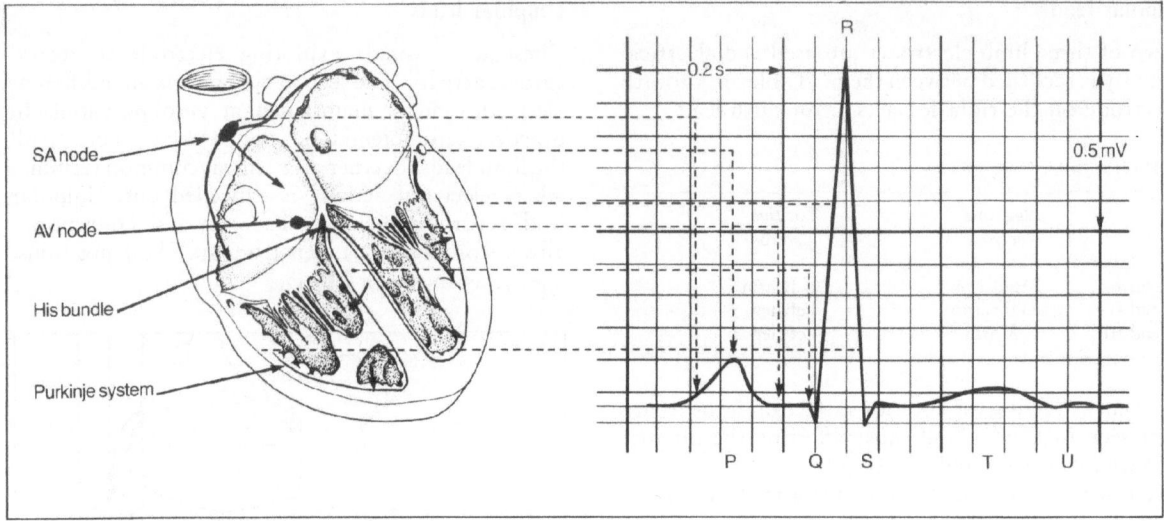

LD-48. *Genesis of the normal ECG*

Sequence of cardiac activation

The relationship between the sequence of cardiac activation and the surface ECG is shown in LD-48. The discharge of the sinus node pacemaker cannot be detected by a surface electrode and is therefore electrocardiographically silent. Activation of the atria occurs by generalized spread from the sinus node through atrial tissue and this is recorded on the ECG as a P wave. Activation of the left atrium occurs in the later part of the P wave but, normally, activity from the individual atria cannot usually be separately identified. Conduction in atrial tissue is relatively rapid and activation is completed within 0.12 second.

Conduction in the AV node is a second electrocardiographically silent event. AV nodal cells conduct very slowly and, although the AV node is small in size, an important delay occurs between activation of the atria and ventricles that permits satisfactory ventricular filling. On the ECG, this delay is represented by the PR interval. Normally, the AV node and His Bundle tissue are the only communications through which activation may pass between the atria and ventricles but, if an accessory pathway is present, the normal delay is absent and premature ventricular excitation (pre-excitation) results. This will be discussed (p. 201).

After traversing the AV node, activation reaches the Bundle of His and spreads very rapidly down the left and right bundle branches to the distal Purkinje system. This is also electrocardiographically silent. The subsequent activation of ventricular muscle is recorded on the ECG as the QRS complex. Spread of activation through ventricular muscle is slower than through the conducting tissues, but is normally completed within 0.10 second.

The sequence of ventricular activation has been extensively studied in animals and in isolated human hearts. The earliest ventricular activation occurs simultaneously at several points on the left ventricular endocardium. Activation then spreads sequentially in three major vectors (as shown in LD-49, opposite).

Initially, activation of the interventricular septum occurs from left to right. This is followed by activation of the free left and right ventricular walls. Finally activation occurs at the base of the heart.

The normal ECG

ECG records are made routinely on graph paper run at 25 mm/s so that 0.5 cm (one large square) equals 0.20 second. Each small square equals 0.04 second. Heart rate can be determined by counting either the small squares between QRS cycles and dividing this into 1500 or the number of large squares and dividing this into 300. Records are calibrated so that 1 mV = 1 cm (LD-48).

The P wave

The P wave results from activation of the atria. It is normally upright in the limb leads (inverted in aVR) less than 2.5 mV in amplitude and lasts less than 0.12 second.

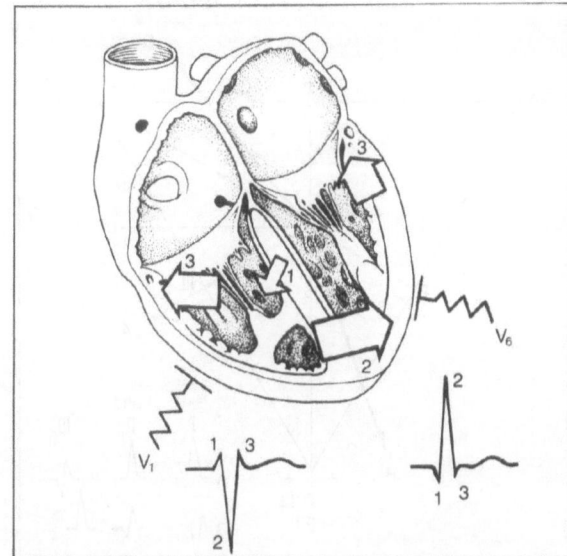

LD-49. *Genesis of the QRS complex. The three major electrical forces of ventricular activation are shown: 1, initial activation is from the left to the right side of the ventricular septum; 2, activation of the free ventricular walls follows, greatly dominated by the left ventricle; 3, the base of the heart is activated last. The genesis of the QRS in V₁ and V₆ is shown with the contribution made by each of these three major forces. Activation approaching the electrode gives a positive deflection and activation leaving the electrode gives a negative deflection*

The PR interval

This is measured from the onset of the P wave to the initial part of the QRS complex, either a Q wave or an R wave. It varies between 0.12 and 0.20 second and is usually shorter at faster heart rates. Most of the interval is taken up by slow conduction through the AV node but some is due to conduction through the atria and the His–Purkinje system.

The QRS complex

This is generated by activation of the ventricles. Q describes an initial negative deflection, R an initial positive deflection and S a subsequent negative deflection. A secondary R wave is usually termed R′ and a totally negative deflection is termed QS. The QRS complex may start with a Q wave that should normally be less than 0.04 second in duration and less than 25% of the amplitude of the complex. A QS deflection may be present in V₁ and V₂ in normal recordings and a QS deflection is usually present in aVR. This is because these leads resemble a right ventricular cavity lead. The duration of QRS should

be less than 0.10 second. The normal amplitudes of QRS will be discussed under Ventricular Hypertrophy (see p. 41).

Different vectors contribute to the various parts of the QRS complex with the result that the configuration of the QRS complex depends upon the site of recording (see LD-49). Although the right and left ventricles are activated simultaneously, the left ventricle is so much larger than the right ventricle that it obscures right ventricular forces and these cannot normally be separately identified.

The T wave

This is the deflection following a QRS complex and reflects ventricular repolarization. Normally upright, it usually has the same sign as the corresponding QRS complex. It is commonly inverted in aVR and V₁. Inverted T waves may be normal in lead III but not in aVF.

The ST segment

This is the part of the record between the S wave and the T wave. It is usually isoelectric, i.e. it has the same potential as the preceding PQ interval. It corresponds to the plateau phase of the action potential.

U waves

These are waves sometimes seen following the T wave. Their basis is not understood.

The QT interval

This is measured from the onset of the QRS complex to the end of the T wave. It is rate dependent, shortening with an increase in heart rate. The approximate upper normal limit is 0.40 second.

Generation of the QRS complex

The genesis of the QRS complex is shown in LD-49. In V₁, septal activation is recorded as a positive deflection because activation is approaching the electrode from the left side of the septum towards the right. The second major vector travels away from the electrode and results in a negative deflection. Activation of the base of the heart at the end of the activation sequence may be recorded as another R wave (R′) depending on the direction taken by the vector and the magnitude of the opposing forces.

The same events recorded from V_6 result in virtually a mirror image complex. The initial septal activation is recorded as a Q wave. Activation of the free left ventricular wall results in an R wave and activation of the base of the heart causes a diminutive S wave. Recordings from V_2 to V_5 give a form of QRS complex intermediate between V_1 and V_6. Similarly QRS configuration in the limb leads varies depending on the mean frontal QRS axis (see below) and the lead recorded (LD-50).

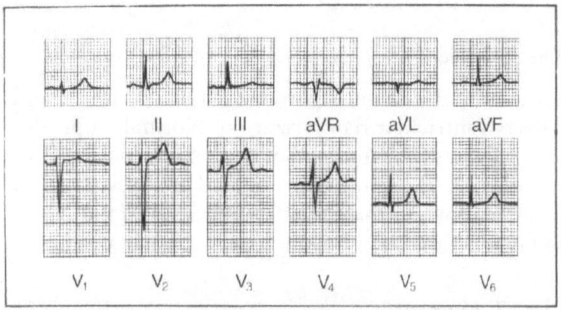

LD-50. *Normal twelve-lead ECG. There is sinus rhythm. PR = 0.16 s. The mean QRS axis is between +60° and +90°. QRS configuration is normal and varies in different leads. Small U waves are present and are best seen in V_2, V_3 and V_4*

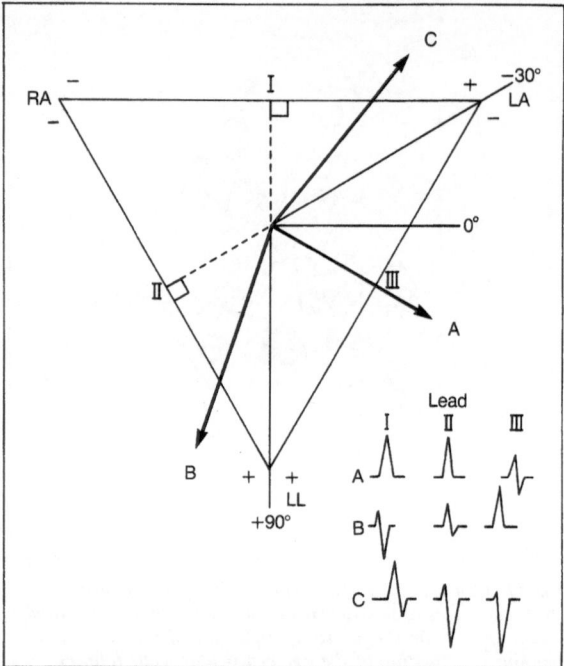

LD-51. *Derivation of mean frontal QRS axis. RA = right arm; LA = left arm; LL = left leg. For details, see text*

Derivation of the mean frontal QRS axis

Cardiac activation occurs in three planes and, like any electrical force, it can be divided into component vectors. The axis of the mean frontal QRS vector is the mean direction of cardiac activation in the frontal plane. Different mean frontal QRS axes result in different QRS configurations. A knowledge of the direction of the vector is therefore essential to an understanding of the ECG.

The three limb leads can be considered to form an equilateral triangle with the heart at its centre (LD-51). By convention, when the direction of the mean frontal QRS axis is parallel to Lead I it is termed 0°. The normal axis lies between −30° and +90°. An axis less than −30° is termed 'left axis deviation' and an axis greater than +90° is termed 'right axis deviation'. Precise derivation of axis is not necessary but derivation of the approximate axis is important and is readily achieved.

As discussed earlier, the limb leads have positive and negative electrodes as shown in Table 7. An electrical force moving parallel to an ECG lead gives a maximal positive potential when moving towards the positive electrode and maximum negative potential when moving towards the negative electrode. When moving perpendicular to a lead, an equiphasic potential occurs. These principles allow derivation of the mean frontal QRS axis by inspection of the limb leads as shown in LD-51.

With a normal mean frontal QRS axis (A in LD-51) the direction of activation is towards the positive electrodes of leads I and II so that the QRS configuration is positive in these leads. Activation is perpendicular to lead III so that the QRS is equiphasic in lead III. If the axis moves towards 0°, the negative electrode of lead III, the QRS in lead III becomes predominantly negative and if it moves towards +90°, the positive electrode of lead III, the QRS in lead III becomes positive.

Right axis deviation

With an axis of +90°, activation is perpendicular to lead I so lead I is equiphasic. Leads II and III give positive deflections. With right axis deviation (B in LD-51), lead I becomes predominantly negative and leads II and III remain positive.

Right axis deviation is common in right ventricular hypertrophy and is associated with block in the posterior fascicle of the left bundle branch.

Left axis deviation

With an axis of $-30°$, the mean frontal QRS vector is perpendicular to lead II so that an equiphasic potential results in lead II. With left axis deviation (C in LD-51), lead II becomes predominantly negative, lead I is positive and lead III negative.

Left axis deviation is associated with block of the anterior fascicle of the left bundle branch.

Axis of the P wave and T wave

The same principles can be used to determine the axis of the P and T waves. In sinus rhythm with normal situs, atrial activation results in an upright P wave in leads I and II. The configuration in lead III varies with the P wave axis. With situs inversus, the P wave axis is abnormal and the P waves are negative in lead I. When atrial activation originates in the AV junction, the P waves are inverted in leads II, III and aVF.

The T wave axis is usually within about $60°$ of the mean QRS axis.

Use of the ECG in diagnosis

ECG changes occur in many conditions. However, their sensitivity and specificity varies and in only some instances are they diagnostic. In many cases the changes are non-specific.

Left ventricular hypertrophy (LVH) (LD-52)

Hypertrophied muscle generates a greater electrical potential than normal muscle so that left ventricular hypertrophy results in large voltages in leads over the left ventricle. However, the magnitude of the electrical signal recorded varies inversely with the square of the distance between the source of the signal and the recording site. This explains some of the discrepancies between the ECG diagnosis of LVH and the pathological findings. For example, large left ventricular voltages are common in thin young people and when present as an isolated abnormality will incorrectly diagnose LVH in at least 15% of cases. Quite marked left ventricular hypertrophy may also be present in patients with a normal ECG, especially in those with thick chest walls.

Commonly used voltage criteria for LVH are:

- $R > 20$ mm in any limb lead
- $R > 25$ mm in V_5 or V_6
- $RV_5 + SV_1 > 35$ mm
- R in aVL > 13 mm

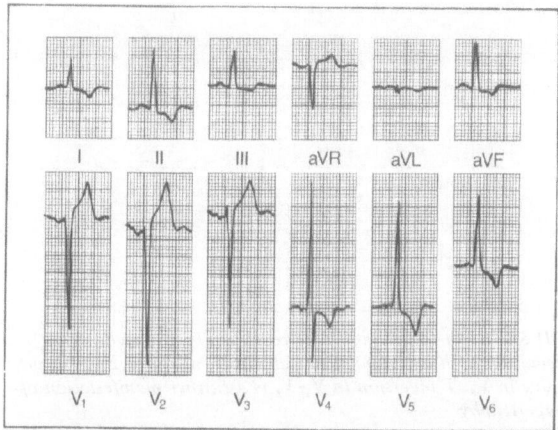

LD-52. *Left ventricular hypertrophy. An abnormally large R wave is present in V_5 and an abnormally large S wave is present in V_1 ($RV_5 + SV_1 = 62$ mm). ST shifts opposite to the QRS direction are well marked and T inversions are prominent. The axis is normal and total QRS duration is normal, though the upstroke time in V_6 is prolonged*

Voltage changes alone are insufficient to make a reliable diagnosis of LVH and the presence of one or more of the additional criteria, listed below, improves the specificity of the ECG changes.

- ST shift opposite to the QRS direction in the precordial leads, provided digitalis has not been given
- Left axis deviation
- Left atrial hypertrophy
- Intrinsicoid deflection in V_5 or V_6 (i.e. the duration of the upstroke of the QRS complex) > 0.04 second
- QRS duration > 0.10 second and < 0.12 second with a partial left bundle branch block (LBBB) pattern

With these additional criteria, only about 60% of cases of LVH will be detected, but the false positive rate is low at about 5%.

Right ventricular hypertrophy (RVH) (LD-53)

Right ventricular hypertrophy causes abnormally large voltages in leads overlying the right ventricle. Commonly used criteria for RVH are:

- R or $R' > S$ in V_1 provided $R > 0.5$ mm and QRS duration is less than 0.12 second
- right axis deviation of greater than $110°$

These findings can occur in normal individuals, about 5% having a dominant R wave in V_1 and about 7%

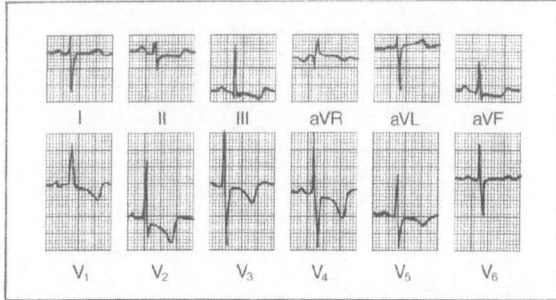

LD-53. *Right ventricular hypertrophy. There is right axis deviation with a dominant R wave in V₁ mirrored by a deep S wave in V₆. T inversion in V₁–V₅ is a further manifestation of hypertrophy*

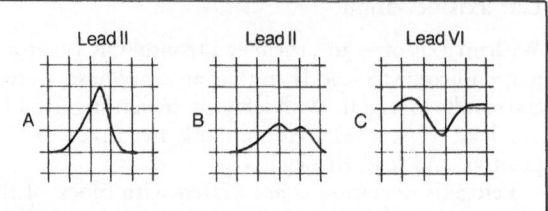

LD-54. *Atrial hypertrophy. A, Right atrial hypertrophy often causes tall peaked P waves; they are often best seen in lead II and are sometimes referred to as P pulmonale. B, Left atrial hypertrophy often causes prolonged and bifid P waves; they are often best seen in lead II and are sometimes referred to as P mitrale. C, left atrial hypertrophy typically causes a large terminal negative force in the P wave in lead V₁*

having right axis deviation, but it is unusual to have both criteria in a normal individual. However, isolated RVH is an uncommon pathological finding and the accuracy and specificity of ECG criteria for RVH are therefore less well established than those for LVH.

In infants the ventricles are of approximately equal thickness at birth. The right ventricle is, therefore, relatively hypertrophied and there is a dominant R wave in V₁ that reduces with age. T waves in the right precordial leads are usually upright for the first 48 hours but thereafter are inverted and remain so until about 14 years. Marked RVH may be associated with reappearance of T inversion in adults or, inappropriately, upright T waves in children.

The presence of complete right bundle branch block precludes an ECG diagnosis of RVH, as large R′ waves are usually present.

ECG changes are frequently absent even with marked RVH, especially in rheumatic heart disease and pulmonary heart disease, although the ECG is usually abnormal when RVH occurs in congenital heart disease.

Right atrial hypertrophy

Right atrial hypertrophy is usually diagnosed if the P wave in a limb lead exceeds 2.5 mm. The P wave is often peaked and may be especially well seen in lead II (LD-54,A).

Left atrial hypertrophy

Left atrial hypertrophy commonly causes prolongation of the P wave beyond 0.12 second, resulting in a bifid P wave (LD-54,B). Left atrial hypertrophy also causes a terminal negative force in the P wave in V₁. When this exceeds 0.04 second in duration and 0.1 mV in amplitude, left atrial hypertrophy is usually present (LD-54,C).

Myocardial infarction

Myocardial infarction is commonly associated with diagnostic changes in the QRS complexes, ST segments and T waves, but in about 20% of patients with infarction diagnostic ECG changes are absent. However, when typical sequential changes of infarction are present they have a specificity of virtually 100%.

Basis for ECG changes of infarction

The occurrence of myocardial infarction results in a central area of necrotic inactive tissue surrounded by an area of myocardial ischaemia. The ECG changes reflect both findings. Though unable to generate electrical potentials, the necrotic area acts as a passive conductor of electrical activity. An electrode over the necrotic area therefore looks through an electrical window into the ventricular cavity. Ventricular activation occurs from endocardium to epicardium, so cavity potentials are wholly negative and an electrode over the infarct records a Q wave that mirrors this cavity potential (LD-55).

When infarction only involves the inner surface of the heart, Q waves can still occur. Activation of the non-infarcted epicardial region is delayed so that initially the cavity potential is recorded giving a Q wave followed by an R wave due to activation of the epicardium (LD-55).

Myocardial ischaemia causes ST and T wave changes. When infarction occurs the adjacent epicardial surface is ischaemic. Ischaemic cells depolarize and therefore have a less negative potential so that in diastole an injury potential exists between ischaemic and normal cells. This results in current flow from epicardium to endocardium (LD-56) and a shift of the ECG baseline in a negative direction. When complete depolarization occurs with ventricular activation, the potential difference is virtually abolished and this is

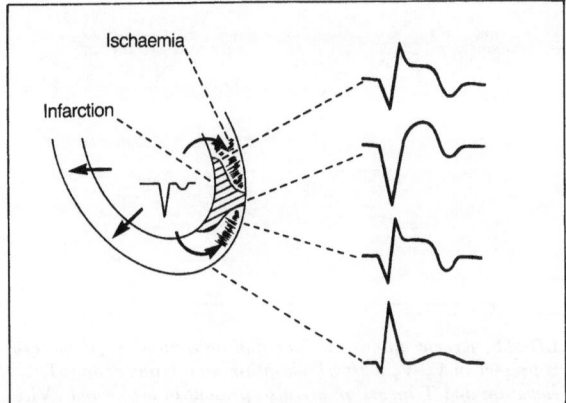

LD-55. *ECG changes of myocardial infarction. For details, see text*

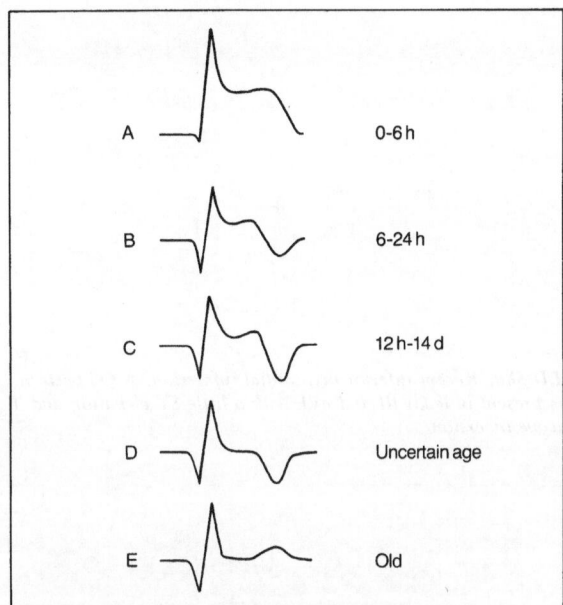

LD-57. *ECG changes of myocardial infarction*

seen on the ECG as apparent ST elevation. In addition, it is likely that some potential differences exist in systole between ischaemic and normal cells and these contribute to a further genuine elevation of the ST segment. ST elevation in one lead may be recorded as ST depression in an opposing lead. This is seen especially with anterior and inferior leads and is termed 'reciprocal ST depression'.

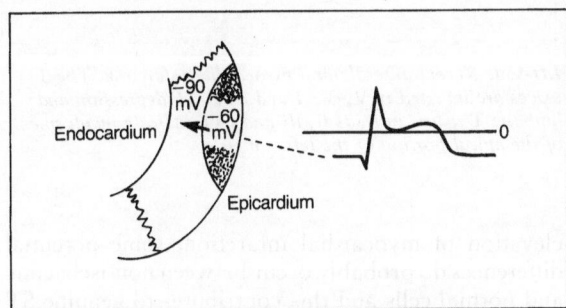

LD-56. *Genesis of ST elevation with epicardial ischaemia. A resting 'injury potential' is present between ischaemic and normal muscle. For details, see text*

The T wave changes of myocardial infarction reflect changes in repolarization and are not well understood.

Sequence of ECG changes in infarction

The typical sequence of ECG changes is shown in LD-57. ST elevation occurs immediately in experimental coronary artery occlusion, but in clinical myocardial infarction the ECG changes may be delayed. ST elevation is rapidly followed by T wave inversion and the development of abnormal Q waves. ST elevation is often initially marked but usually becomes much less marked over 24–72 hours. In inferior infarcts, it usually resolves completely within 2 weeks. In anterior infarcts, chronic ST elevation occurs in about 40% of cases and in some of these is associated with aneurysm formation.

T wave inversion may persist indefinitely or may resolve.

Q waves usually persist indefinitely but may resolve, especially with inferior infarcts, leaving no subsequent trace of infarction on the ECG. Infarction can occur without diagnostic Q waves developing and the term 'subendocardial infarction' is sometimes used, in such cases. This is not a good term, because most infarcts have a predominantly subendocardial site and Q waves are often recorded from them as shown in LD-55.

Localization of infarction

Infarction at different sites is recorded on different leads of the ECG. Infarction involving the inferior surface causes changes predominantly in leads II, III and aVF (LD-58a). Anterior infarction is seen in precordial leads and in leads I and aVL (LD-58b).

The term 'anteroseptal infarction' is often used when the changes are confined to V_{1-3} in the precordial leads (LD-58c) and the term 'anterolateral infarction' is used when the changes are in V_{4-6} (LD-58d).

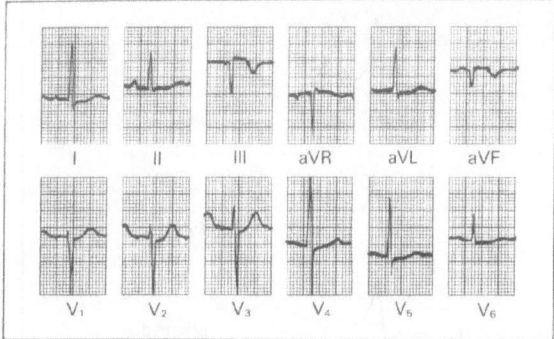

LD-58a. *Recent inferior myocardial infarction. A QS pattern is present in leads III and aVF with a little ST elevation and T wave inversion*

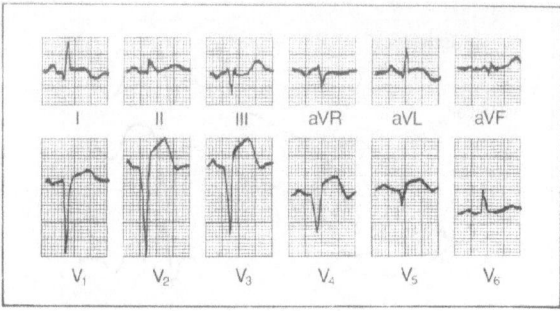

LD-58b. *Recent anterior myocardial infarction. A QS pattern is present in V_2–V_5 with ST elevation and T inversion. ST elevation and T inversion are also present in lead I and aVL as these leads reflect anterior changes*

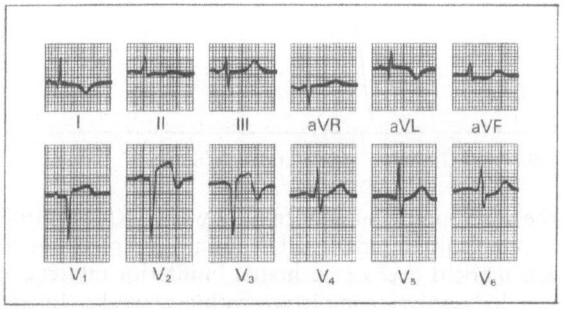

LD-58c. *Recent anteroseptal myocardial infarction. A QS pattern is present in chest leads V_1–V_3 with ST elevation. The T waves are inverted in V_2 and V_3 and in leads reflecting the anterior surface of the left ventricle, I and aVL. The broad deep Q in aVL is also significant*

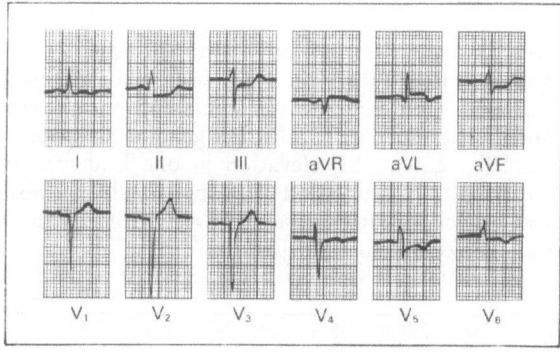

LD-58d. *Recent anterolateral myocardial infarction. The T waves are inverted in V_4–V_6, I and aVL. ST depression and biphasic T waves in leads II, III and aVF indicate involvement of the apical portion of the left ventricle*

True posterior infarction affects the posterior surface of the heart where routine leads are not recorded. A dominant R wave is seen in right precordial leads, especially V_1, due to loss of the usual opposing forces. When special recordings are made over the posterior chest, typical Q waves with ST and T wave changes are present.

Myocardial ischaemia

Coronary blood flow is distributed preferentially to the epicardium so that when myocardial ischaemia occurs it tends primarily to affect the endocardium. Ischaemia results in depolarization of the endocardial cells, an injury potential develops and current flows from endocardium to epicardium. This causes an upwards shift in the ECG baseline. With complete depolarization, the potential difference is abolished and apparent ST depression occurs. As with the ST

elevation of myocardial infarction, some potential differences do probably occur between non-ischaemic and normal cells and this contributes to genuine ST depression. Occasionally, myocardial ischaemia is associated with St elevation as in Printzmetal's angina where coronary artery spasm is probably the main aetiological factor. Myocardial ischaemia may also cause T wave inversion.

Pericarditis

In many cases of pericarditis there is generalized ST elevation that is characteristically concave upwards (LD-59). In some, the ECG remains normal or shows non-specific changes. The absence of sequential changes and the generalized abnormality usually distinguish these changes from those of acute myocardial infarction.

Occasionally, slight ST elevation may be a normal

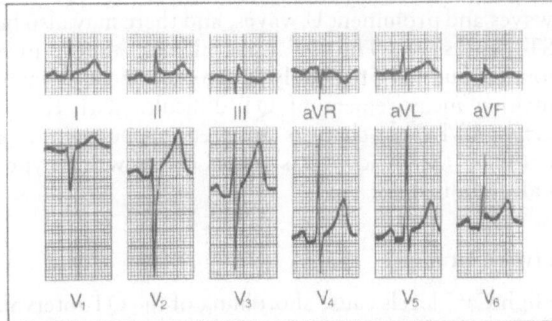

LD-59. *Pericarditis. There is widespread ST elevation, concave upwards, with upright T waves*

finding. Its persistence through several records in the absence of other signs of disease should distinguish it from other causes of ST elevation.

Bundle branch block

Rapid activation of the heart depends upon an intact conduction system. If conduction is impaired in either of the bundle branches, the duration of QRS is prolonged beyond the upper limit of normal (0.10 second). Slight prolongation, between 0.10 and 0.11 second, is termed 'partial bundle branch block' and prolongation beyond 0.12 second is termed 'complete bundle branch block'.

These conduction abnormalities, like others, may be either permanent or intermittent.

Also, the ECG pattern of partial bundle branch block is frequently not due to abnormal conduction but to right or left ventricular hypertrophy.

Right bundle branch block

In right bundle branch block, activation of the right ventricle is delayed. Activation of the septum and the left ventricle are not affected (LD-60). The initial QRS configuration is therefore normal, but is followed by delayed activation of the right ventricle (Force 3). This occurs in the absence of opposing left ventricular forces and is recorded as a large secondary R wave (R') in the right precordial leads and as a large S wave in left precordial leads. The abnormal pattern of right ventricular depolarization is associated with abnormal repolarization, so that T wave inversion in the right precordial leads is a normal finding in right bundle branch block.

The normal pattern of left ventricular activation in right bundle branch block allows the identification of myocardial infarction, but precludes the diagnosis of right or left ventricular hypertrophy.

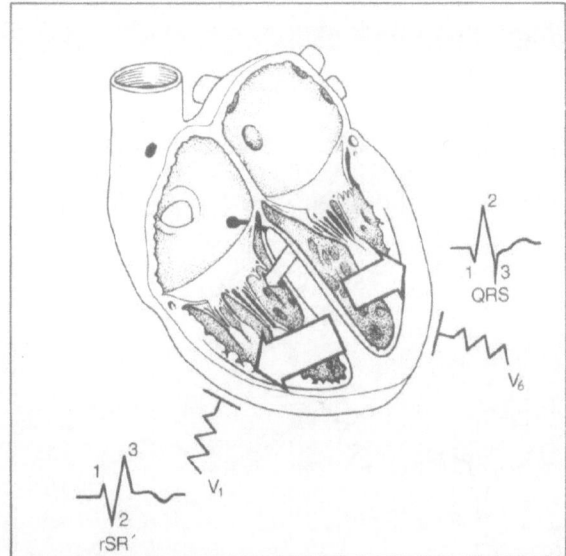

LD-60. *ECG pattern of right bundle branch block. For details, see text*

Left bundle branch block

In left bundle branch block, the pattern of left ventricular activation is abnormal, but activation of the right ventricle is normal. Activation of the septum occurs from right to left instead of from left to right. The initial forces of the QRS complex are therefore reversed, resulting in a Q wave in V_1 and an R wave in V_6 (LD-61a). Activation of the left ventricle occurs slowly by spread through muscle, producing a broad slurred S wave in V_1 and a broad slurred R wave in V_6. Although activation of the right ventricle is usually obscured by left ventricular forces, an initial R wave may be present in V_1 (Force 2), and the initial Q wave (Force 1) may be absent.

As with right bundle branch block the abnormal pattern of depolarization is associated with abnormal repolarization, so T inversion in left precordial leads is a normal finding with left bundle branch block.

The presence of left bundle branch block precludes the ECG diagnosis of both left ventricular hypertrophy and myocardial infarction.

When a broad QRS is identified, the QRS configuration in V_1 most readily distinguishes right and left bundle branch block, being largely positive in the former and largely negative in the latter (LD-61b).

ST and T wave changes
Ionic changes

ECG changes may occur with abnormal ionic concentrations, but these are seldom diagnostic.

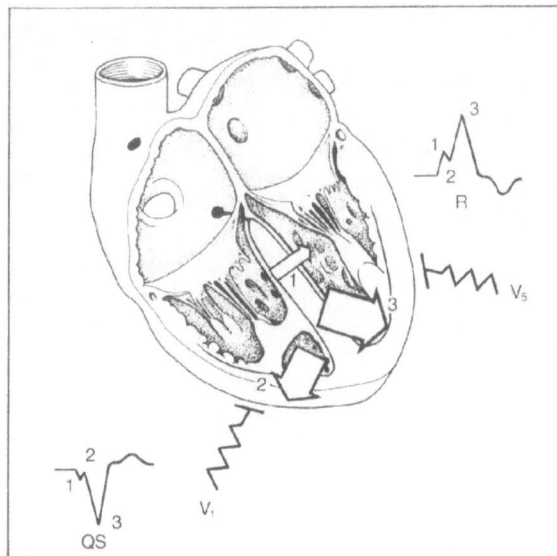

LD-61a. *ECG pattern in left bundle branch block. For details, see text*

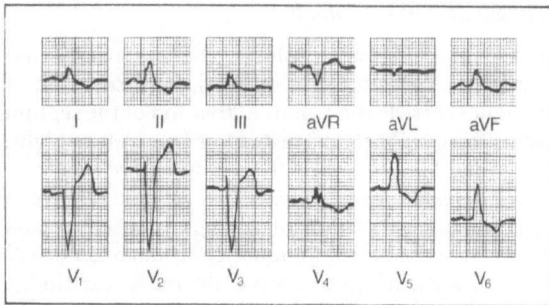

LD-61b. *Left bundle branch block. The QRS duration is prolonged to 0.16 s. There is an initial r wave in V_1 as is often the case, but the main deflection is a large broad S wave. In V_5 and V_6 there are broad R waves. T inversion is secondary to abnormal depolarization*

Hyperkalaemia

With K^+ at 5.5 mmol/l, tall peaked T waves occur in about 20% of patients and this is the earliest ECG abnormality in hyperkalaemia. With higher levels, ECG abnormalities are much more common. The QRS complexes broaden in a non-specific manner and the P waves become reduced in amplitude and may disappear. With very high levels, cardiac arrest may occur with asystole or ventricular fibrillation.

Hypokalaemia

Low K^+ levels are associated with low amplitude T

waves and prominent U waves, and there may also be ST depression. The QT interval may appear prolonged, but this is probably due to prominent U waves making measurement of QT difficult. With $K^+ < 2.7$ mmol/l these changes are seen in about 70% of patients; the incidence is much lower when hypokalaemia is mild.

Hypercalcaemia

High Ca^{2+} levels cause shortening of the QT interval.

Hypocalcaemia

Low Ca^{2+} levels are associated with prolongation of the QT interval.

Digitalis

Digitalis commonly causes ST depression with or without T wave inversion. In most patients a characteristic pattern is present as shown in LD-62, but many have atypical changes. Excess digitalis may cause dysrhythmias that can take almost any form (see p. 210).

Quinidine

Quinidine causes a decrease in amplitude or inversion of T waves and prolongation of the QT interval. ST depression may be present.

Non-specific changes

Many patients have changes in the ST segments and T waves that do not conform to a specific pattern. Other evidence to suggest left ventricular hypertrophy, conduction abnormality, myocardial ischaemia, drug administration or ionic abnormalities should be looked for, but in many cases no explanation will be

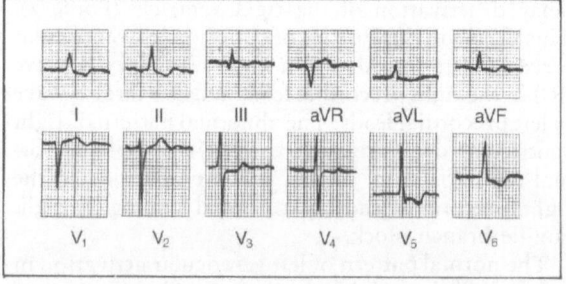

LD-62. *Digitalis effects. Atrial fibrillation is present, so there are no P waves. Downsloping ST depression with T inversion, typical of digitalis, is present*

forthcoming. Such changes are referred to as non-specific ST–T wave changes.

Approach to the electrocardiogram

Interpretation of the ECG should be approached systematically and deductively rather than with the hope of recognizing a pattern. The following steps are a guide:

- determine the rate
- determine the rhythm by identifying the P waves and their relationship to the QRS complexes
- measure the PR interval
- identify the axis of P waves, QRS complexes and T waves
- check the configuration, duration and magnitude of P waves
- check the configuration, duration and magnitude of QRS complexes
- check the ST segment and T waves
- correlate all the information and reach a conclusion

RADIOLOGY

Radiological examination is an essential part of the investigation of the cardiovascular system. It reveals vital information about the nature of the thoracic cavity, the size and shape of the heart, the position of the great vessels and the vascularity of the lung fields without which no considered opinion should be given.

Of the various techniques that are available, the ordinary chest X-ray, often referred to as a plain film, is the one most commonly used. This is known as the postero-anterior (PA) view because the patient stands with the anterior chest wall in contact with the plate and the X-ray is taken from behind.

A cardiac series of X-rays is made up of a postero-anterior film together with left and right anterior oblique views taken at 45° to the median plane while the oesophagus, which has an intimate posterior relationship to the heart, is outlined with a barium swallow. If oblique views are not available, a lateral view will provide additional information about the constituent parts of the cardiac silhouette.

Other methods include:

- fluoroscopy
  This is observation of the heart under continuous X-ray screening and is used to study pulsation, intracardiac calcification and prosthetic valve motion.
- angiocardiography
  Here an injection of radio-opaque contrast medium is used to visualize the interior of the chambers and vessels.

The postero-anterior X-ray

The cardiac silhouette

The constituent parts that make up the borders of the normal cardiac silhouette in the postero-anterior view (X-1) are from above downwards (arrows) as follows.

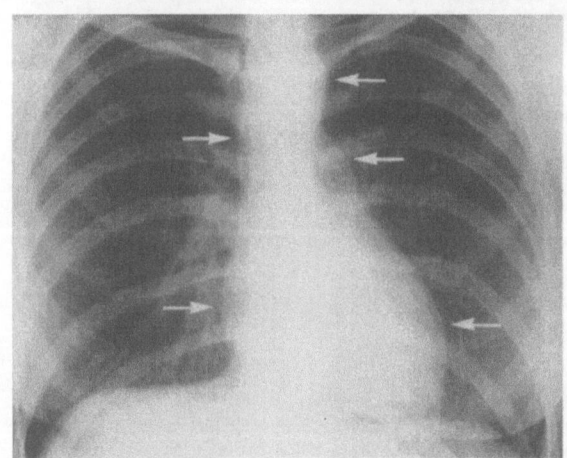

X-1.

On the right side

- the superior vena cava
- the right atrium

On the left side

- the aortic arch
- the pulmonary trunk
- the left ventricle

The right ventricle forms the greater part of the anterior surface of the heart but is not normally apparent on PA films, being flanked on one side by the right atrium and on the other by the left ventricle.

Similarly, the ascending aorta, a prominent part of the supracardiac shadow, does not normally contribute to the right border in health. In practice, however, it is so often enlarged, especially in older patients, that (arrow) it is frequently seen to overlap the shadow produced by the superior vena cava (X-2).

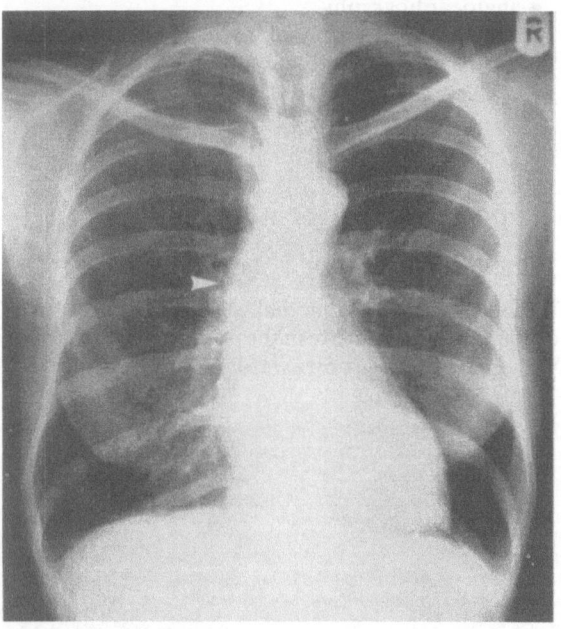

X-2.

The pulmonary circulation

The PA X-ray can also give valuable information about the pulmonary circulation. It is important to remember, however, that the appearance of the lung fields depends greatly upon the exposure of the film. A soft, grey, underexposed film gives a false impression of congested vessels, whereas a hard, black, overexposed film suggests that they are constricted (X-3a, b). For this reason, great care must be taken with the interpretation of vascular shadows in chest X-rays, particularly when assessing the significance of anything other than fairly gross changes.

Increased pulmonary blood flow causes dilatation of the main pulmonary arteries and their branches. It is seen to spread outwards from the hilar vessels into the lung fields and is more obvious on the right side than on the left because the cardiac shadow obscures the left hilum (X-4).

When pulmonary blood flow is decreased, the pulmonary vascular markings on plain X-ray films are less obvious than normal.

In pulmonary arterial hypertension, the main branches of the pulmonary arteries enlarge while those in the peripheral lung fields remain relatively normal. If the pressure remains high for many years, the arteries nearest the hilum become greatly dilated and those in the periphery constrict, giving an appearance that has been likened to pruning of the vascular tree.

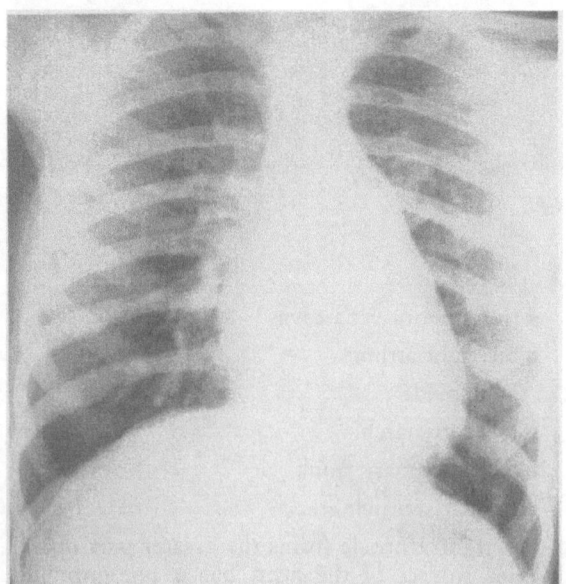

X-3a.

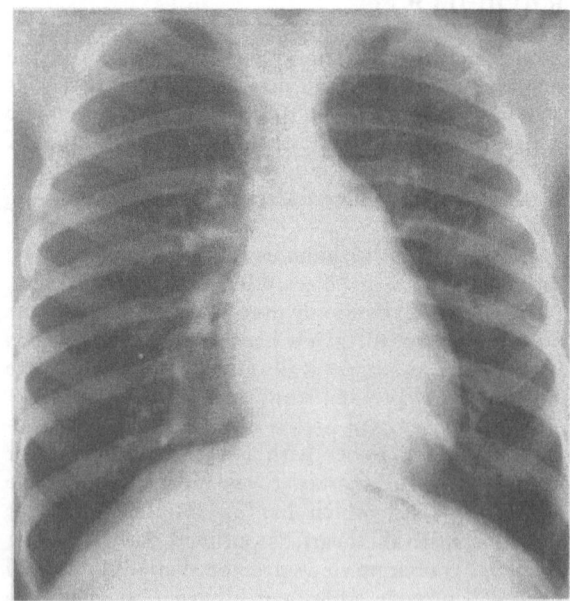

X-3b.

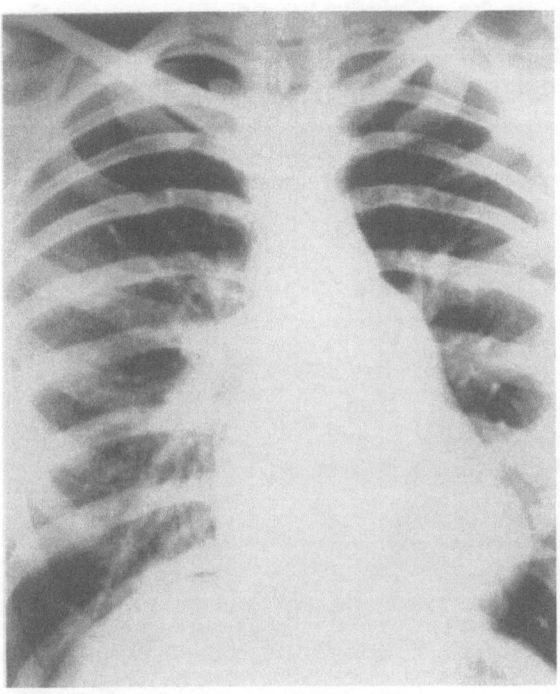

X-4.

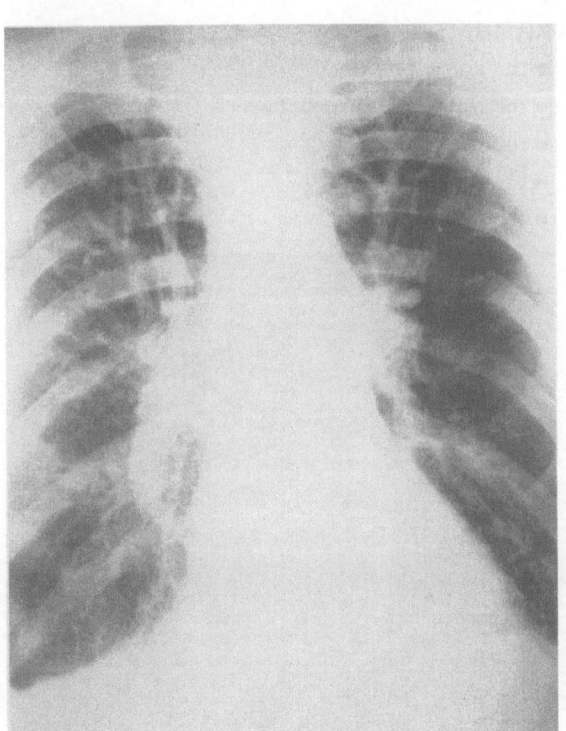

X-5.

By contrast with these pulmonary arterial abnormalities that radiate from the hilar regions, evidence of pulmonary venous hypertension is most readily detected in the upper lobes where the pulmonary veins, which are usually invisible because of gravitational flow, stand out as obvious vertical shadows when they become engorged (X-5).

Pulmonary oedema

Pulmonary oedema is of two kinds:

- acute
- chronic

Acute pulmonary oedema causes diffuse opacities that extend in a wedge shape from both hilar regions to produce a characteristic picture aptly referred to as 'bat's wing' or 'butterfly' shadows (X-6). Sometimes this is more marked on one side than the other.

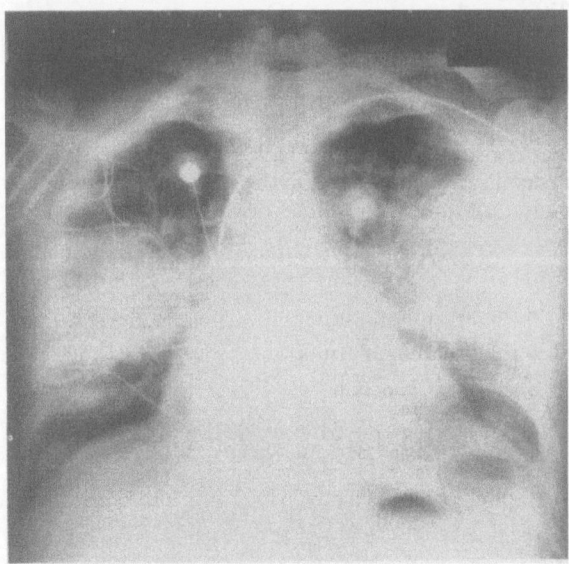

X-6.

Chronic interstitial pulmonary oedema is seen as a haziness around the vascular shadows (X-7). In severe cases, thickening of the interlobular septa shows up as thin horizontal lines (Kerley's B lines) extending inwards for a few centimetres from the periphery at the bases of the lungs just above the diaphragm.

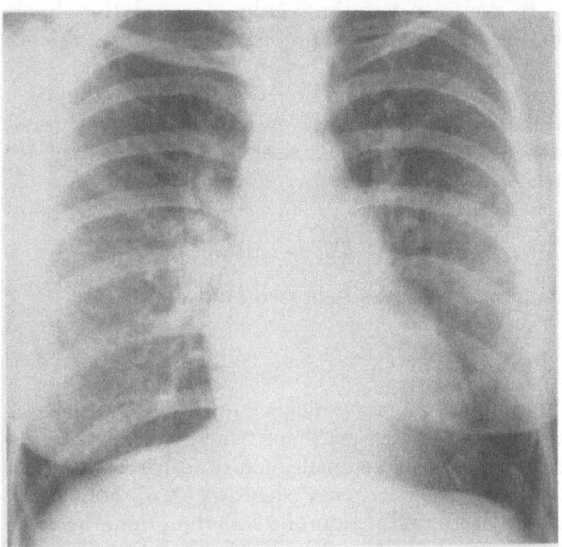

X-7.

Right anterior oblique X-ray

The constituent parts that make up the borders of the normal cardiac silhouette in the right anterior oblique view (X-8) are from above downwards (arrows) as follows.

Anteriorly

- the ascending aorta
- the pulmonary trunk
- the right ventricle

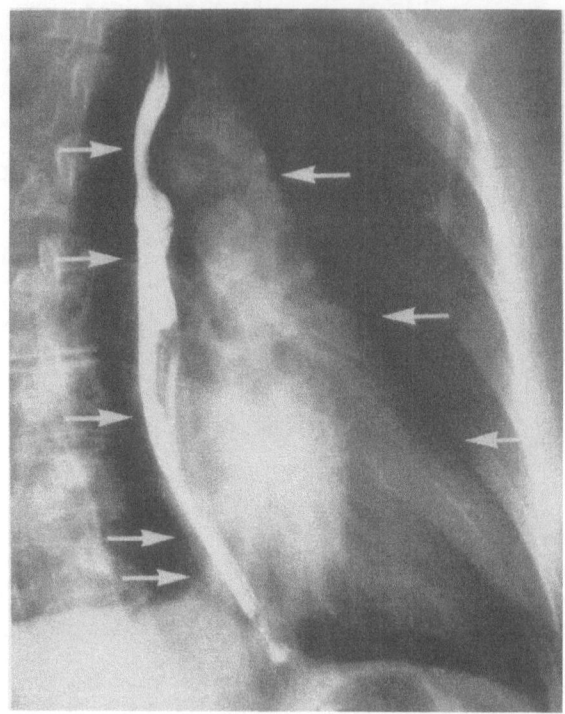

X-8.

Posteriorly

- the aortic arch
- the right main bronchus
- the left atrium
- the right atrium
- the inferior vena cava

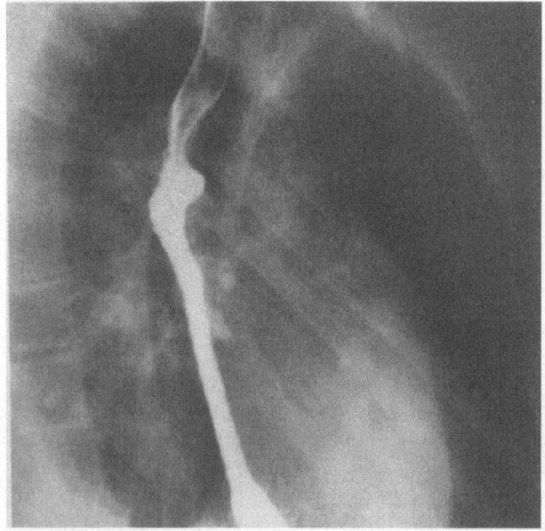

X-9a.

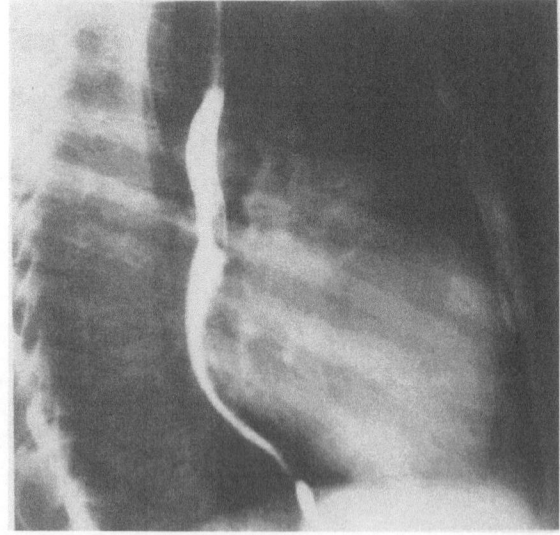

X-9b.

50

The left atrium forms most of the posterior surface of the heart, and the oesophagus is in contact with it throughout most of its retrocardiac course (X-9). When the left atrium is enlarged, the oesophagus is displaced backwards and this can be demonstrated by opacifying the oesophagus with a barium swallow (X-9).

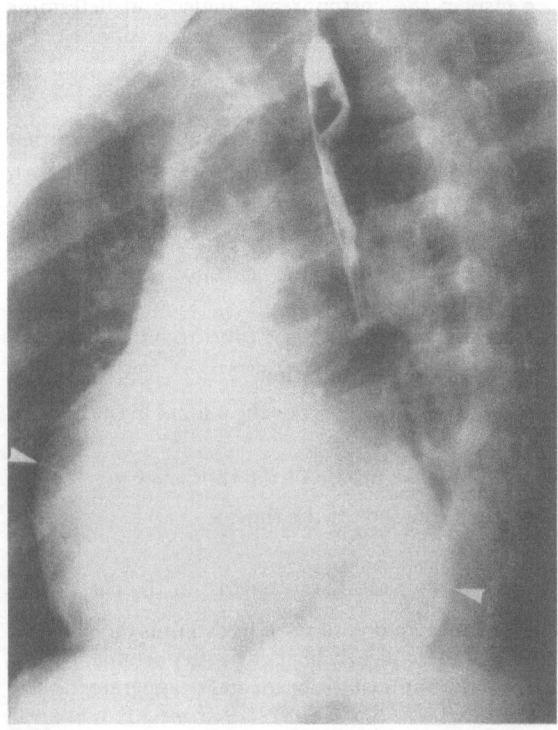

X-11.

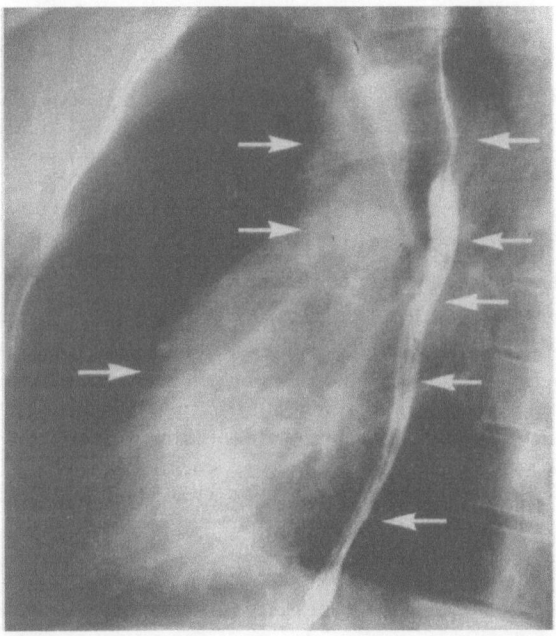

X-10.

Left anterior oblique X-ray

The constituent parts that make up the borders of the normal cardiac silhouette in the left anterior oblique view (X-10) are from above downwards as follows.

Anteriorly

- the ascending aorta
- the pulmonary trunk
- the right ventricle

Posteriorly

- the aortic arch
- the left pulmonary artery
- the left main bronchus
- the left atrium
- the left ventricle

In this view, the ventricles, which, like the septa, lie at an angle of 45° to the median plane, are seen end-on (cf. LD-11). An enlarged right ventricle, therefore, projects upwards and forwards; an enlarged left ventricle projects downwards and backwards (X-11).

The examination of cardiac X-rays

When looking at an X-ray, it is important to develop a method and to follow it scrupulously on every occasion. The temptation to concentrate on obvious things, such as an opacity in the left upper lobe or an aortic aneurysm, should be resisted at all costs. Their turn will come; and meantime the danger of missing other less obvious abnormalities will have been avoided by the painstaking application of a chosen routine to the whole picture.

A suggested method for looking at chest films is:

- assess the correctness of exposure (neither too black nor too white)
- make sure that the patient has been standing in the correct position when the film was taken
  Significant rotation can be excluded by confirming that the tracheal shadow is in the midline and that the clavicles and shoulder girdles appear symmetrical.
- examine the ribs, the scapulae, the sternum and the spine
  Assess here the nature of the thoracic cage.

- inspect the costophrenic angles and determine the shape and height of each side of the diaphragm
- look for the stomach gas bubble
- scan the lung fields for major abnormalities that might influence the heart and great vessels
- finally, study the cardiac silhouette and the pulmonary vascular tree in detail

The size and shape of the heart on X-ray films may be influenced by:

- the distance of the X-ray tube from the chest wall
- the phase of respiration
- rotation of the heart or the patient in the median plane
- the bony structure of the thoracic cage
- other contents of the thorax

The distance of the X-ray tube from the chest wall

This should be 2 m (at least 6 feet). Films taken closer than this, as frequently happens with portable X-rays, increase the angle of the beam and exaggerate the size of the heart.

Heart size is judged as the ratio of the maximum width of the cardiac silhouette to the maximum width of the thorax. This should not exceed 50%, although the size of normal hearts varies widely within this limit.

The phase of respiration

By varying the position of the diaphragm and the angle of the ribs the phase of respiration may alter the length, breadth and depth of the thoracic cavity and consequently the appearance of the heart within it. For this reason, all films should be taken with the breath held in full inspiration.

Rotation of the heart

Rotation of the heart around its vertical axis or rotation of the patient with a normally placed heart causes distortion of the soft tissue shadows made by the heart and great vessels on the X-ray plate (X-12a, b).

The bony structure of the thoracic cage

This affects the relative positions of its contents in both health and disease. Generally speaking, tall thin people tend to have narrow vertical hearts and short squat people tend to have hearts that look broader and lie more horizontally. If the bony structure is deformed, as for example when the sternum is depressed or the spinal column twisted by kyphoscoliosis, the cardiac contour may be grossly distorted (X-13).

Other contents of the thorax

These may exert pressure or traction upon the heart and may alter its location or obscure its outline.

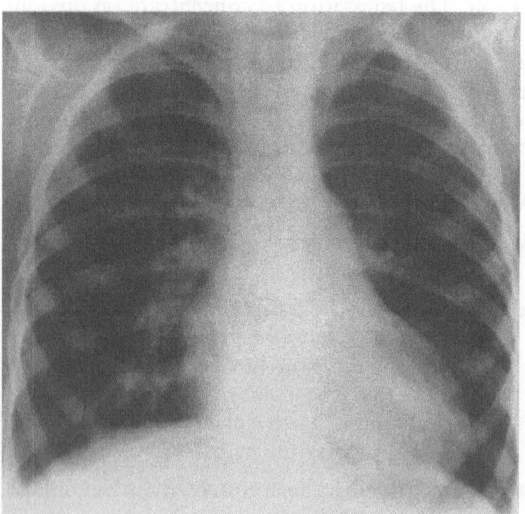

X-12a.

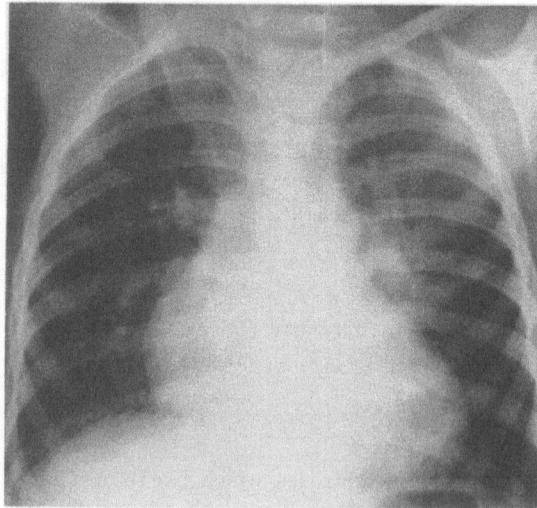

X-12b.

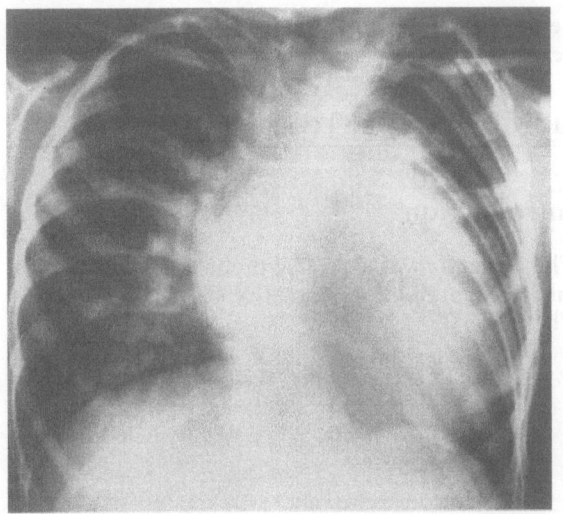

X-13.

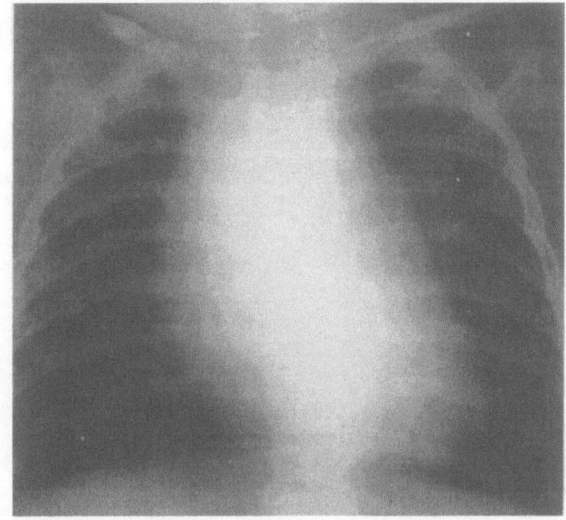

X-14.

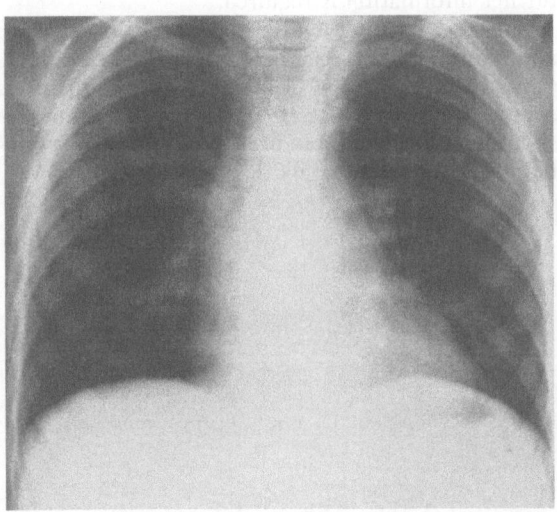

X-15a.

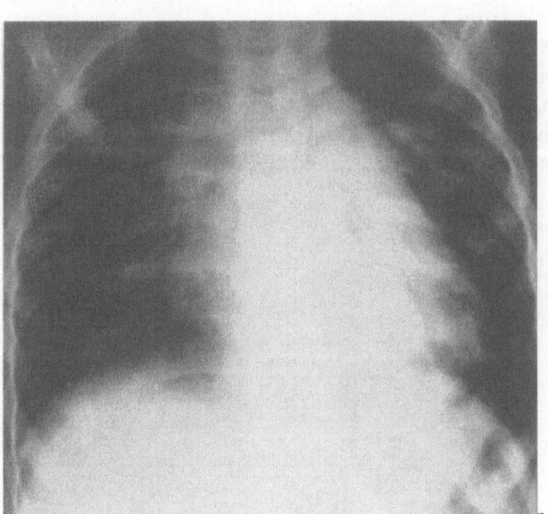

X-15b.

Young children

In babies and young children the X-ray appearance of the heart is often difficult to assess because of the relatively flat diaphragm, the horizontal ribs, the thymic shadow (X-14) and the considerable variation that may occur with respiration (X-15a, b).

Summary

When studying the cardiac silhouette remember that
- normal hearts vary greatly in size
- X-rays cannot differentiate between enlargement due to dilatation and enlargement due to hypertrophy

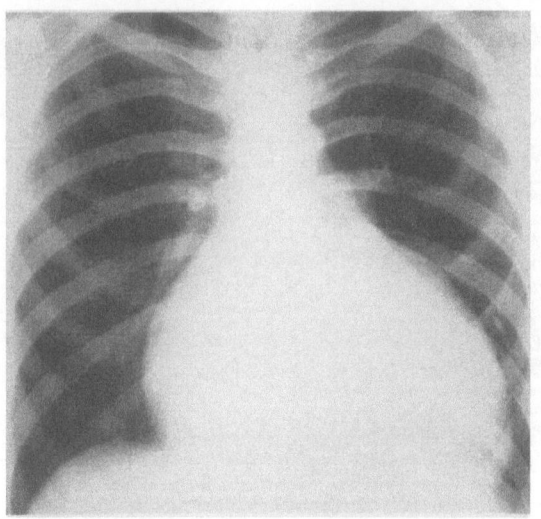

X-16.

The shape of the heart may indicate:

- generalized cardiac enlargement (X-16)
- enlargement of a particular chamber or vessel (arrows) (X-17a, right atrium; b, pulmonary trunk)

With practice, various characteristics will be recognized that suggest or confirm a diagnosis, but *the guiding principle when interpreting X-rays is never to read too much into them.* They should be regarded merely as pieces of a jigsaw which, when taken to-

gether with the history, physical examination, ECGs, echoes etc. will help to complete the overall picture.

SPECIAL INVESTIGATIONS

Introduction

The evaluation of a cardiac problem should always take account of information from four basic sources. These are:

- the clinical history
- the physical examination
- the routine chest X-ray, possibly including special views
- the electrocardiogram

Correlation of this information should usually allow a diagnosis or a differential diagnosis to be made.

Thereafter, the physician must decide either, that he has already determined the nature of the abnormality and can advise about its management or, that further information is required.

If further information is required, several invasive and non-invasive special investigations are available that may provide it. Unnecessary investigations should be avoided and non-invasive techniques should always be used in preference to invasive ones because they are safer and less expensive.

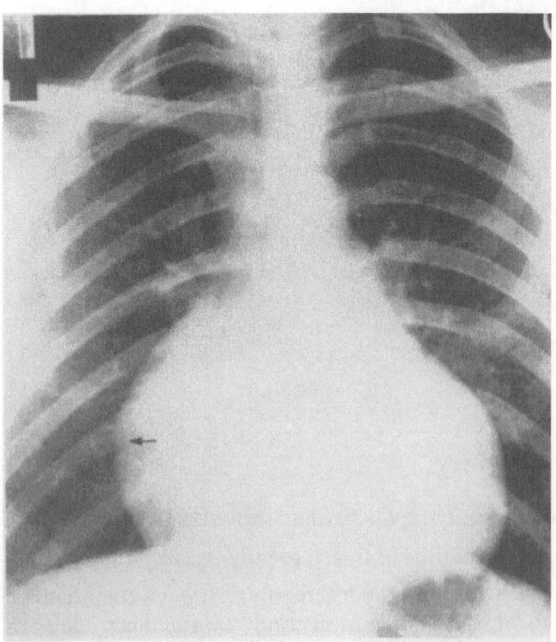

X-17a.

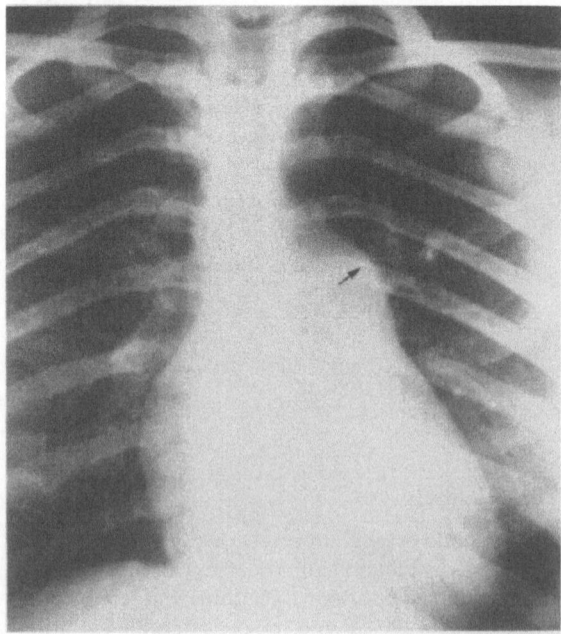

X-17b.

Each investigative technique has particular merits and limitations and these will be discussed in turn.

Non-invasive investigations

X-ray screening (fluoroscopy)

This can be a useful non-invasive investigation in some circumstances but it requires an experienced observer to be of value. Information can be obtained on the following:

- intracardiac calcification
- pericardial calcification
- prosthetic valve function
- pulsation and its absence

Intracardiac calcification – mitral and aortic valves

Screening can positively identify calcification within the aortic or mitral valves. When the patient has clearcut features of obstruction to left ventricular outflow, this information may be sufficient to identify the aortic valve as the site of the obstruction, though the presence of calcification does not necessarily indicate that the obstruction is severe.

Mitral valve calcification can also be identified and, if severe, would preclude mitral valvotomy in a patient with mitral stenosis. Calcification of the mitral valve is seen not infrequently in older patients and does not necessarily indicate severe mitral valve disease.

Pericardial calcification

Pericardial calcification can often be seen in the plain lateral or PA chest X-ray but, in constrictive pericarditis, screening may reveal it when plain films do not. However, calcification can occur without significant pericardial disease and its diagnostic value is therefore limited.

Prosthetic valve function

Screening can be invaluable if malfunction of a prosthetic valve is suspected. When a prosthetic valve is obstructed, excursion of the ball or disc may be seen to be restricted and if clinical features of obstruction are also present, this would be sufficient confirmatory evidence to advise reoperation. When the valve has become detached, as may occur in subacute bacterial endocarditis for example, demonstration of its abnormal mobility can again be diagnostic. Severe malfunction can be present, however, with normal appearances on X-ray screening and, in these circum-

stances, a normal finding is unhelpful and may be misleading.

Left ventricular aneurysm and pericardial effusion

X-ray screening is of little value in assessing left ventricular function or in the diagnosis of left ventricular aneurysms, as these may not be visible. Also, a pericardial effusion cannot be reliably distinguished from a dilated, poorly contracting heart and is much more reliably diagnosed by echocardiography.

Echocardiography

Echocardiography is a non-invasive method of investigating the dimensions of the heart and the movements of the structures inside it. An ultrasonic beam is used to examine a narrow segment of tissue, the depth and width of which depends upon the type of beam used.

Ultrasound waves are thought to be harmless to the tissues, and the technique, which has been developing over nearly 30 years, is now reliably standardized. It has the advantage of being safe and readily repeatable, and has sufficient diagnostic accuracy to make cardiac catheterization unnecessary in many cases. The quality of results, however, depends on the skill and experience of the recordist and the interpreter who should have some knowledge of what they are looking for in each case, because some parts of the heart are much more difficult to visualize than others.

The patient reclines on a couch, turned slightly to the left side, and is encouraged to relax. A transducer is held against the chest wall, the standard position being in the fourth left intercostal space near the sternal edge. It transmits an ultrasonic beam, some of which is reflected each time the beam crosses an interface between different tissues as it penetrates the chest. Good results depend on finding an 'acoustic window', and thus avoiding dissipation of the beam's energy by bone or lung tissue.

The reflected echoes are displayed on a screen and a permanent record is recorded along with an ECG. This method is known as 'M-mode echocardiography'.

The results, although sometimes diagnostic as in mitral stenosis, atrial myxoma or pericardial effusion, are considered in conjunction with the clinical findings, ECGs, X-rays, etc.

Normal patterns (LD-63)

With the transducer directed along line A, the recording will appear as shown in segment a, representing the left ventricular wall just apical to the tips of the mitral valve cusps. Similarly, B–b shows the move-

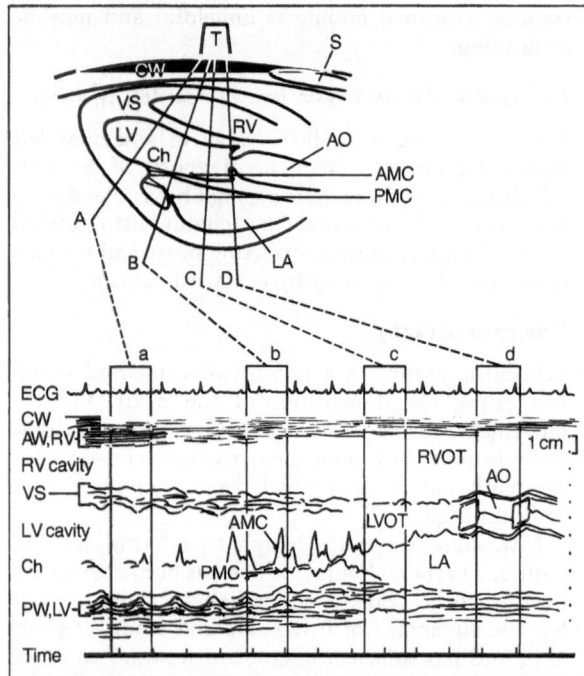

LD-63. *Continuous sweep recording from transducer position A to position D (apex to base). Key: T = transducer; S = sternum; CW = chest wall; RV = right ventricle; AW,RV = anterior wall, right ventricle; VS = ventricular septum; LV = left ventricle; CH = chordae; PW,LV = posterior wall, left ventricle; AMC = anterior mitral cusp; MV = mitral valve; PMC = posterior mitral cusp; LVOT = left ventricular outflow tract; RVOT = right ventricular outflow tract; LA = left atrium; Ao = aorta. For other details, see text*

ment of the mitral cusps in the LV, C–c the LV outflow tract, and D–d the aortic valve and left atrium.

By steadily angling the transducer from position A through D, a continuous recording is produced that shows the continuity of the ventricular septum (VS) with the anterior wall of the aorta and, of the anterior mitral cusp with the posterior wall of the aorta (cf LD-11 and 17).

The left ventricle

Standard LV measurements are made just apical to the tips of the mitral valve cusp echoes (LD-64). The technique has limited value because the ventricle is visualized reliably only as far as the papillary muscles and so is not helpful nearer the apex.

The end-systolic and end-diastolic diameters, wall-thickness and amplitude of wall motion can be measured. They have proved of value in the follow-up of valvar disease, but are not reliable in cases where

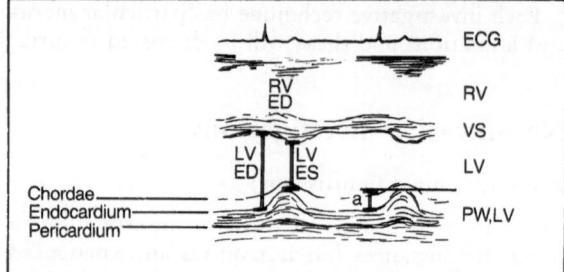

LD-64. *Left ventricle. Key: ED = end-diastole; ES = end-systole; a = amplitude of wall motion; other abbreviations as in LD-63. For other details, see text*

there may have been localized wall damage, as in myocardial infarction.

Variations in wall movement may indicate abnormalities, such as reduction of motion in an infarcted area with compensatory exaggeration of motion in other areas.

Movement of the VS away from the LV immediately following the R wave of the ECG (paradoxical motion) in association with a large RV, indicates the presence of an RV volume overload, e.g., in atrial septal defect. LV volume overload, e.g., in aortic incompetence, will often produce an exaggerated normal septal motion with an enlarged LV.

Dilatation due to cardiomyopathy is suggested by a large LV with thin wall measurements.

The normal mitral valve

The pattern of mitral valve cusp motion is shown in LD-65. The section CD shows the cusps closed in systole. At point E the cusps are thrown fully open at the onset of diastole. EF shows the anterior cusp

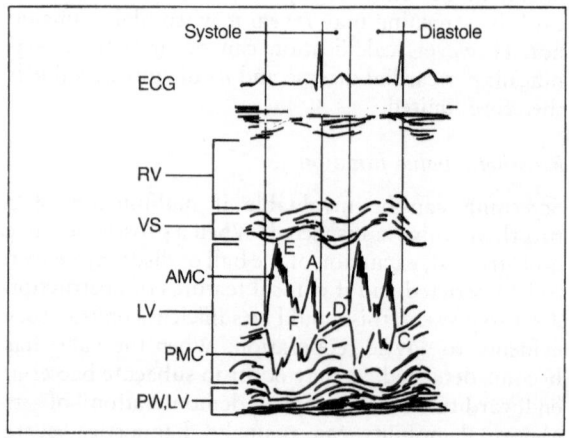

LD-65. *Normal mitral valve. Key: as in LD-63. For other details, see text*

floating back towards the closed position, to be thrown open again at A by the force of atrial contraction. This is followed by an abrupt return to the closure point C, as ventricular systole commences.

It should be noted that the posterior cusp traces out a pattern that is a small mirror image of the anterior cusp.

Mitral stenosis

The finding of a normal mitral valve echocardiogram excludes the diagnosis of mitral stenosis. The features necessary for this diagnosis are:

- reduction of cusp separation
    due to adhesion of the cusps at the commissures
- cusp thickening
    due to distortion or calcification from the rheumatic process
- reduction in the EF slope
    due to slow LV filling through the stenosed valve orifice
- reduction in DE measurement
    due to reduced mobility of the anterior cusp

The measurement DE is a good indication of whether the anterior cusp is sufficiently mobile to benefit from valvotomy or is calcified and distorted with only poor movement, suggesting the need for valve replacement (LD-66).

Prolapse of mitral valve cusps

In many cases of clinically suspected prolapse, one of two echo patterns may be seen that represent the cusps billowing towards the atrium in systole. The majority show late systolic buckling, but about a third appear as pansystolic bowing (LD-67).

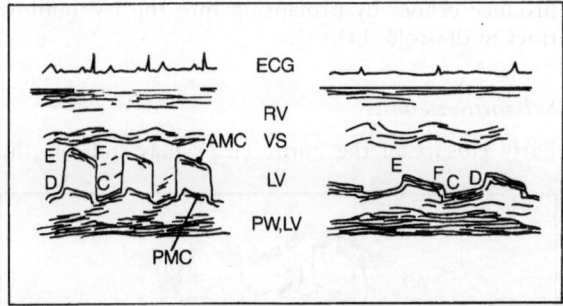

LD-66. Mitral stenosis. Left, *mitral stenosis with pliable cusps suitable for valvotomy.* Right, *severely stenosed immobile mitral valve with thickened cusps not suitable for surgery.* Key: as in LD-63. For other details, see text

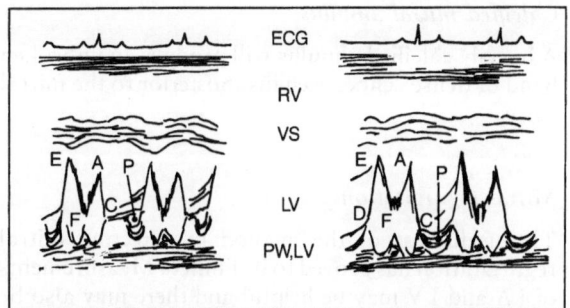

LD-67. *Prolapse of mitral valve cusps. Left, P = late systolic buckling. Right, P = pansystolic bowing. Key: as in LD-63. For other details, see text*

Left atrial myxoma

The characteristic layers of dense echoes from a myxoma are seen between the mitral cusps in diastole and the EF slope is reduced due to slow filling of the LV through the obstructed orifice. Echoes of the tumour may be identified also in the LA (LD-68).

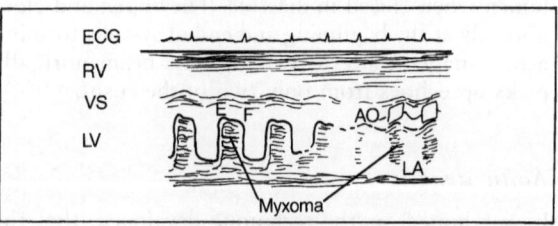

LD-68. *Sweep from left ventricle to left atrium to show atrial myxoma. Key: as in LD-63. For other details, see text*

Vegetations of the mitral valve

These can be detected on the anterior or posterior cusp in many cases of subacute bacterial endocarditis and are characterized by dense and ragged echoes that stand out against an otherwise normal valve pattern. The vegetations may prolapse into the atrium during systole (LD-69).

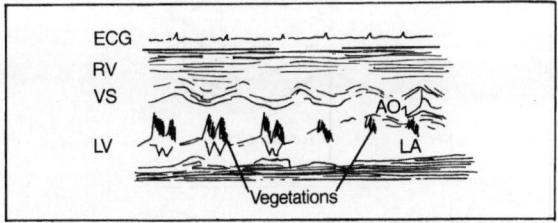

LD-69. *Sweep from left ventricle to left atrium showing vegetations on the anterior cusp prolapsing into left atrium. Key: as in LD-63*

Calcified mitral annulus

A heavily calcified annulus will produce an unbroken band of dense echoes seen just posterior to the mitral cusps.

Mitral regurgitation

The usefulness of the method in detecting mitral regurgitation has proved to be limited. Measurements of LA and LV may be helpful and there may also be evidence of LV volume overload as shown by a large LV and exaggerated VS motion. Partial closure of the aortic cusps in systole may be noted in cases of gross mitral regurgitation.

The aortic valve

The undulation of the echoes from the parallel walls of the aorta is due to the movement of the base of the heart relative to the transducer. The cusps, not always easy to visualize, can be seen as a single line in mid-lumen when closed in diastole. They open and close abruptly at the beginning and end of systole, forming a box-shaped pattern (LD-70). The beam normally picks up echoes from only two of the cusps.

Aortic stenosis

It was hoped, as the technique developed, that the measurement between the open aortic cusps would give an accurate assessment of the degree of stenosis. This has not proved to be so, but it is accepted that thickening or duplication of the echoes implies distortion, stenosis or calcification. Identification of LV hypertrophy also aids assessment (LD-71).

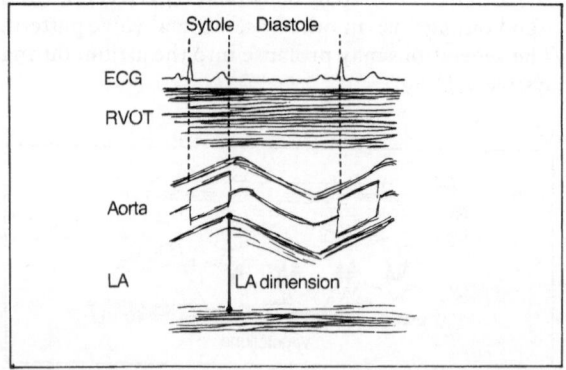

LD-70. *Normal aortic valve. Key: as in LD-63. For other details, see text*

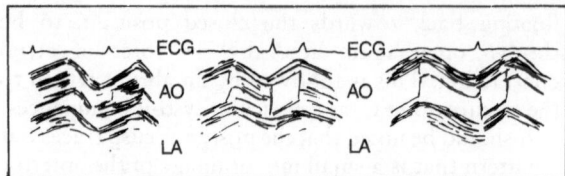

LD-71. *Aortic stenosis.* Left, *thick echoes in calcification.* Centre, *duplication of diastolic echoes suggesting stenosis.* Right, *eccentric diastolic closure line suggesting a bicuspid aortic valve. Key, as in LD-63*

Aortic incompetence

This condition is recognized echocardiographically by the effects it may produce in the LV. There may be early closure of the mitral valve, fine vibration on the anterior cusp echo, if the regurgitant jet strikes it (a possible explanation of the Austin–Flint murmur), or signs of LV volume overload (LV-72).

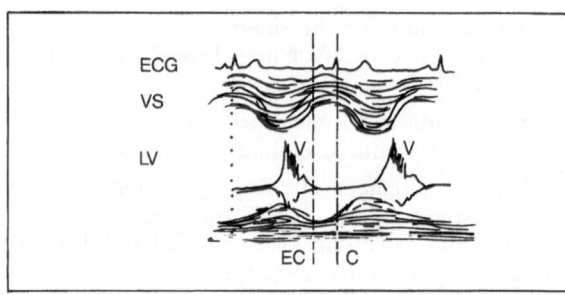

LD-72. *To show the effects of gross aortic regurgitation in the left ventricle. Key: C = normal closure point; EC = early closure of mitral valve; V = vibrations on anterior mitral cusp; VS = ventricular septum*

Vegetations on the aortic valve

These produce strong echoes, usually seen in the aortic lumen during diastole, but occasionally noted between the open cusps in systole. In some cases they produce echoes by prolapsing into the LV outflow tract in diastole (LD-73).

Subaortic stenosis

Early closure of the aortic cusps may indicate the

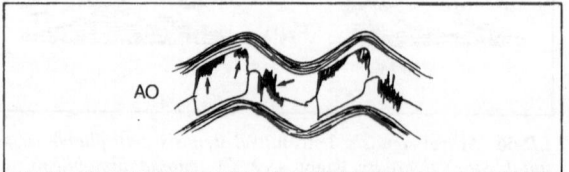

LD-73. *Aortic vegetations (arrows)*

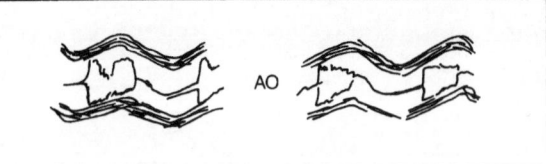

LD-74. Left, *subaortic stenosis*. Right, *effect on aorta of gross mitral regurgitation*

presence of subaortic stenosis and may also be found in gross mitral regurgitation (LD-74).

Hypertrophic obstructive cardiomyopathy (HOCM)

Echocardiography has been of great value in the diagnosis of HOCM and in screening relatives of patients with this condition. In those who have the disease, it should be possible to demonstrate some or all of the following features:

- asymmetric septal hypertrophy (i.e., VS thick and AW,LV normal)
- systolic anterior movement of the mitral cusps (SAM)
- midsystolic aortic cusp closure
- reduction of LV outflow tract dimension (LD-75)

Pericardial effusion

Echocardiography can identify even a fairly small pericardial effusion, which is recognized as an echo-free space between the ventricular walls and the relatively immobile stronger echo of the pericardium. In a very large effusion, it may be difficult to identify cardiac landmarks because the heart swings about in the fluid. This excessive movement may cause apparent variations in cardiac response to depolarization (LD-76).

Prosthetic valves

Biological valves, usually of human or porcine tissue,

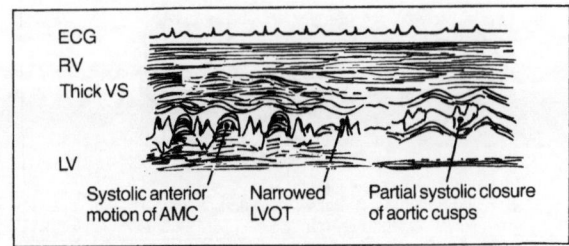

•**LD-75.** *To show the features of hypertrophic obstructive cardiomyopathy. Key: as in LD-63*

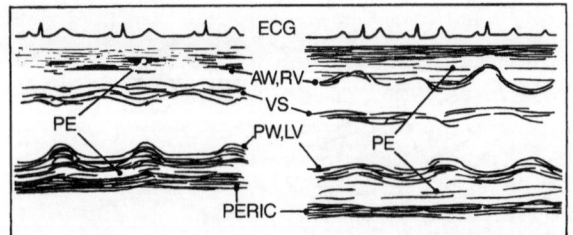

LD-76. *Pericardial effusion. Left, small effusion. Right, large effusion. Key: PERIC=pericardium; PE=pericardial effusion; other abbreviations as in LD-63*

have no particularly characteristic echo patterns, but serial measurements of chamber size may be of use in follow-up. The condition of non-biological valves, such as ball-in-cage or tilting-disc valves, can be assessed by using time intervals from phonocardiographically recorded heart sounds to valve opening or closing on a simultaneously recorded echocardiogram. These studies may detect early signs of valve wear or abnormal movement due to thrombus formation. For the best results in such cases, the transducer is placed at the apex (LD-77).

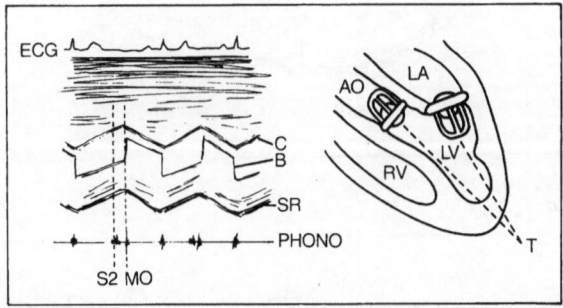

LD-77. Left, *echo pattern of mitral ball-in-cage prosthesis*. Right, *to show apical view of mitral and aortic prostheses. Key: S2=second heart sound; MO=mitral opening; C=cage; B=anterior opening of ball; SR=suture ring; T=transducer position; other abbreviations as in LD-63*

Pulmonary and tricuspid valves

These valves are difficult to visualize and, although some useful observations have been made, their echocardiographic evaluation has tended to lag behind that of more accessible structures.

Cross-sectional echocardiography

This development of cardiac ultrasonics allows the heart to be viewed in cross-section from various angles. It displays the anatomy and motion of the parts at the moment of observation, hence, the expression 'real-time', used to describe it.

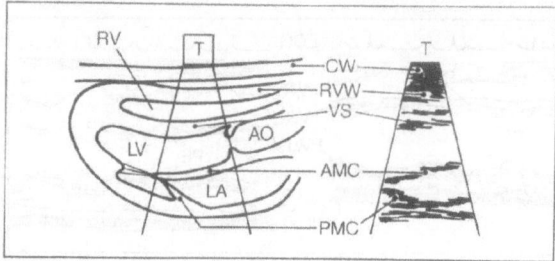

LD-78. *Long axis view of left ventricle at the level of the mitral cusps. Key: T = transducer; RVW = right ventricle wall; other abbreviations as in LD-63*

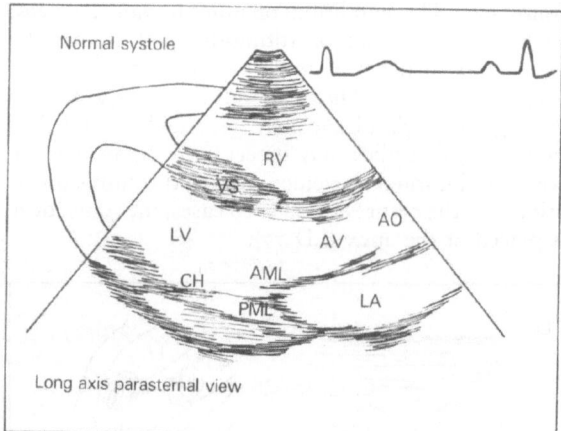

a

LD-79. *Showing the detail now obtainable in two-dimensional echocardiography. a, The aortic cusps are open and the mitral cusps are closed. b, The mitral cusps are now open and, characteristically, the aortic cusps are visible only where they are in apposition*

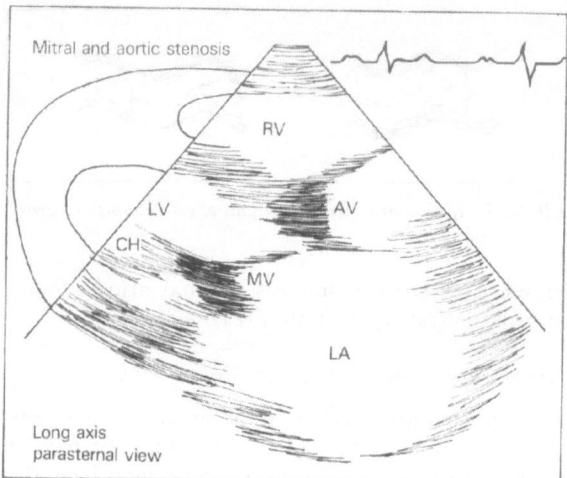

LD-80. *A case of mitral and aortic stenosis demonstrating the thickened mitral and aortic cusps, the grossly enlarged LA and the hypertrophied LV*

The advance has been achieved by using a sector scanner that enables a transducer to oscillate rapidly through an arc. The resulting echoes are displayed on a screen and can be videotaped or photographed to provide a permanent record. The transducer can be placed on different parts of the chest wall and its angle varied to study cross-sections of the heart. The images shown in LD-78, LD-79 and LD-80 are long axis views. Those recorded when the transducer is turned through 90° are known as short axis views (LD-81). Views obtained from the apex of the heart (LD-82 and LD-83) show all four cardiac chambers (Cf. LD-11, p. 9).

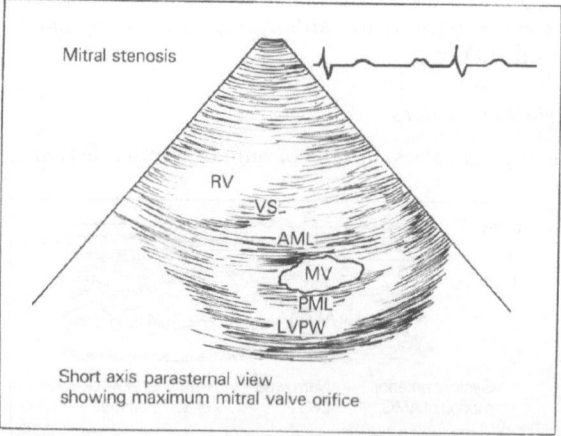

LD-81. *The area of the stenosed mitral valve orifice can be measured in the short axis view (same case as shown in LD-80)*

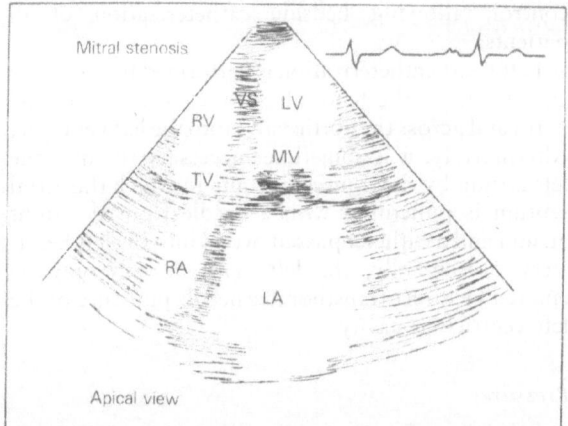

LD-82. *A third view of the mitral valve: this time seen from the apex. It demonstrates the thickened cusps and the large LA*

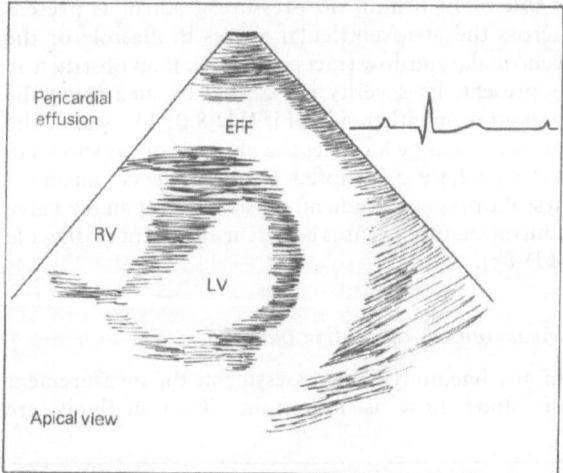

LD-83. *A large pericardial effusion (EFF)*

Congenital cardiac malformations

In skilled hands, paediatric echocardiography has been shown to be of value in the diagnosis of congenital malformations and such is the potential of the method that gross development abnormalities of the fetal heart have been identified at an early stage *in utero.*

Future developments

The development of more sophisticated two-dimensional echocardiographic scanning techniques is already well advanced and will undoubtedly result in a further increase in the role of this technique in cardiac diagnosis.

Phonocardiography

This is a useful technique for documenting auscultatory findings but is seldom used in clinical diagnosis. It may be combined with external recordings of the carotid pulse from which systolic time intervals can be derived. These intervals have been used in research to assess cardiac function but have little practical value.

Nuclear angiography

Recent developments indicate that nuclear angiography may play an increasing role in diagnosis and assessment of cardiac performance. A radioactive tracer (usually labelled with technetium 99m) is injected into a peripheral vein and the amount and distribution of radiation within the heart is detected with a scintillation camera. Two techniques have been developed.

(1) First-pass radionuclide angiocardiography.

In the first-pass technique, the rapid injection of a radioactive bolus into a peripheral vein is followed by analysis of radiation as the bolus passes for the first time through the cardiac chambers. It is possible to measure the size and shape of each ventricle, segmental wall motion and the ejection fraction. Intracardiac shunts can also be detected and quantified by examining pulmonary radiation.

(2) Equilibrium-gated blood pool imaging.

With the equilibrium-gated blood pool method, events on the electrocardiogram are used to define parts of the cardiac cycle. Following injection of an ionic tracer, radiation over the heart is repeatedly assessed over many heart beats at the same part of the cardiac cycle. The pattern of radioactivity is evaluated by a computer. This technique requires an ionic tracer that fills the entire intravascular compartment uniformly for a long period. In practice, the patient's own erythrocytes labelled with Tc 99m achieve this objective. Activity from the ventricles can be separated by examining the heart in the left anterior oblique projection and, as with the first-pass technique, chamber volumes, segmental wall motion and ejection fractions can be evaluated.

The equilibrium-gated blood pool technique has the advantage over the first-pass technique that multiple studies can be performed over several hours after only one injection. This is useful in studying the effect of drugs on cardiac function. It is less useful than the first-pass technique in assessing the right ventricle, because superimposed images from more than one chamber can be a problem.

Ambulatory ECG monitoring

This technique makes prolonged ECG monitoring possible by using a portable, miniature taperecorder that records the patient's ECG for 24 hours. The record can subsequently be analysed at high speed and abnormal rhythms can be documented. It is a valuable investigation when intermittent dysrhythmias are suspected of causing recurrent palpitation or syncopal attacks. Identification of the abnormal rhythm allows specific treatment to be prescribed. Also, 24 h recording can be useful in excluding intermittent dysrhythmias as a cause of symptoms, should symptoms occur while the rhythm is normal.

Exercise testing

This will be discussed in the section on Coronary Heart Disease (see p. 131).

Invasive investigations

Cardiac catheterization

Although cardiac catheterization is now a relatively safe procedure, it should not be performed unnecessarily. Many patients can be referred for cardiac surgery on the basis of clinical assessment and information derived from non-invasive techniques.

Catheterization may be indicated if the nature, severity and aetiology of the abnormality cannot be determined by other means. It may be indicated to exclude important cardiac disease and, in some instances, is required to evaluate the results of surgery. One of the most common current indications is as part of the evaluation of coronary artery disease.

Procedure

The patient usually receives light premedication and, under local anaesthesia, a catheter is passed from an arm or leg vein to the right atrium. Thereafter, with X-ray fluoroscopy, the catheter can be manipulated into the right ventricle and the main pulmonary artery. From the main pulmonary artery, the catheter can be advanced and wedged in a small pulmonary artery. From this wedged position, a pulmonary artery wedge (PAW) or pulmonary capillary wedge (PCW), pressure can be recorded that measures the left atrial pressure indirectly through the capillaries and pulmonary veins with sufficient accuracy for most clinical purposes. Recently, flow-guided balloon-tipped catheters have been used without fluoroscopic control, allowing bedside catheterization of ill patients.

Left heart catheterization is performed by passing a catheter from the femoral or brachial artery to the aorta and across the aortic valve into the left ventricle. Alternatively, it is sometimes necessary to enter the left atrium by the transeptal route in which the atrial septum is punctured with a needle from the right atrium and a catheter passed over it into the left heart. Very occasionally, the left ventricle can only be entered by direct transthoracic needle puncture of the left ventricular cavity.

Pressures

Pressures are recorded in the cardiac chambers and great vessels, and blood samples are taken for oxygen saturation. Normal pressure values are shown in Table 8. In health, no pressure gradient is present across the atrioventricular valves in diastole or the ventricular outflow tracts in systole. If an obstruction is present, its severity is assessed by measuring the pressures on either side of it (LD-84). The site of the pressure change localizes the obstruction, as shown in LD-84 where a stenosed aortic valve is causing a systolic pressure gradient. Obstruction at an AV valve (mitral stenosis) causes a pressure gradient in diastole (LD-85).

Measurement of cardiac output

In any haemodynamic assessment, the measurement of blood flow is important. Two methods are

---

TABLE 8   Normal haemodynamic values

		Range
Pressures: mmHg		
Right atrium		0–8
Right ventricle	systolic	15–30
	end-diastolic	0–8
Pulmonary artery	systolic	15–30
	diastolic	5–16
	mean	16–22
Pulmonary artery wedge	mean	6–15
Left atrium	mean	4–12
Left ventricle	systolic	90–140
	end-diastolic	4–12
Aorta	systolic	90–140
	diastolic	60–90
	mean	70–105
Cardiac Index l/min per m²		2.8–4.2
a-v O₂ difference ml/100 ml blood		3.0–5.0
Pulmonary vascular resistance		1–3 u

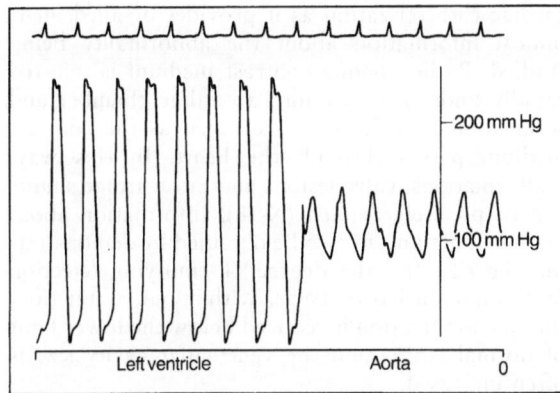

LD-84.

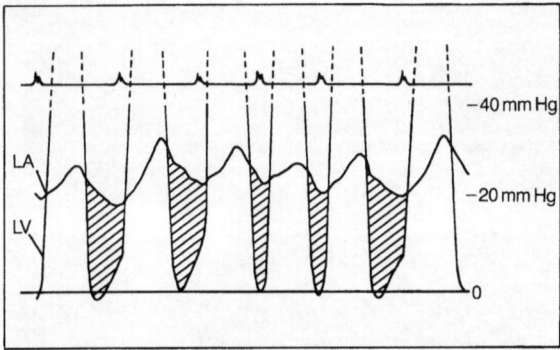

LD-85.

available, using either the Fick Principle or the Indicator Dilution technique.

In 1878 Adolf Fick enunciated that 'the total uptake or release of a substance by an organ is the product of blood flow to the organ and the arteriovenous concentration of the substance'. If the Fick Principle is applied to the lungs, then blood flow to the lungs can be derived from knowledge of the arteriovenous oxygen difference and oxygen uptake. Arteriovenous (a-v) oxygen difference can be derived from the oxygen content of pulmonary arterial and systemic arterial blood, and oxygen uptake can be measured from a collection of expired air:

$$\frac{\text{cardiac}}{\text{output}} = \frac{O_2 \text{ uptake}}{\text{a-v } O_2 \text{ difference}}.$$

With the indicator dilution technique, a known amount of indicator is added to the blood and the blood volume is then derived by measuring the concentration of indicator. Usually, indocyanine green dye is used as the indicator, but the same principle can be applied to thermal dilution when

changes in temperature are measured after injection of a known amount of cold saline at known temperature. At cardiac catheterization, a known volume of indicator is injected and blood is withdrawn at a constant rate from a downstream sampling site through a cuvette that instantaneously measures the concentration of the indicator. In this way, a plot of concentration against time is obtained (LD-86).

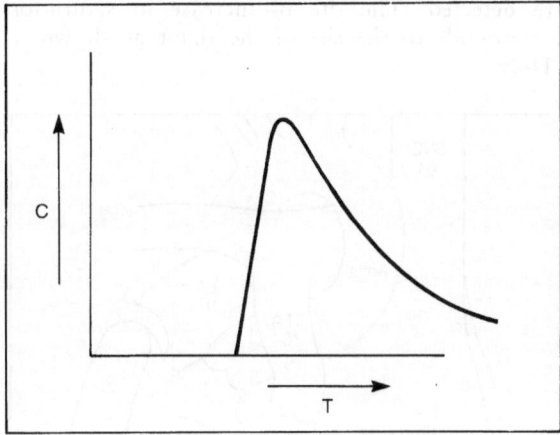

LD-86.

Cardiac output can be derived from knowledge of these variables and measurement of the area under the curve by planimetry.

Valve area

Measurement of blood flow or cardiac output is important in assessing the severity of valve stenosis. The pressure gradient across a stenosed valve depends upon blood flow through it, the higher the blood flow the bigger the pressure gradient. An estimate of valve orifice size or valve area can be derived from a hydraulic formula incorporating values for pressure difference and blood flow.

Pulmonary vascular resistance (PVR)

Pressure in the pulmonary circulation is dependent on pulmonary blood flow and PVR. Very high pulmonary blood flow may occur with left to right shunts and may cause elevated pulmonary artery pressure even in the absence of pulmonary vascular disease. Pulmonary vascular resistance can be derived from the formula:

$$PVR = \frac{\text{mean PA} - \text{mean LA pressure (mmHg)}}{\text{cardiac output (l/min)}}.$$

Normal values are less than 3 units. When pulmonary vascular disease is present, values for PVR rise.

Shunt detection

A left to right intracardiac shunt is usually detected by measuring the oxygen saturation of blood within the right heart chambers. If oxygenated blood is entering the right heart chambers, elevated oxygen saturations are detected. The site of increase in saturation corresponds to the site of the shunt as shown in LD-87.

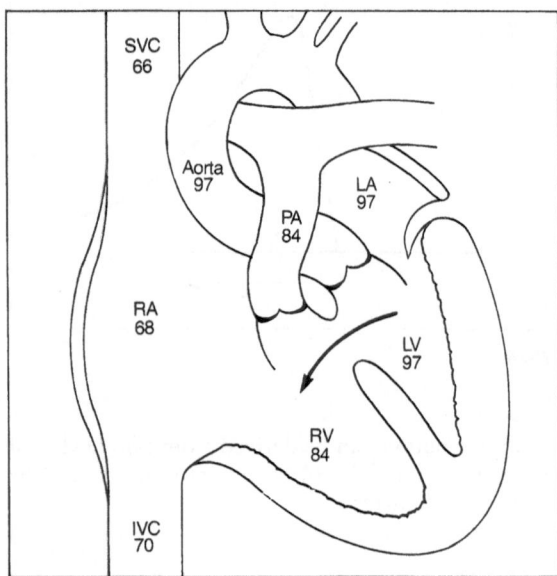

LD-87.

The shunt can be quantified by applying the Fick Principle.

With significant shunts, pulmonary blood flow may be twice systemic blood flow or greater.

Right to left shunts can be detected in a similar fashion by measuring the oxygen saturation of blood in the left heart chambers. For example, a right to left shunt due to reversed flow through a persistent ductus arteriosus would result in desaturated blood in descending aorta but fully saturated blood in ascending aorta.

Right to left shunts can also be detected by indicator dilution techniques and by angiocardiography.

Angiocardiography

Angiocardiography is usually an integral part of cardiac catheterization as it provides detailed anatomical information about the abnormality being studied. Radio-opaque contrast medium is injected rapidly under pressure into a cardiac chamber and serial films or cine films are taken as the contrast medium passes through the heart. In this way, malformations, valve lesions and intracardiac shunts can be precisely defined (X-18). Information about cardiac function can also be obtained by demonstrating the size and the degree of emptying (ejection fraction) of the left ventricle. With impaired function, the ejection fraction is reduced below the lower limit of normal (50%) and the ventricular cavity size is often increased.

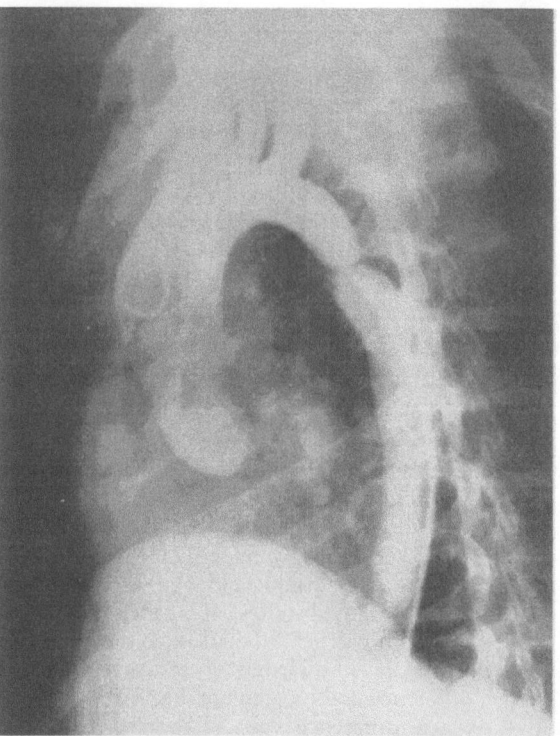

X-18. *Angiographic appearance in coarctation of the aorta. An area of discrete obstruction is seen distal to the left subclavian artery*

Coronary arteriography

With recent developments in coronary artery surgery, coronary arteriography is now a common investigation. It is usually performed either by the Sones' technique, using a brachial arteriotomy approach, or by the Judkin's technique, using a percutaneous femoral artery puncture and preshaped catheters. In the hands of skilled investigators, both can give good visualization of the coronary arteries. Because of the tortuosity of the coronary arteries and their tendency to overlap in any given projection, multiple views are required and cine film is taken to allow analysis at slow speed.

Intracardiac electrograms

Recording of intracardiac electrical potentials can be useful in the investigation of conduction abnormalities and disorders of rhythm. An electrode catheter can be passed from the femoral vein across the tricuspid valve to record electrical activity from the bundle of His.

A catheter in this position also records atrial and ventricular activity, giving a characteristic His Bundle electrogram (LD-88). Abnormal AV conduction gives abnormal atrial – His (AH) or His – ventricular (HV) times. When AV block is present, the site of block can be determined as either distal or proximal to the His bundle, depending on the presence or absence of a His bundle potential. Recordings from the His bundle and other sites within the heart can document the activation sequence in disorders of rhythm and can be useful in identifying the nature and mechanism of the various tachycardias.

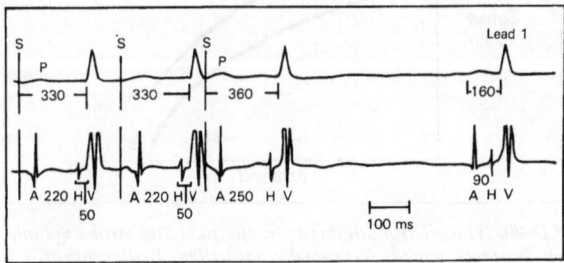

LD-88. *His bundle electrogram (HBE). A catheter placed across the tricuspid valve can record atrial (A), His bundle (H) and ventricular (V) activity. The normal AH interval is 50–120 ms and the HV interval is 35–55 ms. With atrial pacing (S) the PR interval is prolonged to 350 ms due to a prolonged AH of 220 ms. The third S is premature and PR is further prolonged due to relative refractoriness of the AV node. With recovery (the last complex) the PR interval is normal*

Complications of catheterization

Cardiac catheterization can have complications but, in experienced hands, the incidence should be low. The introduction of a venous catheter may cause thrombophlebitis and arterial catheterization may result in vascular occlusion requiring surgical exploration. Dysrhythmias are not infrequent, but are seldom life-threatening. The catheter may perforate

the heart. Injection of contrast medium may result in extravasation of contrast within the myocardium. Lengthy procedures involve considerable exposure to ionizing radiation. Fatal complications do occasionally occur. All these considerations emphasize that catheterization must never be advised unnecessarily.

HEART FAILURE

When clinicians refer to heart failure, they usually have in mind a collection of clinical features resulting from the heart's inability to fulfil its normal circulatory function. These clinical features are largely manifestations of congestion within the tissues of the body. Hence, the term 'congestive cardiac failure' is widely used. It is sometimes applied to signs of congestion in the systemic circulation alone (i.e. as a synonym for right heart failure) or to signs of congestion in both the systemic and pulmonary circulations.

'Right' and 'left heart failure' are preferable terms. They indicate that certain clinical features are due largely to the malfunction of one side of the heart or the other. These terms also have shortcomings, however, because some signs are due to disordered function of both sides of the heart. The right and left hearts cannot be considered in isolation. A change in cardiac output from one side must inevitably be followed by a similar change in cardiac output from the other side. If this did not happen a vast quantity of blood would soon accumulate in either the pulmonary or systemic circulation.

Heart failure may occur suddenly and unexpectedly, as in acute myocardial infarction, or it may be chronic, as in valve disease or as a consequence of hypertension. As noted above, the failure may affect either side or both sides of the heart; but whereas persistent (chronic) left heart failure may ultimately lead to right heart failure, the converse is rarely true.

Causes

The heart may fail because the myocardium is diseased and is not contracting properly or because it has been subjected to an excessive workload. An excessive workload may either be a 'volume load' or a 'pressure load'.

Volume loads

When a 'volume load' is imposed, the heart must

expel more blood than normal in response to increased circulatory demand in such conditions as anaemia and hyperthyroidism or when pregnancy is complicated by heart disease. This is sometimes referred to as 'high output failure'. An increased 'volume load' can also be associated with a normal or even a low cardiac output if structural abnormalities compel the heart to expel blood in wasteful directions in such conditions as aortic, mitral or tricuspid regurgitation, atrial or ventricular septal defects and arteriovenous shunts.

Pressure loads

These are imposed by disorders that increase the resistance or impedance to outflow of blood from the cardiac chambers. Stenosis of valves imposes a pressure load on the chamber responsible for pumping blood through the stenosed valve; hypertension in the systemic or pulmonary circuit imposes a pressure load on the left or right ventricle.

Determinants of cardiac output

Cardiac output is the product of heart rate and stroke volume.

Three factors govern stroke volume:

- preload
- afterload
- myocardial contractility

An increase in preload or myocardial contractility increases stroke volume. An increase in afterload decreases stroke volume.

Preload

In simple terms, this is the volume of blood available for ejection by the ventricles during systole. It is determined by the length of the ventricular myocardial fibres at the end of the diastole, the end-diastolic ventricular volume. As the ventricle does not empty completely with each contraction, even in health, this is the sum of the end-systolic ventricular volume plus the venous return to the ventricle from the atrium during diastole. Increased venous return therefore augments preload and this in turn improves stroke volume (LD-89).

Afterload

This is the resistance or impedance to the outflow of

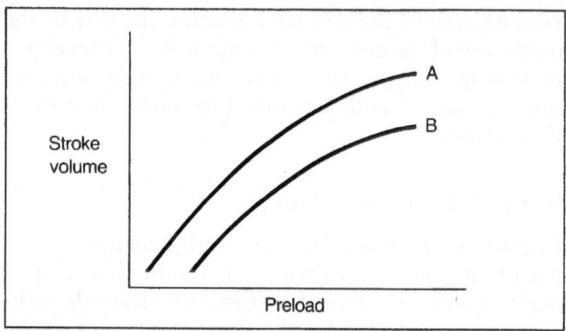

LD-89. *The relationship between preload and stroke volume at constant afterload: A, normal contractility; B, diminished contractility*

blood from a ventricle. In the absence of ventricular outflow tract obstruction, afterload is largely dependent on the peripheral vascular resistance, which is governed by arteriolar tone. An increase in arteriolar tone increases afterload and decreases stroke volume (LD-90).

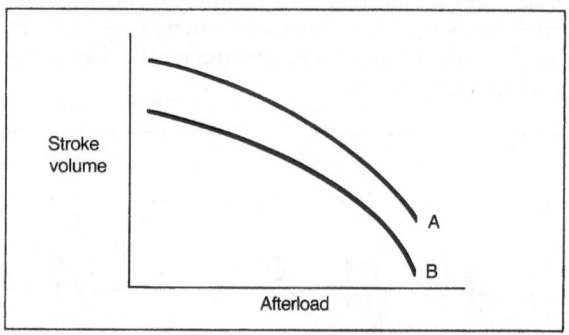

LD-90. *The relationship between afterload and stroke volume at constant preload: A, normal contractility; B, diminished contractility*

Myocardial contractility

When preload and afterload are kept constant, stroke volume can still be modified by a third factor termed 'myocardial contractility' – an index of the intrinsic functional state of the myocardium. Sympathetic stimulation enhances contractility: myocardial disease depresses it.

In practice, preload, afterload and contractility cannot be considered in isolation. They are constantly interacting and modifying cardiac output. For example, when the myocardium is diseased, even a large increase in preload causes relatively little augmentation of stroke volume (LD-89). When contractility is poor, a small increase in afterload substantially reduces stroke volume (LD-90).

Circulatory responses

When heart failure develops, various compensatory responses occur in an attempt to improve cardiac output and maintain blood pressure. These responses modify preload, afterload and myocardial contractility.

The most immediate response is mediated by an increase in sympathetic tone triggered by the falling pressure, which is an inevitable consequence of the failing cardiac output. The cardiac β-sympathetic receptors are stimulated to increase heart rate and myocardial contractility. Stimulation of the α- and β-receptor sites in the arterioles produces a variable result. There is dilatation of coronary and cerebral arterioles but constriction of renal, splanchnic and skin arterioles. Consequently, blood flow to essential organs is preferentially preserved. Venous tone is increased by sympathetic stimulation. This augments venous return to the heart and increases preload.

However, preload is increased to a much greater extent by a second important response, i.e. sodium and water retention by the kidney. The renal response takes several days to develop after the onset of heart failure. At least three factors are responsible for the saline retention. Glomerular filtration is reduced, but this is probably not very important. After a few days, the secretion of aldosterone is increased, promoting the absorption of sodium from the distal tubule. The most important factor, however, and the mechanism is incompletely understood, is saline retention from the proximal tubule.

The third response is myocardial hypertrophy, i.e. an increase in the size of individual cardiac muscle fibres. Hypertrophy develops in response to increased myocardial wall tension and takes several months to develop. As Laplace's law indicates that tension in the ventricular myocardium is proportional to the systolic pressure within the ventricular cavity multiplied by its radius, hypertrophy develops in response to increases in preload or afterload.

Detrimental effects

Although the circulatory responses to heart failure are initially beneficial, ultimately they are detrimental if failure is severe and prolonged.

The arteriolar vasoconstriction mediated by the sympathetic nervous system increases afterload. This depresses stroke volume, particularly if contractility is poor (LD-90). The greater tension within the myocardium, resulting from increased preload or afterload, leads to a rise in myocardial oxygen demand. If this is not met, contractility is reduced and further increases

in preload can have little or no benefit in improving stroke volume (LD-89).

When the failing left ventricle becomes incapable of expelling the blood presented to it during diastole, left ventricular end-diastolic pressure rises. The increased pressure is transmitted through the mitral valve to the left atrium, pulmonary veins and pulmonary capillaries, resulting in pulmonary congestion. If the hydrostatic pressure within the pulmonary capillaries exceeds the osmotic pressure of the plasma proteins, fluid exudes from the capillaries into the interstitial lung tissue and causes pulmonary oedema.

Similarly, when the right ventricle fails, the venae cavae become distended with blood under high pressure. As pressure increases, the abdominal viscera become enlarged and congested and peripheral oedema develops in the dependent parts.

Clinical features

Left heart failure

Signs and symptoms of left heart failure develop when the outflow of blood from either the left ventricle or the left atrium is obstructed or when the left ventricle cannot cope with the workload placed upon it. Under these circumstances, the left atrial pressure rises. This is transmitted to the lungs and pulmonary congestion develops. Pulmonary congestion due to sudden malfunction of the left heart, e.g. following myocardial infarction, can occur even before saline retention by the kidneys develops. However, in longstanding left heart failure, saline retention is the main contributor to pulmonary congestion. The commonest causes of left heart failure are systemic hypertension, myocardial infarction and mitral and aortic valve disease.

Pulmonary congestion causes breathlessness. If left heart failure is mild, pulmonary congestion and breathlessness occur only during exercise. In contrast, patients with severe left heart failure complain of breathlessness during slight exertion or even at rest. Assuming that non-cardiac causes of breathlessness have been excluded, it is therefore possible to assess the degree of left heart failure by enquiring about those activities that provoke breathlessness or dyspnoea, the unpleasant sensation of breathlessness.

A characteristic feature of dyspnoea due to heart disease is 'orthopnoea', i.e. breathlessness worsened by lying down. Orthopnoea occurs because the venous return to the heart is increased by adopting the supine position. Orthopnoea may present as attacks of acute nocturnal dyspnoea, when the patient awakes with severe breathlessness. Sudden, severe left heart failure causes the clinical picture of 'acute pulmonary oedema', when the patient gasps for breath, sweats and is often terrified. He will insist on sitting upright and may cough up frothy bloodstained sputum.

The main signs of left heart failure are pulmonary crepitations: high-pitched, crackling sounds heard best with the diaphragm of the stethoscope. Only crepitations occurring after coughing are abnormal. In mild heart failure, they are only audible at the bases of the lungs. Signs of hydrothorax may also be detected.

Other signs, more obviously caused by the failing left ventricle, are a third heart sound, a fourth heart sound and pulsus alternans. Both third and fourth heart sounds are low-pitched and heard best with the bell of the stethoscope over the apex of the heart. The third sound occurs in early diastole, the fourth sound in late diastole. In tachycardia, the additional sound is often referred to as a 'gallop rhythm'. A third heart sound can be physiological, especially in young people, and is not necessarily of pathological significance.

Pulsus alternans is characterized by alternating large and small volume arterial pulses.

When the diagnosis of left heart failure is in doubt, a chest X-ray is of value. It is a more sensitive method of detecting pulmonary congestion than clinical examination.

The electrocardiogram gives no guide to the severity of heart failure but may help in determining its cause.

Right heart failure

Signs and symptoms of right heart failure develop when the right ventricle cannot cope with the workload placed upon it or, much less commonly, when outflow of blood from the right atrium or the right ventricle is obstructed. In either circumstance, the right atrial pressure rises and this raised pressure is transmitted to the venous side of the systemic circulation, which becomes engorged with blood.

Right heart failure is often a consequence of left heart failure – the raised pressure having been transmitted backwards through the pulmonary capillaries to the pulmonary arteries and so to the right heart.

Right heart failure also results from pulmonary disease, particularly from chronic bronchitis and emphysema.

In right heart failure, the jugular veins become distended. The liver becomes congested and may be palpably enlarged and tender as its pain-sensitive capsule is stretched. Hepatic congestion usually causes slight elevation of the serum bilirubin. Renal congestion causes proteinuria.

Peripheral oedema is a common feature of right heart failure. It is a consequence of reduced renal perfusion and of increased capillary pressure secondary to systemic venous congestion. Oedema is most noticeable in dependent parts of the body where the subcutaneous tissues are lax, i.e. the ankles of those who are up and about, the back of the thighs or the sacrum of those who are confined to bed.

Less specific features of heart failure are fatigue and lassitude, presumably caused by a low cardiac output. In advanced cases of failure, patients develop cahexia and may become confused.

SECTION II

History and Physical Examination

GENERAL PRINCIPLES OF TAKING A HISTORY

Taking a good history is by far the most important part of any medical examination. It is the foundation upon which everything else depends. Basically, you must discover the answer to two simple questions:

- what is the patient complaining about?
- for how long has the complaint been present?

This may sound easy enough, but nowadays so many patients have told their story so many times, to so many people and answered so many questions about it, that the original complaint may be difficult to determine.

All too often one hears what the patient thinks is wrong, what some other doctor thinks is wrong or what diagnostic label has been attached at some other hospital or clinic.

Also, the patient's reluctance to be precise frequently makes it difficult to determine the exact duration of symptoms and their relationship to each other. Such questions as, how long is 'a long time' and how recently is 'a short time', are frequently required.

Method

When taking the detailed history from a patient with suspected heart disease, the standard method should be followed.

Information volunteered by the patient is collected first.

The examiner merely interferes to contain those who are too talkative and to keep them to the point.

Only when insufficient information has been obtained in this way should prompting be used to complete the picture.

Information obtained by prompting is often less valuable than that which has been given spontaneously. A technique that does not suggest the answer must be developed. For example, if no mention has been made of breathlessness and the examiner thinks, having heard the rest of the story, that this seems odd, the prompt should be 'how about your breathing', rather than 'are you troubled by breathlessness'.

Direct questions should not be asked.

Human nature being what it is, suggestions conveyed by direct questioning are often incorporated into a patient's story, sometimes quite unwittingly, with the result that the unadulterated truth may never be told again. So, if a patient does not complain of chest pain, do not suggest it to him. If he does complain of chest pain, do not ask whether it is a tight crushing pain or one that feels as though a needle was stabbing into his chest; let him try to describe it.

These rules are especially important in cardiology, where important and highly significant diagnoses often have to be made on the history alone when physical examination and special tests reveal no abnormality.

The history as a yardstick for physical findings

Most disease processes cause fairly characteristic symptoms that can be regarded as variations on a theme. When the history has been taken correctly, the physical examination nearly always confirms what the story has suggested to the examiner. In this regard, history taking can be used as a yardstick for physical examination: unexpected findings should be the exception rather than the rule. If you are constantly finding things that were not expected, there is something wrong with the way you are taking the history.

For example, the natural history of mitral disease is completely different from that of aortic valve disease and the difference will be reflected in the patient's story. One will usually have known about the presence of heart disease for many years; to the other it often comes as a complete surprise.

A middle-aged woman suffering from mitral stenosis will tell of 20 or 30 years' disability with gradually increasing breathlessness and fatigue. This is often punctuated by episodes of mild heart failure caused by intercurrent chest infection or the onset of atrial fibrillation. With appropriate treatment, these are but temporary setbacks in a long story of chronic ill health. A middle-aged man with aortic stenosis, on the other hand, will have seemed in perfect health until the appearance of grave symptoms that herald the onset of severe heart failure.

The mitral valve has behind it only the left atrium, which may fail because of some temporary haemo-dynamic upset and may do so many times over a period of many years. The aortic valve has the full contractile force of the left ventricle behind it. It does not fail until it is nearing the end of its ability to sustain a greatly increased workload and rarely does so more than once or twice.

Having listened to the history, the patient is examined not to find out which valve is involved, but to confirm which valve is involved.

The way the story is told is also most important. It tells the examiner a lot about the patient as well as what may or may not be causing the trouble. Those patients whose precordial pain is the result of anxiety rather than an indication of heart disease, frequently dramatize their symptoms in striking contrast to the matter of fact way in which patients with serious coronary heart disease tell of the anginal pain that limits their activities and threatens their lives.

Assessment of the cardiac grade

Assessment of the cardiac grade is an important part of the history of patients with heart disease. It acts as a rough measure of incapacity and as a way of monitoring progress either in the natural course of events or in response to treatment. Also, the rapidity with which it changes is a useful guide to cardiac reserve.

The cardiac grade is expressed as Grades I to IV according to criteria laid down by the New York Heart Association.

Grade I denotes no incapacity

Grade II denotes incapacity on strenuous exertion

Grade III denotes incapacity on normal exertion

Grade IV denotes incapacity on less than normal exertion or even at rest (heart failure)

The classification is usually based on the history of breathlessness; less often on the severity of effort pain. Difficulties may arise, especially where symptoms are due not so much to heart disease as to the fear of it, but despite such limitations, the cardiac grade is of considerable value and should be recorded routinely on each visit to the hospital or clinic.

Special circumstances

Some patients are unable to give a history and some give doubtful testimony.

Infants and small children, and those who are comatose or confused, are examples of the first category. The elderly and infirm, and those with mental instability of one sort or another, are examples of the second.

Obtaining a good history is so important that when it cannot be obtained from the patient, it must be obtained from others. With infants and small children the mother is obviously the first choice. The spouse will usually keep things right when an adult witness seems unreliable. Close family or near neighbours can nearly always help with the elderly and infirm.

PAIN

Chest pain is a common complaint and, although it is often assumed to be due to heart disease, this is frequently not the case, because it has many different causes. True cardiac pain is usually caused by myocardial ischaemia or infarction and less often by pericarditis. It produces characteristic symptoms that can be easily recognized if one asks about:

- the site of the pain
- the nature of the pain
- radiation of the pain
- what brings it on
- what makes it worse
- how long it lasts
- what relieves it

Ischaemic pain

Site and radiation

Chest pain due to ischaemia most often starts in the middle of the chest behind the sternum. It can start slowly and build up or be severe from the onset. It may or may not spread. If it does, it may spread to:

- the arms (especially the left arm) and may cause tingling or a feeling of heaviness. Sometimes both arms are involved and occasionally only one part of one arm is involved
- the neck, gums and angle of the jaw
- the shoulders
- the back between the scapulae

Occasionally there is no central chest pain, only pain at one or other of these sites of radiation (e.g. watch-strap angina).

Nature of the pain

When a patient with cardiac pain is asked to describe it, he often grimaces, clenches his fist and holds it over the middle of the sternum. This emphasizes that tightness or a feeling of constriction is experienced and some patients do not think of it as pain. Stabbing or jabbing transitory pain in the region of the left nipple is a common symptom that is not due to heart disease. It is often described by patients who think they have heart disease or are afraid that they might have heart disease.

Precipitating factors

Chest pain due to heart disease occurs when the heart is receiving less oxygen than it needs. This explains why the pain (angina pectoris) usually develops on exertion, in cold or windy weather or after a heavy meal.

To estimate the nature and severity of disability, find out if the pain occurs on:

- hurrying or running
- climbing hills or stairs
- walking quickly on the level
- walking slowly on the level
- at rest or in bed

Excitement and emotional upset may also trigger-off chest pain due to heart disease. A few patients who do not have chest pain on effort are incapacitated by emotionally induced pain. Anger, fear or excitement while watching films, boxing or football matches often causes such pain.

How long does the pain last and what relieves it

Angina of effort goes away quickly if the precipitating factor is removed. Patients will usually have discovered for themselves that slowing down or stopping relieves the pain in a minute or two. Some may say that their symptoms have improved, when all that has happened is that they have learned from experience what circumstances cause pain and have subconsciously adapted their way of life to avoid them as much as possible.

Glyceryl trinitrate taken sublingually nearly always relieves angina pectoris, but is less effective in other types of chest pain. If this has not been tried, it can be used as a therapeutic test. Other drugs, such as β-blockers or nifedipine, also reduce the frequency and severity of attacks in most cases.

Prolonged pain that lasts for 20 minutes or more is unlikely to be caused by transient ischaemia and suggests myocardial infarction.

Pericardial pain

This resembles ischaemic pain in some ways but

- is often sharp or aching in character
- may radiate to the upper abdomen and less commonly to the arms
- is frequently aggravated by movement, such as taking a deep breath, coughing, swallowing or lying flat in bed

DYSPNOEA

Dyspnoea is best defined as inappropriate breathlessness. Everyone can and does become breathless. How breathless, depends on the amount of exertion and their degree of fitness. Dyspnoea occurs when the breathlessness is out of proportion to the amount of exertion.

To establish the degree of disability, one must enquire if there is undue breathlessness when

- hurrying or running
- climbing hills or stairs
- walking quickly on the level
- walking slowly on the level
- at rest

Questions also need to be asked about breathlessness at night. Can the patient lie flat in bed or how many pillows are needed to prevent breathlessness?

Some patients wake breathless from sleep. They are compelled to sit up and often get up and go to a window for air. Their breathlessness is often associated with a feeling of choking or constriction in the throat and a fear of death. This is a serious symptom known as paroxysmal nocturnal dyspnoea and is caused by transient left heart failure. Such attacks of acute breathlessness may also occur during the day.

FATIGUE

Many patients with heart disease complain of non-specific symptoms. These include fatigue and lack of energy due to poor cardiac output and diminished cardiac reserve. Initially, they feel unduly tired by the end of a busy day. Eventually, they are unable to cope even with normal activities.

Such symptoms, like pain and breathlessness, are helpful when assessing the degree of disability, but being common psychosomatic complaints are often more difficult to evaluate.

COUGH

Coughing, a prominent symptom in respiratory disease, is also a feature of some cardiovascular disorders.

When taking a history from a patient with a cough, the points discussed below should be kept in mind.

Duration

A cough that has been present for many years is more likely to be due to respiratory disease than by cardiac disease. However, heart disease can be caused by chronic lung disease (see Cor Pulmonale p. 176) and in such cases a longstanding cough is the rule.

A cough that is associated with congestion of the lungs caused by left heart failure is likely to be acute and of shorter duration. It may be accompanied or worsened by an intercurrent respiratory infection.

Sputum

It is useful to know whether or not the cough produces sputum (is productive). If it is, find out:

- if it is profuse or scanty
- what it looks like: watery and frothy or thick and sticky
- what colour it is: green, yellow or brown
- if it is bloodstained
- if the symptoms are relieved by coughing up sputum

In cardiac disease, sputum is either absent or scanty. When present it is often frothy. As a rule it is not coloured, although blood may be present in some cases.

In acute respiratory infections, such as bronchitis or pneumonia, cough is often at first unproductive and later becomes profuse and purulent. In pneumonia, early red-bloodstaining later turns to a rusty brown.

In chronic respiratory infections, sputum is usually thick and sticky and, especially during exacerbations, purulent and coloured yellow or green. Only very occasionally is it bloodstained. Getting rid of a good quantity of sputum, either unaided or with the help of a physiotherapist, often temporarily relieves both the cough and the dyspnoea.

Aggravating factors

All coughs may be increased on exertion, but cough due to cardiac disease is noticeably worsened on completion of the exertion.

Lying down flat may make a cardiac patient start to cough, especially in a cold bed.

In chronic bronchitis or bronchiectasis, changes in temperature, such as moving from a warm to a cold room, provoke fits of coughing. Similarly, dusty or smoky atmospheres aggravate coughing in patients with respiratory disorders.

In chronic bronchitis, too, the cough is often worst on rising in the morning.

Type of cough

It is always useful to hear a cough, if this is possible.

Many coughs are described by patients as a 'smoker's cough', but this self-assessment should never be accepted without further evaluation.

A loose or productive cough suggests bronchitis or bronchiectasis.

A short, sharp, irritating cough suggests pulmonary congestion due to cardiac or infective causes. When caused by a painful disorder, such as pneumonia or pleurisy and occasionally in pericarditis, the cough is very short and obvious attempts are made to suppress it.

A loud, hacking cough is often due to pharyngitis, but also occasionally reveals a neurotic or hysterical personality.

A hard, echoing cough, often described as 'brassy' and characteristic of a mediastinal tumour or an aortic aneurysm, is easily recognized and once heard is unlikely to be forgotten.

HAEMOPTYSIS

A patient who has coughed up blood, even a small quantity of it, is likely to be anxious and concerned. When confronted by such a patient, the physician should keep the following facts in mind.

Duration and quantity

In most cases due to heart disease, haemoptysis comes suddenly, lasts only a short time and is often associated with dyspnoea or cough. Prolonged haemoptysis is much more likely to be associated with chronic respiratory disorders such as bronchiectasis, tuberculosis or bronchial neoplasm.

A really large gush of blood has only one, relatively rare, cardiac cause – rupture of an aortic aneurysm. Quite large quantities may occasionally be produced in some cases of mitral stenosis, but more commonly haemoptysis of cardiac origin consists of small amounts of blood, often tiny flecks, coughed up as part of the sputum. Blood, evenly spread through copious frothy sputum, is seen in acute pulmonary oedema.

Associated features

Pain

Haemoptysis associated with pleural type chest pain (catching on breathing) is most likely to be due to pulmonary consolidation or infarction or a recent rib fracture.

Sputum

The associated sputum, if any, is important. Profuse bleeding with little sputum suggests arterial rupture, either from a bronchopulmonary anastomosis in mitral stenosis, an aneurysm or a pulmonary arteriovenous angioma. Occasionally, a brisk bleed without accompanying sputum occurs in bronchiectasis.

Copious frothy sputum, tinged pink, has already been referred to above, as characteristic of pulmonary oedema.

Copious purulent or sticky sputum mixed with varying quantities of blood suggests a respiratory infection.

Bleeding elsewhere

It is important to find out if the haemoptysis is part of a generalized haemorrhagic diathesis or if the patient is receiving anticoagulant drugs. Finally, one has to make sure that the blood came from the lungs and not from the mouth, nose or pharynx.

Haemoptysis or apparent haemoptysis is not infrequently produced artificially by mentally disturbed patients. In these circumstances it is important to establish that the patient actually coughed up the blood from the lungs or bronchi.

Previous history

This must be taken with care, to find out about possible cardiac or respiratory disease, keeping in mind the possibility of embolism from recent venous thrombosis.

OEDEMA

Oedema may be defined as an increase in interstitial fluid within the extravascular compartment. It may be generalized throughout the body or localized to certain parts of it.

In cardiovascular disease, the oedema fluid gravitates to the most dependent parts: the ankles in those who are up and about, the sacrum in those who are confined to bed.

When oedema is suspected the following questions should be asked:

- has there been a recent gain in weight
- which part of the body is swollen
    the periorbital tissues – puffy eyes
    the hands – rings too tight
    the abdomen – waist band too tight
    the ankles – shoes too tight
- has the patient been subject to allergies or lived in the tropics

Ankle swelling

This is usually the most important and earliest sign of oedema due to cardiovascular disease. Questions are designed to differentiate it from other causes of oedema and to determine its severity. Ask if:

- one or both ankles are involved
- the patient has varicose veins
- any other parts of the body are swollen
- it is present all the time or only in the evenings
- it has extended up the calves
- it is related to the menstrual cycle

PALPITATION

When a patient complains of 'palpitation' the first thing to do is to establish that this means an abnormal awareness of the heart beat.

Symptoms

Ask the patient to imitate what is felt, either by beating the chest or tapping out the rhythm on the table top. Many find this difficult. It may help to ask whether the rhythm is regular or irregular 'like the morse code'; is it an occasional 'bump' or a sustained rhythm. Ask also:

- how fast it is: has anyone felt the pulse during an episode
- how does it start: is the onset sudden or gradual
- how does it stop: does it pass off gradually or stop abruptly
- how long does it last
- how frequently does it occur

Associated features

The following information is helpful:

- are there associated symptoms, such as dyspnoea, chest pain, light-headedness or syncope
- do episodes cause sweating or anxiety
- does polyuria occur

Precipitating factors

Ask if any precipitating factors have been recognized:

- are they related to stress, fatigue, exercise, alcohol, meals
- do they occur more commonly at rest or in bed

Relieving factors

Ask if the patient can or has tried to terminate the palpitation by vagal stimulation, such as, gagging, the Valsalva manoeuvre, ocular pressure or carotid sinus massage, or if any other means of avoiding or stopping them has been discovered.

Associated conditions

Ask about features that might suggest the presence of underlying heart disease, either rheumatic, ischaemic, thyrotoxic or hypertensive.

Medications

Find out if the patient is receiving medication that might cause palpitation or increased awareness of the heart's action. Ask also about medication used to treat the palpitation.

SYNCOPE

Syncope or fainting occurs for a variety of reasons, most of which are unconnected with diseases of the cardiovascular system.

The patient usually complains of 'blackouts' and it is essential first to establish what is meant by this, e.g. is there actual loss of consciousness or only altered consciousness.

Symptoms

Once it has been established that the patient has actually lost consciousness, the following questions should be asked:

- how long does the loss of consciousness last
- how often has it occurred
- is there any warning of the attack
- does palpitation occur at any time
- has the patient been injured in an attack
- has there been incontinence or tongue biting
- have there been neurological symptoms
- are all episodes identical
- have there been minor episodes when complete loss of consciousness does not occur

Precipitating factors

Having found out about the nature of the attacks, the next thing to do is to find out what causes them:

- have any precipitating factors been identified
- are they related to posture, head movement, coughing, micturition or exertion
- have episodes occurred at rest, in a chair or in bed

Eyewitness account

Patients who have lost consciousness may remember little about events that immediately preceded the attack and nothing about what happened during it. An eyewitness account may be most helpful in determining:

- if the patient was genuinely unconscious
- if convulsions occurred
- if the face changed colour
- how long the episode lasted
- if anyone checked the patient's pulse during an episode

Associated conditions

When considering the aetiology of syncopal attacks it is useful routinely to exclude certain well-known causes such as:

- a simple vasovagal attack
- epilepsy
- paroxysmal dysrhythmias
- postural hypotension, possibly caused by drug therapy

FEVER

Febrile conditions may cause headache, anorexia, lassitude and malaise (feeling generally unwell). Patients with fever may also complain of shivering while the temperature is rising, a feeling of warmth while it is high and sweating while it is falling. Tachycardia and the large volume pulse that often accompany fever may be experienced as palpitations (a consciousness of the heart's action).

It should be kept in mind that patients' perception of fever varies enormously and the absence of febrile symptoms does not exclude pyrexia. This is particularly true in cardiovascular disorders, e.g. in myocardial infarction where fever is common but symptoms due to fever are rare.

HEADACHE

Headache may be a feature of cardiovascular disease (see p. 105). When taking the history from a patient complaining of headache the questions enumerated below should be asked.

Site

Is it localized and if so where?
Tension may produce pain at the vertex or in the temporal area.
Disorders of the neck may produce occipital headache.
Lesions below the tentorium tend to produce occipital headache and lesions of cerebral hemispheres frontal headache.

Timing

Was the onset abrupt, as in subarachnoid haemorrhage?

Are there periods without headache, as in migraine, or is it constant, as when the intracranial pressure is raised?

At what time of day is the headache worst?
The headache of hypertension or raised intracranial pressure occurs immediately on waking. Tension headaches will develop during the day.

Does it occur on weekdays or at weekends?
Headache from hypertension or raised intracranial pressure will be aggravated by sleeping late at weekends.
Tension may be associated with the working week.

Is it related to any other factor?
Alcohol or glyceryl trinitrate, for example, can precipitate headache.

Is there a history of head injury?
Headache may last several months after head injuries. There may be an intracerebral haematoma.

Type of pain

Tight or gripping headache will suggest tension, throbbing suggests a vascular cause and scalp tenderness can be associated with cranial arteritis or possibly tension.

Associated symptoms

Visual disturbance:

- migraine may produce flashing lights
- papilloedema may lead to blurred vision
- intracranial lesions may lead to diplopia or visual field defects
- vomiting may signify migraine or raised intracranial pressure

Photophobia or neck stiffness are seen in subarachnoid haemorrhage or meningitis.

Neurological symptoms, such as hemiparesis, will signify intracranial disease.

Pallor, sweating and palpitations occur with the paroxysmal headache of pheochromocytoma.

LIMB PAIN

Two types of limb pain are complained about in peripheral vascular disease:

- intermittent claudication
- rest pain

Intermittent claudication

The nature of the pain

The pain occurs in the leg muscles on walking. It is felt as a tightness that may produce limping (claudication) and rapidly increases until it becomes so severe that the patient has to stop. After a short rest the pain disappears.

The site of the blockage

The muscles most commonly affected are the calf muscles due to a block in the superficial femoral artery. Claudication of the thigh and buttock is associated with a block in the common iliac artery and, if bilateral, with an aortic bifurcation block. If there is associated impotence in the male, the condition is termed the Leriche syndrome. Claudication of foot muscles indicates blockage of vessels below the knee.

Natural history

When claudication first starts, the distance that can be walked before the onset of pain may be variable. The pain is especially incapacitating when climbing stairs or hills or when walking against a wind. The condition may progress in one of three ways.

- It may clear up altogether when a collateral circulation becomes established
- The claudication distance may get shorter and then stabilize at a distance related to the adequacy of collateral blood supply
- Progressive deterioration may occur

Rest pain

This is a burning pain felt in the forefoot, especially in bed at night, because when the patient gets warm, the non-obstructed vessels dilate and this tends to siphon off blood from the obstructed limb. Also, warmth in the affected foot increases tissue metabolism and increases the need for blood at a time when less blood is available. The pain may be eased by putting the foot out of the bed to cool off and lowering it.

As the condition progresses, the patient may have to sit up all night with the foot on a cold floor. Gangrene may finally supervene.

LIMB COLDNESS

Many patients complain of cold limbs in our so-called temperate climate. As the skin vessels regulate the body temperature, coldness of a limb may be merely a response to a fall in body temperature. It may indicate a vascular problem, but before diagnosing vascular disease one should exclude such things as the cold limbs found in women where the coldness is related to a layer of subcutaneous fat that acts as an insulator.

Vasospastic disease

In vasospastic arterial disease or Raynaud's syndrome, the hands are most commonly affected. The fingers become white, cold and painful because of severe vasoconstriction. Later, the colour changes to blue and then red. The coldness can be very severe and is a problem especially in winter.

Occlusive arterial disease

Occlusive arterial disease may also produce a cold limb. This coldness to some extent reflects the degree and extent of the ischaemia. It can be felt by drawing the back of the hand downwards from the warm zone to the cold one and by comparing the two limbs. In acute ischaemia caused by embolism or thrombosis, the sudden onset of coldness is very noticeable to the patient and is accompanied by pain and pallor.

LIMB WEAKNESS

Patients with peripheral vascular disease often complain of weakness in a limb. This weakness is due to loss of muscle power and may result from loss of muscle itself, loss of nervous control or loss of blood supply. All these elements may be present to a greater or lesser degree in peripheral vascular disease. For example, in aorto-iliac disease pain occurs in the buttocks and leg muscles on exercise. This tends to limit muscle movement and increases the atrophy caused by the deficient blood supply. The limbs are weak and become noticeably wasted and thin. In femoropopliteal disease, the muscle weakness affects the calf and foot.

In chronic arterial disease the degree of weakness depends on the extent of the occlusion and the amount of collateral circulation. In acute arterial occlusion, weakness occurs rapidly with pain, pallor, paraesthesia and coldness.

GENERAL PRINCIPLES OF EXAMINATION

Always examine the heart, arteries and veins in a systematic manner.

Remember that the normal circulation can change quite rapidly because of nervous and humoral influences. Emotion and exercise can greatly increase the cardiac output. It may, for example, double with excitement. Remember also that both the anatomy and the physiology of the heart and circulation alter with age.

General approach

It is usually convenient to examine the patient lying in bed or on a couch propped up at an angle of about 30–45°, although some physical signs are easier to elicit when the patient lies flat, stands or squats. Make sure you are on the patient's right-hand side.

You should note the patient's demeanour, watching out for dyspnoea and for signs of anxiety such as deep sighs or the excessive axillary sweating so commonly seen in anxious adolescents. Look carefully at the patient's general complexion for such abnormalities as pallor, pigmentation, the 'café-au-lait' tinge sometimes associated with advanced infective endocarditis, for unusual distribution of body hair and for the characteristic features of many diseases that incidentally involve the cardiovascular system:

- myxoedema
- thyrotoxicosis
- acromegaly
- myopathies
- Paget's disease
- various congenital syndromes such as
  Down's
  Marfan's
  Hurler's
  Turner's

The face and head

Inspect the face and head with particular care. Characteristic nodules may be felt in the occipital aponeurosis in acute rheumatic fever.

The cheeks

Look at the cheeks for the 'malar flush' of longstanding mitral stenosis and pulmonary arterial hypertension: dilated venules are seen in the cyanosed skin. Severe aortic valve disease may be associated with a rather pink-and-white complexion; the complexion is muddy in haemochromatosis and brick-red in severe polycythaemia. In systemic lupus, a characteristic butterfly rash is sometimes seen across the cheeks and nose. In scleroderma, the skin is shiny and firmly attached to the underlying tissues, particularly those of the brow and nose.

The mouth

For a variety of reasons, the lips are often blue, so inspect the inside of the mouth for central cyanosis which is best seen in the buccal mucous membrane opposite the molar teeth. If this area appears cyanosed, it is central in origin.

Central cyanosis is not clinically detectable until the P_aO_2 is less than about 50 mmHg. Cyanosis is the result of too much reduced haemoglobin in the blood: if the patient's haemoglobin level is normal (15 g/dl), central cyanosis is seen only when there is more than 5 g/dl of reduced haemoglobin. Central cyanosis, therefore, suggests that about one third of the cardiac output bypasses the lungs through a shunt that is either anatomical (e.g. cyanotic congenital heart disease) or physiological (e.g. a ventilation/perfusion ($\dot{V}/\dot{Q}$) abnormality in the lungs).

With polycythaemia, which may complicate cyanotic congenital heart disease or severe anoxic pulmonary heart disease, cyanosis is deeper.

If Marfan's syndrome is suspected, look for the high arched palate.

The neck

Observe the arterial and venous pulses (see pp. 81, 83). Examine the neck for enlargement of the thyroid and auscultate for systolic bruits, not only over the thyroid but also over the carotid and vertebral arteries on each side.

The eyes

If you suspect aortic valve disease, look for Argyll–Robertson pupils. If you suspect Marfan's syndrome, look for the shimmering iris caused by lens dislocation. The scleral conjunctiva may contain congested vessels in polycythaemia and may be icteric if the liver is damaged. Look for a corneal arcus. Examine both retinae with an ophthalmoscope for the changes of hypertension and diabetes.

The hands

Inspect the hands for evidence of rheumatoid arthritis or arachnodactyly (Marfan's syndrome).

Look at the palms for the pallor of anaemia or the erythema of liver failure or hypercapnia. Note rare lesions such as the Janeway lesions (erythematous patches) of infective endocarditis or the pigmented creases of Addison's disease.

Look at the fingers for evidence of Raynaud's phenomenon or the tightly bound-down skin of scleroderma. Palpate for tender Osler's nodes in the pulps of all ten digits. Look at the nails for subungual splinter haemorrhages, koilonychia and abnormal capillary pulsation. Look carefully for finger clubbing, found in cyanotic congenital heart disease and sometimes in pulmonary heart disease and infective endocarditis.

If you suspect acute rheumatic fever, look for nodules in the tendon sheaths on the back of the clenched fist. Nodules of various types are sometimes found on the back of the elbows in acute rheumatic fever, rheumatoid arthritis and gout.

The abdomen

The abdomen should be examined. In particular, the liver should be percussed and palpated and the spleen palpated. Hepatic enlargement is common in right heart failure and an enlarged tender spleen may be a feature of infective endocarditis. The pulsation of the abdominal aorta is often visible in the epigastrium and the aorta can almost always be palpated. In elderly people, the abdominal aorta may be kinked and dilated or may be aneurysmal.

If the patient has right-sided heart failure or constrictive pericarditis, ascites may be present.

Auscultation of the abdomen may disclose arterial bruits. These usually arise in the aorta but are occasionally the result of a renal artery stenosis, in which case they are heard on the appropriate side of the midline.

Oedema

Cardiac oedema moves by gravity to the most dependent parts. In ambulant patients it is therefore most severe in the ankles and may get worse as the day progresses. When patients are lying in bed, the oedema will be present in the sacral area or the backs of the thighs. When it is gross, it may involve the genitalia. Look for it in these sites and confirm its presence by 'pitting'.

Legs

Examine the legs not only for oedema but also for evidence of peripheral arterial disease and varicose veins. If you suspect Marfan's syndrome look for unstable or dislocated patellae and a long patellar tendon. There may also be pes cavus. Luetic aortic valve disease may be accompanied by neurosyphilis and the tendon reflexes at the ankle may be abnormal.

Urine

Always examine the urine for the presence of protein or sugar and look at the centrifuged deposit under the microscope for red cells, white cells and casts.

THE THORACIC CAGE

Inspection

Before you reach for your stethoscope, inspect the thoracic cage. Note sternal deformities such as:

● protrusion ('pigeon breast')

● depression ('funnel chest')

Pigeon breast in children is sometimes associated with congenital heart disease when there has been a large left to right shunt. Severe sternal depression produces physical signs (cardiac displacement, murmurs) that may falsely suggest heart disease.

Inspect the thoracic spine. Severe scoliosis may displace the heart and give a misleading impression of its size. A thoracic spine that is unduly straight, may also cause a misleading appearance of the cardiac silhouette on the chest X-ray.

Some thoracic skeletal abnormalities are associated with mild mitral incompetence. Ankylosing spondylitis is sometimes associated with aortic incompetence.

Palpation

Look carefully for any pulsations and palpate them.

The apex beat

Try to identify the apex beat by inspection or palpation and relate its position to the intercostal spaces and midclavicular line. If it is greatly displaced, refer it to the anterior or mid-axillary lines. Identify the apex beat with the patient either lying flat or propped up a little, but tilted neither to one side nor to the other.

With atrial hypertrophy or obstructive cardiomyopathy, the apical impulse may feel bifid and this abnormality is best felt with the patient lying towards the left side.

An obvious 'tapping' single beat is often felt in mitral stenosis and is a 'palpable' first heart sound.

Ventricular heaves

Examine for the characteristic sustained heave of ventricular hypertrophy.

The heave of left ventricular hypertrophy can be felt by the hand placed flat and firmly over the apex beat as a movement of the ribs and other structures of the chest wall downward and outward to the left. When the left ventricular hypertrophy is severe, there may also be systolic retraction in the intercostal spaces nearer the left sternal border.

The heave of right ventricular hypertrophy is felt by the hand laid flat along the left sternal edge. You can see and feel your hand being lifted by the sternum and left sternocostal joints with each systole. The impulse is directed forward and slightly upward.

Coarctation of the aorta

If you suspect coarctation of the aorta, examine for the tortuous and dilated arteries that carry the collateral blood flow in the dorsal intercostal spaces and subscapular regions. They are best looked for by having the patient strip to the waist, bend over the back of a chair and hold the front of the seat with his hands. If the lighting is arranged so that it falls tangentially between the scapulae, the tortuous arteries are seen pulsating in the light and shade.

Auscultation

Auscultate the lung bases during deep respiration to detect the post-tussive, fine crepitations that may indicate pulmonary oedema. Remember, however, that a chest X-ray may show pulmonary congestion when no crepitations can be heard.

Percussion

In congestive cardiac failure percussion of the lung bases may give evidence of pleural effusions.

Percussion of the heart is of little or no value.

THE ARTERIAL PULSE

Each of eight accessible arteries has its own particular usefulness in the assessment of heart and peripheral vascular disease. Examine carefully:

- the temporal
- the carotid
- the brachial
- the radial
- the femoral
- the popliteal
- the posterior tibial
- the dorsalis pedis pulses

The temporal artery

The temporal artery may be tender or obliterated in temporal arteritis.

The carotid artery

This gives the best indication of arterial wave form. In elderly women the right common carotid artery is sometimes kinked and it is important not to confuse this with an aneurysm.

Coarctation of the aorta causes a slow swelling pulsation of the carotid arteries visible above the clavicles and of the aortic arch visible in the suprasternal notch.

Corrigan's sign is a striking, jerky, visible pulsation of the carotid artery associated with severe aortic incompetence.

The carotid pulses are absent in the arteritis known as Takayasu's disease.

One or other carotid artery may be less easily palpable and may be the site of a bruit in peripheral arterial disease or dissecting aneurysm of the aorta.

The brachial artery

This is auscultated during sphygmomanometry. If it is arteriosclerotic, it may be seen as obviously kinked and contracting with each pulse ('locomotor brachialis').

The radial artery

This is the most convenient to palpate for most purposes because it is always accessible with a patient fully clothed.

The pulses in the legs

These are absent or reduced with obliterative arterial disease and in coarctation of the aorta, which causes a delay in the femoral pulse when it is compared with the brachial. If the coarctation is severe, the femoral pulses may be absent.

During the dissection of an aortic aneurysm, one or more of any of these pulses may disappear either temporarily or permanently.

Examination of the pulse

Palpate the radial (and sometimes the carotid) artery for four aspects of the arterial pulse:

- the rate
- the rhythm
- the pulse pressure
- the shape of the pulse wave

The traditional examination for the 'state of the arterial wall' is a ritual that yields no valuable information. Palpate the pulses on both sides.

Rate

Time the pulse rate with a watch, preferably over 1 minute and certainly over not less than a quarter-minute. If the heart rate is fast or irregular, auscultate the heart sounds to determine the rate of cardiac contraction.

Tachycardia is normal in infants and children and at any age during and after exercise. It is also associated with excitement or anxiety, fever, thyrotoxicosis and other hyperkinetic circulatory states such as occur with severe anaemia, circulatory shock, severe hypoxia and hypercapnia, and large arteriovenous shunts. It may also be caused by a dysrhythmia.

Bradycardia sometimes occurs after acute myocardial infarction and also occasionally accompanies viral illnesses or raised intracranial pressure. Complete heart block or high grade AV block also cause bradycardia.

Rhythm

Sinus arrhythmia

When a patient breathes slowly and deeply, sinus arrhythmia is usually noticeable, the pulse rate speeding towards the end of inspiration and slowing during early expiration. It is found commonly in children and occasionally in the elderly at normal respiratory rates.

Irregular pulse

If the pulse is irregular and the patient does not seem to have sinus arrhythmia, ask yourself whether the pulse is basically regular with occasional or repetitive irregularities, or totally irregular without any pattern at all. The commonest cause of an occasionally irregular pulse is ectopic beats (extrasystoles, premature contractions).

The commonest cause of a totally irregular pulse is atrial fibrillation, although very frequent ectopic beats may give the impression of total irregularity. If the pulse is totally irregular and also fast, the pulse rate at the wrist may be less than the ventricular rate estimated by cardiac auscultation. The difference is called a 'pulse deficit'. The ventricular rate is, of course, the important one.

Pulsus bigeminus

When the beats are 'coupled' (pulsus bigeminus), the cause is almost always an ectopic beat following each normal beat. This is sometimes associated with digitalis overdosage.

Pulse pressure

A rough estimate of the pulse pressure can be made by palpation of an artery. This has been traditionally referred to as the pulse 'volume', because there is an indirect relationship between the pulse pressure and the left ventricular stroke volume that initiates the pulse. The term 'volume', as in 'a low volume pulse', should probably not now be used when the pulse pressure can be accurately measured by sphygmomanometry.

Increased pulse pressure

The pulse pressure is raised ('bounding') in hyperkinetic circulatory states (e.g. fever, pregnancy, emotion, exercise). It is also increased in aortic incompetence, large central left-to-right shunts and peripheral vasodilatation.

Decreased pulse pressure

The pulse pressure is low (pulsus parvus) in heart failure or obstruction to left ventricular outflow (e.g. aortic stenosis). The peripheral pulse may be impalpable in shock or hypothermia. During acute

attacks of asthma and sometimes when ventricular filling is restricted by a pericardial effusion or constrictive pericarditis, the pulse pressure is noticeably less during deep inspiration (pulsus paradoxus).

Pulsus alternans

A regular rhythm with a regular alternation of pulse pressures (pulsus alternans) may be present in left ventricular failure. This may be detected when taking the blood pressure. As the pressure in the cuff falls, the Korotkoff sounds are noted suddenly to double in rate.

Shape of the arterial wave form

You should assess the shape of the arterial wave form (pressure pulse) by palpation of the carotid artery because it is the accessible pulse nearest to the aortic root. The further from the aortic root the pulse is felt, the more it is distorted. Feel for the carotid artery just medial to the upper medial edge of the sternomastoid muscle in the neck. Remember that carotid palpation is almost always uncomfortable for the patient; also, that stimulation of the carotid sinus by palpation can cause syncope. Never palpate both carotid arteries simultaneously.

Assess the speed of both the rise and the fall of the pressure pulse and any obvious notches in the wave form.

Anacrotic pulse

A slow rising pulse with a delayed peak (plateau or anacrotic pulse) is associated with aortic valve stenosis; in severe stenosis the pulse pressure is low as well (pulsus parvus et tardus).

Water-hammer pulse

An abnormally rapid upstroke ('water-hammer') and an abnormally rapid downstroke ('collapsing') of the wave form is associated with aortic valve incompetence or peripheral vasodilatation.

Corrigan's pulse of severe aortic incompetence (both water-hammer and collapsing) is exaggerated if the pulse pressure is increased further by gravity. Lift the patient's whole arm above his head with the first three fingers of your hand lying flat across the palmar aspect of his forearm just above the wrist. The abrupt flicking sensation of the pulse is greatly exaggerated by this manoeuvre.

A fasting rising and fast falling pulse without a high

pulse pressure gives the pulse wave a jerky quality, as in severe mitral incompetence or obstructive cardiomyopathy. A high pulse pressure by itself can cause a sensation of a collapsing pulse, as, for example, in complete heart block when a large stroke volume is caused by the long ventricular diastole.

Pulsus bisferiens

A double impulse (pulsus bisferiens) or the presence of several palpable notches on the carotid pressure pulse ('carotid shudder') is associated either with combined aortic stenosis and incompetence or, occasionally, with obstructive cardiomyopathy.

VENOUS AND HEPATIC PULSATION

The jugular venous pulse

The jugular venous pulse can provide valuable information, but many people find the pulsations difficult to interpret. They are seen to the best advantage if the patient sits propped up comfortably at an angle of about 30° to the horizontal, with the head resting so that the neck muscles are relaxed. Ignore the external jugular vein. Look instead for the pulsations of the internal jugular veins, which lie deep to the sternomastoid muscle. Adjust the position of the head so that skin wrinkles are smoothed out. Arrange the lighting so that it falls tangentially on the lower part of the sternomastoid and the nearby skin and soft tissues. Look at the shadows cast in that area to spot the slowly swelling and subsiding outward pulsations of the internal jugular vein.

When you have identified these pulsations, decide how far up the neck they reach. Measure the distance between their highest point and the manubriosternal joint ('sternal angle', 'angle of Louis') in centimetres. If you cannot see the pulsation, lower the patient little by little until you do. If the pulsations reach the angle of the jaw, sit the patient upright and measure again. If the pulsations still reach the angle of the jaw when the patient is sitting upright, you cannot make an accurate clinical estimate of the height of the pulsations.

The distance between the highest point of internal jugular venous pulsation and the manubriosternal joint is the jugular venous pressure measured in

centimetres of blood. A distance greater than about 3 cm is abnormal.

Wave form

Look again at the pulsations of the internal jugular vein for the wave form of the venous pulse. The normal venous pulse has two main waves, an *a* (atrial) wave and a *v* (ventricular) wave. With atrial fibrillation there is no atrial contraction so there is no *a* wave.

Giant *a* waves may be present in tricuspid or pulmonary stenosis or in severe pulmonary arterial hypertension. Occasional giant *a* waves ('cannon waves') occur when the right atrium contracts against an intermittently closed tricuspid valve as happens in some dysrhythmias – for example, in complete heart block.

Sometimes there is a wide, slowly swelling, venous pulse wave that is single. This is the characteristic physical sign of tricuspid incompetence usually associated with right ventricular dilatation and right heart failure. If you press on the abdomen and raise the intra-abdominal pressure, the reflux of blood into the inferior vena cava is impeded and reflux into the superior vena cava and the internal jugular vein is increased. This hepatojugular reflux raises the venous pressure in the neck and may help to identify the venous pulse.

Hepatic pulsation

Moderate to severe tricuspid incompetence causes reflux down the inferior vena cava with every ventricular systole so that the liver, which acts as an extension of the right atrium, is often enlarged and pulsating. This hepatic pulsation is often palpable. It is intrinsic pulsation, so the movements are felt at right angles to each other. Feel for the anterior movement by palpating the enlarged liver with your hand laid across the right hypochondrium.

To feel the sideways pulsation, clench your fist so that the proximal metacarpophalangeal joints are flexed at right angles and your four fingers are held together. Place the first phalanges of your fingers so that they fit snugly into the patient's right lower intercostal spaces about the mid-axillary line over the enlarged liver. Keep your wrist and hand steady and vary the pressure applied to the patient's intercostal spaces. At a critical pressure you will feel and see pulsations superimposed on the movements of respiration. Pulsations are systolic and coincide with the jugular venous pulsations of tricuspid incompetence.

AUSCULTATION OF THE HEART

The stethoscope

Competent cardiac auscultation needs a long period of ear training and an efficient stethoscope with both bell and diaphragm chest pieces.

The diaphragm transmits high pitched sounds more efficiently than the bell. The bell transmits low pitched sounds more efficiently than the diaphragm. Not all stethoscopes have efficient bells, so make sure that yours has. Also make sure that it has suitable tubing with a lumen of about 3 mm (one eighth of an inch), that the tubes are no longer than about 25 cm (10 inches) and that the ear pieces fit your ears to exclude extraneous sound. If you cannot hear as well as your peers with your stethoscope, try another one and if that is no better consult a trained instructor. Each must find by trial and error the stethoscope that suits him or her best.

The approach to auscultation

Cardiac sounds are difficult to hear, not only because they are often very soft, but also because their frequencies lie very close to the limits of human hearing. When auscultating you must concentrate as hard as you can. Listen deliberately and systematically for what you expect to hear and also to detect the absence of anything that you would normally expect to hear.

Cardiovascular sounds are vibrations caused by a turbulent blood flow or by sudden changes in the velocity of blood flow within the heart and great vessels.

The opening and closing of valves produces sudden changes of velocity and momentary turbulence that cause short sounds, such as heart sounds. More prolonged turbulence – for example, that arising from blood flow across valves or through holes – produces longer sounds called 'murmurs' or 'bruits'. These cardiac sounds have three properties and you should always listen for each

- length
  This is related to the length of the systole or diastole in which it occurs.
- pitch (high or low)
  This is related to the frequency of the vibration; high pitch or high frequency like the sound made by a violin; low pitch or low frequency like the sound made by a double bass.

- timbre
  This is associated with the harmonic content of the sound; e.g. the difference in quality between a note of the same pitch played by an oboe and a violin.

Areas of auscultation

The turbulence that creates heart sounds and murmurs is carried downstream from the site that produces the turbulence. This explains the 'areas of auscultation' of the four heart valves (LD-91–94).

Heart sounds

The normal heart sounds are heard all over the precordium. The first heart sound is usually loudest at the apex and the second heart sound loudest at the base.

The first heart sound can sometimes be heard as a split sound, the result of asynchronous closure of the mitral and tricuspid valves. The second heart sound is normally split because of the sudden closure of first the aortic and then the pulmonary valve. Auscultation at the pulmonary area during slow continued respiration will allow you to appreciate that the second heart sound is normally only single during the phase of full expiration. During the inspiratory phase the increased volume of blood entering the right ventricle delays the closure of the pulmonary valve and postpones the pulmonary component of the second heart sound. During expiration the splitting narrows again.

This normal movement of the splitting of the second heart sound is best heard in young people in the erect position. Try to 'tune in' to this splitting every time you start to auscultate.

In children and younger adults, the physiological third heart sound is heard in early diastole at the apex and gives a triple rhythm to the cardiac cadence. It is short, low-pitched and muffled. A similar sound is sometimes heard in presystole before the first heart sound. This is the atrial sound (fourth heart sound) and is abnormal, usually the result of atrial hypertrophy. When a triple rhythm is present and the heart rate is fast, the cadence is referred to as a 'gallop' rhythm.

How to auscultate

You cannot listen critically to more than one thing at a time. Concentrate on listening separately for high pitched and low pitched sounds. Do not attempt to assess the cadence of heart sounds while you are listening for murmurs.

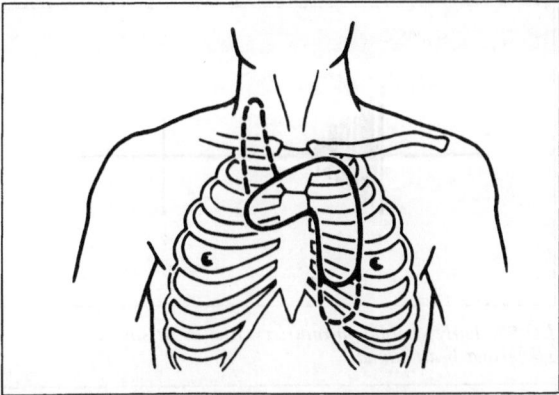

LD-91. *Aortic area auscultation (the area indicated by the dashed line shows the direction of radiation)*

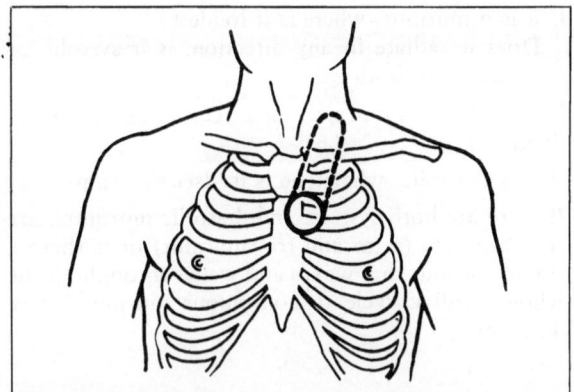

LD-92. *Pulmonary area of auscultation (the area indicated by the dashed line shows the direction of radiation)*

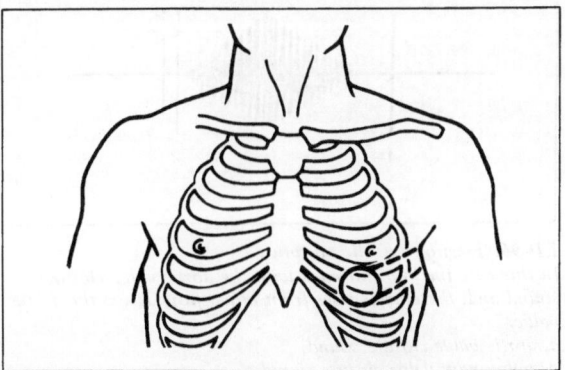

LD-93. *Mitral area of auscultation (the area indicated by the dashed line shows the direction of radiation)*

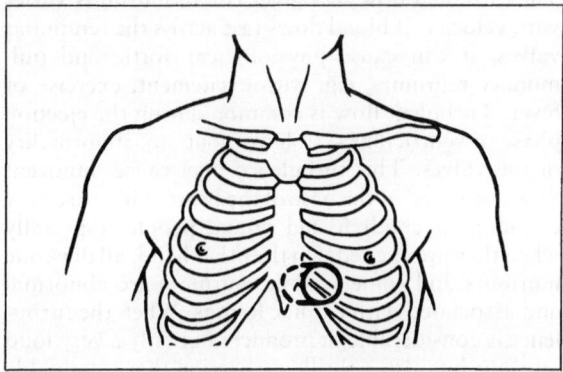

LD-94. *Tricuspid area of auscultation (the area indicated by the dashed line shows the direction of radiation)*

You should concentrate so hard that when you are 'tuned in' for low pitched sounds you will not be able to hear high pitched sounds unless they are very loud. There are many easily heard murmurs whose frequency is well above the threshold of human hearing. These may be comparatively loud and they tend to 'capture the ear'. You must try to ignore them and concentrate intently on other parts of the cardiac cycle for the soft sounds that are difficult to hear. Identify the constituent sounds of the cardiac cycle in a sequential manner and then assemble the various components of the pattern into a whole.

Start with the diaphragm of the chest piece at the pulmonary area and listen for the splitting of the high pitched second sound until you can hear it: you will then be able easily to identify the lower pitched first heart sound. Allow the basic cadence of the sound to become imprinted on your mind and then move the stethoscope centimetre by centimetre to other areas of the precordium. At each site you must listen with the diaphragm for high pitched sounds and with the bell

for low pitched sounds. You should have a rest between each spell of concentrated listening.

After each spell of concentrated listening you should put to yourself the questions in the following catechism.

Do I hear the first heart sound?
   If so, is it loud or soft or is it varying in loudness; is it single or is it split?

Do I hear the second heart sound?
   If so, is it loud or soft, split or unsplit and does the splitting 'move' normally during respiration?

Do I hear any other heart sound?
   If so, is it a third heart sound in early diastole or a fourth heart sound in presystole (an atrial sound)?

Do I hear any other short sound that is not one of these heart sounds, e.g. a clicking sound?
   If so, is it systolic or diastolic, and at what point in systole or diastole is it heard?

Is there any other sound?
   If so, is it a murmur or pericardial friction?

If it is a murmur, where is it loudest?

    Does it radiate in any direction; is it systolic or diastolic, or both?

If it is systolic, is it of ejection or regurgitant type? (see diagram)

If it is diastolic, what type is it? (see diagram)

If there are both systolic and diastolic murmurs, are they separate (a 'to and fro' murmur) or is there a single murmur that waxes and wanes throughout the whole cardiac cycle (a continuous murmur)? (see diagram)

Murmurs

The turbulent flow that gives rise to murmurs varies with velocity. If blood flows fast across the semilunar valves, it can cause physiological aortic and pulmonary murmurs, e.g. with excitement, exercise or fever. Turbulent flow is common during the ejection phase of ventricular systole without any abnormality of the valves. This turbulence may cause 'innocent flow murmurs' at the base of the heart. These are very common in children and young people, especially when they are excited. On the other hand, all diastolic murmurs and some systolic murmurs are abnormal and associated with cardiac lesions. When the turbulence is considerable, it produces not only a very loud murmur but also a thrill, a vibration that is palpable on the surface.

Systolic murmurs

Systolic murmurs are associated with blood flow during ventricular systole, either forwards during ejection through a semilunar valve, or backwards through an incompetent atrioventricular valve. Another kind of ejection systolic murmur is the result of high velocity blood flow through a septal defect from a high pressure left heart chamber into a low pressure right heart chamber, e.g. through a ventricular septal defect.

    There are four types of systolic murmur classified according to their time during systole (LD-95–98).

Early systolic murmurs

These usually sound like a rather rough, indistinct first heart sound and have no pathological significance (LD-95).

Ejection murmurs

These are caused by the ejection of blood with increased velocity across normal aortic or pulmonary

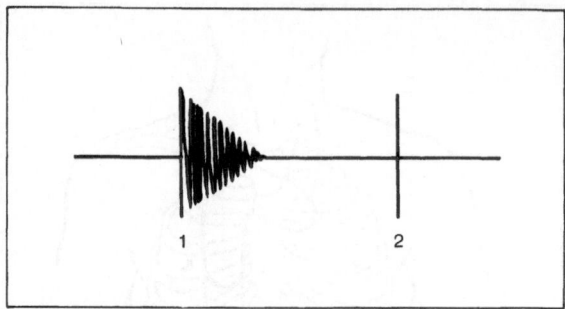

LD-95. *Early systolic murmur:* 1 = *first heart sound;* 2 = *second heart sound*

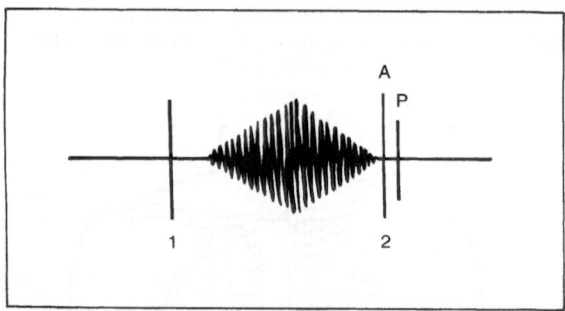

LD-96. *Ejection systolic murmur.*
In this case the murmur ends with the aortic valve closure sound and, therefore, arises from blood flow across the aortic valve.
a, aortic valve closure sound;
p, pulmonary valve closure sound

valves or by the ejection of blood with normal velocity across abnormal aortic or pulmonary valves.

    They have a characteristic appearance when recorded on a phonocardiogram, being diamond shaped with the apex of the diamond corresponding to the point of maximum velocity of ejection across the valve (LD-96). The murmur is short and brusque, with a rapid crescendo and diminuendo. A clear gap may be heard between the first heart sound and the onset of the murmur. The relationship of the end of the murmur to the aortic and pulmonary valve closure sounds depends upon which valve gives rise to the turbulence: when it arises at the aortic valve, the murmur ends with the aortic closure sound and the pulmonary closure sound may still be heard, but if it arises at the pulmonary valve, the murmur ends with the pulmonary closure sound and the aortic component, which comes earlier, may be hidden in the murmur.

    Ejection systolic murmurs are often loudest at the aortic or pulmonary area and may radiate to the carotid area of the neck.

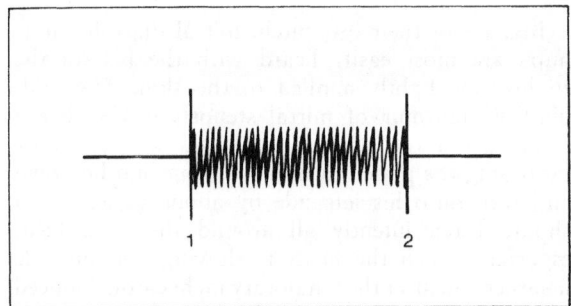

LD-97. *Pansystolic murmur*

Regurgitant murmurs

The regurgitant flow from ventricle to atrium in mitral or tricuspid incompetence gives rise to fairly uniform turbulence throughout the whole of systole. LD-117 shows the relationship between the pressure gradient responsible for the turbulent flow and the shape of the murmur.

On auscultation, the murmur sounds as if it occupies the whole of systole (pansystolic) from the first heart sound to the second heart sound, which it may even obliterate. When pansystolic murmurs are soft, they may sound 'blowing', but when loud, the timbre can resemble an ejection systolic murmur; sometimes they sound musical (LD-97).

The pansystolic murmur of mitral incompetence is best heard at the apex and may radiate out to the left axilla. The pansystolic murmur of tricuspid incompetence is loudest internal to the apex at the lower left sternal edge, may radiate to the midsternal area and may increase with inspiration.

Late systolic murmurs

Phonocardiograms of late systolic murmurs show that they start about the middle of systole and continue up to the second sound. Sometimes they are immediately preceded by one or more sharp high-pitched midsystolic clicks; sometimes the click is audible (LD-98). Occasionally the click is the domi-

nant auscultatory feature and the murmur is very soft. These murmurs are frequently misdiagnosed as early diastolic murmurs, the click being mistaken for the second heart sound. They are most commonly associated with mitral incompetence caused by a prolapsing valve cusp or with papillary muscle dysfunction.

Diastolic murmurs

The three types of diastolic murmur (LD-99–101) are named according to the point in diastole at which each starts.

Diastolic murmurs are always abnormal and are therefore very important. The two common diastolic murmurs are associated with aortic incompetence and mitral stenosis. Although they may be difficult to hear, with practice they should not be difficult to distinguish, because apart from the fact that they both occur in diastole, they have no other features in common. They are different in timing, site, pitch and timbre. They are made easier to hear by different manoeuvres, with the patient in different positions and by using different chest pieces of the stethoscope.

Early diastolic murmurs

The turbulence responsible for early diastolic murmurs is associated with regurgitation of blood backwards into the ventricle across an incompetent semilunar valve, usually the aortic valve.

The murmur immediately follows the second heart sound (LD-99). It is relatively high-pitched and often resembles a breath sound in pitch and timbre. Early diastolic murmurs can therefore best be heard when the patient has emptied his lungs and stopped breathing. Occasionally the timbre is rougher or even musical. The murmur is a diminuendo one, related to the pressure gradient responsible for the turbulent flow. It may be loud or soft, long or short.

You should listen for an early diastolic murmur with the diaphragm of the stethoscope firmly applied at the aortic area or down the left sternal border.

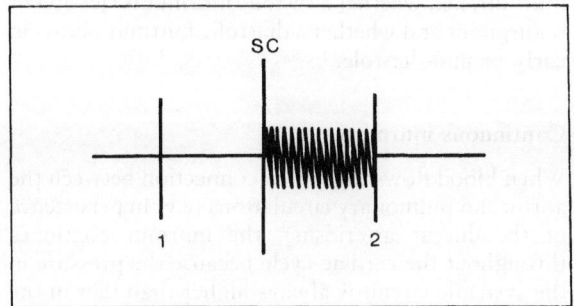

LD-98. *Midsystolic click (SC) and late systolic murmur*

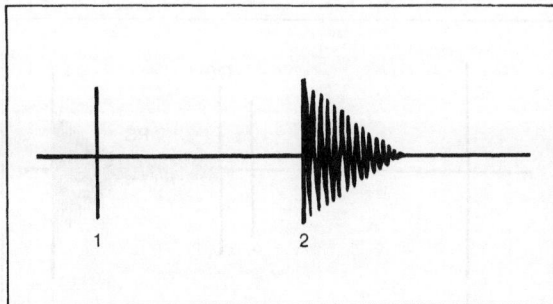

LD-99. *Early diastolic murmur*

Make the patient lean forward, tell him to take a deep breath in, blow it right out and stop breathing. You should then listen intently to early diastole, as these murmurs are often hard to hear.

Mid-diastolic murmurs

These murmurs start well after the second heart sounds, and on auscultation the silent gap is so obvious that the murmur seems to start in mid-diastole (LD-100).

Mid-diastolic murmurs are caused by the turbulent flow of blood through a narrowed atrioventricular valve. The relationship between the shape and duration of the murmur of mitral stenosis and the pressure gradient between the left atrium and the left ventricle is shown in LD-118.

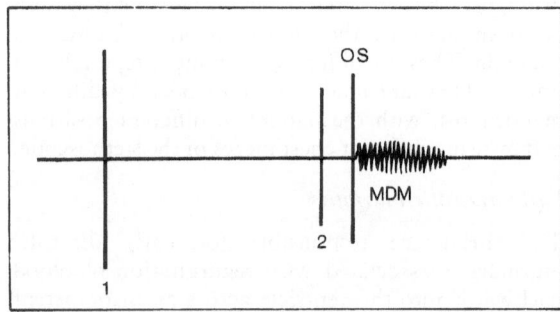

LD-100 *Mid-diastolic murmur (MDM): OS = opening snap of the mitral valve*

Mid-diastolic murmurs have a very low pitched and rumbling quality that is difficult for beginners to hear because they are unused to such low pitched sounds. The pitch resembles that of the faint rumble of distant thunder or the sound of double basses playing pianissimo. When mid-diastolic rumbling murmurs are short, they may be confused with third heart sounds as they have much the same pitch. When they are long, and there is sinus rhythm, they end in presystolic accentuation (a presystolic murmur) (LD-101).

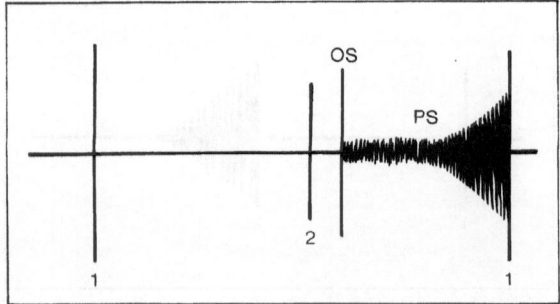

LD-101. *Mid-diastolic murmur with presystolic accentuation (PS)*

Because of their low pitch, mitral diastolic murmurs are most easily heard with the bell of the stethoscope lightly applied to the skin. The mid-diastolic murmur of mitral stenosis is best heard round about the apex. You should seek for it by exercising the patient a little, making him lie down and turn onto his left side by about 30–45°. You should listen intently all around the apex beat, especially when the heart is slowing and diastole lengthening, after the temporary tachycardia induced by the exercise.

Presystolic murmurs

In sinus rhythm, the turbulent flow across a narrowed atrioventricular valve is increased when the atrium contracts. This increased turbulence is responsible for the presystolic accentuation of the diastolic murmur heard in mitral or tricuspid stenosis (LD-101).

Timing murmurs

When you have identified a murmur as either systolic or diastolic, you have already taken a large step towards the diagnosis. Although the trained auscultator can tell one from the other at once, the student has greater difficulty and must make use of whatever help he can in timing.

Some students find it helpful to palpate the carotid pulse, for its upstroke coincides more or less with the first heart sound. Also, if the chest piece of the stethoscope lifts when it is applied to the apex, it will do so during systole. The two heart sounds, however, are the best guide to systole and diastole and whenever you have lost the timing, you should return to the pulmonary area, or wherever the two heart sounds are clearest, and then, having identified the second sound, 'inch' towards the site where the murmur is loudest: a murmur coming before the second sound being systolic and one coming after it diastolic.

The next decision to make is the type of the murmur, i.e., whether a systolic murmur is ejection or regurgitant and whether a diastolic murmur occurs in early or mid-diastole.

Continuous murmurs

When blood flows through a connection between the aortic and pulmonary circulations (e.g. in persistence of the ductus arteriosus), the murmur continues throughout the cardiac cycle because the pressure in the systemic circuit is always higher than that in the pulmonary circuit. Arteriovenous shunts at any site also produce this type of murmur (LD-102).

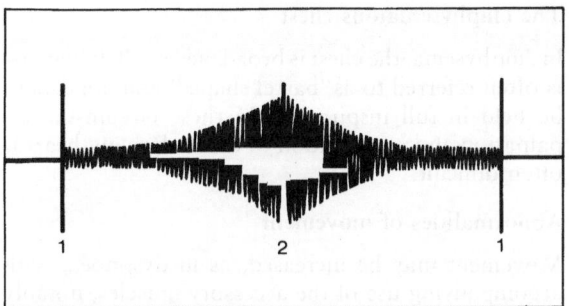

LD-102. *Continuous murmur*

'To and fro' murmurs

When an ejection systolic murmur is followed by an early diastolic murmur, as in combined aortic stenosis and incompetence, the murmurs are sometimes described as 'to and fro' murmurs (LD-103). They should not be confused with continuous murmurs.

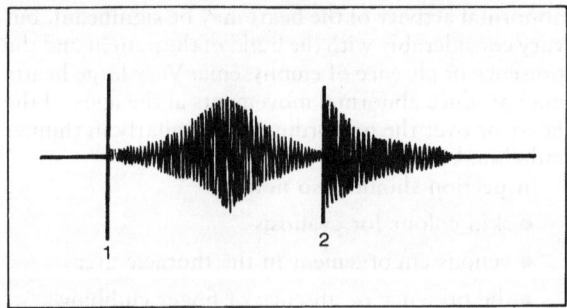

LD-103. *'To and fro' murmur*

Loudness of murmurs

The loudness of cardiac murmurs may be graded on a scale 1–4 or on a scale 1–6. The simple four-grade scale corresponds roughly to the degrees 'mild', 'moderate', 'considerable' and 'gross'.

Pericardial friction

The fibrinous exudate of pericarditis causes friction sounds as the heart contracts and relaxes. These sounds may be heard in systole or diastole or both, but are unlikely to be confused with murmurs because their timbre is usually quite different. Like pleural rubs, they are often crunching or scratchy sounds, and have been likened to footsteps in the snow.

THE BLOOD PRESSURE

Measure the blood pressure by sphygmomanometry (aneroid manometers are more convenient for domi-

ciliary practice but tend to go wrong more easily). Make sure that the cuff is wide enough and long enough to fit snugly around the arm and put it on carefully so that when the pressure is raised the pad does not 'herniate' from below the cuff. A fat arm needs a large cuff. If the rubber bladder will not encircle the arm, centre it over the artery. A child's arm needs a special narrow cuff. Fallacious blood pressures can be recorded if these points are not remembered.

The blood pressure is usually recorded with the patient either sitting or lying on a couch. The cuff should be level with the heart but the level of the manometer is of no consequence. The arm should be supported.

There may be a difference of a 5–10 mmHg between the blood pressure in the arms of normal people.

Technique

Having arranged the cuff satisfactorily, identify the position of the brachial artery by palpation and place the chest piece of the stethoscope over it. Inflate the cuff until either the mercury column rises to the top of the manometer or the radial pulse disappears. Lower the pressure in the cuff by releasing the valve gently and allowing the mercury column to fall slowly while you auscultate. The pressure at which the Korotkoff sounds are first heard as soft muffled thuds is taken as the systolic blood pressure. As the mercury column falls, the sounds become louder and tapping in character, then suddenly become muffled again. This point of change is called 'Phase 4' and is usually taken as the diastolic blood pressure.

As the pressure in the cuff continues to fall, the sounds eventually disappear (Phase 5); occasionally Phase 5 is zero pressure. Sometimes there is little difference between them.

Record the systolic blood pressure and also the pressure at Phase 4 and Phase 5.

Count the pulse rate at the time you take the blood pressure and record that as well because tachycardia may give a misleadingly high blood pressure. Sometimes the sounds disappear some mmHg below the systolic pressure only to reappear again above the diastolic pressure. This is called the 'auscultatory gap'. To avoid mistakes, the pressure cuff must therefore be fully inflated at the start.

On standing, the systolic blood pressure usually rises and certainly should not fall more than a few mmHg. If postural hypotension is suspected, for example, in elderly patients or patients having treatment for arterial hypertension, the blood pressure should be measured immediately after the patient has stood up. A fall of 20 mmHg or more is significant. In patients who are receiving adrenergic neuron-blocking drugs for the treatment of hypertension, postural hypotension is often markedly accentuated by very mild exercise.

THE RESPIRATORY SYSTEM

Examination of the chest in a patient with suspected heart disease is necessary because:

- it helps to exclude coexisting respiratory disease that may either complicate or even be the cause of the heart disease
- it differentiates respiratory from cardiac disorders
- it assists in the assessment of heart disease

The examination should be carried out in the standard manner and include:

- inspection
- palpation
- percussion
- auscultation

The details of these techniques can be ascertained elsewhere, but the following comments emphasize aspects of the examination that may have a bearing on heart disease.

Inspection

With the thorax fully exposed and the patient sitting at an angle of about 45°, look for:

- asymmetry of structure
- the emphysematous chest
- abnormalities of movement

Asymmetry of structure

Deformities of the thoracic cage may alter the position of the heart and great arteries within the mediastinum and if severe may affect its function.

Relatively minor deformities such as depressed sternum, pigeon breast, anteroposterior flattening and thoracic scoliosis may cause abnormal cardiac signs and appearances. Major deformities such as severe kyposcoliosis may eventually lead to heart failure.

Precordial bulging, usually affecting the left anterior chest more than the right, indicates that the heart has been enlarged since early childhood and suggests a probable congenital cause.

The emphysematous chest

In emphysema, the chest is broadened in all diameters, is often referred to as 'barrel shaped' and appears to be held in full inspiration. In these circumstances, palpation and auscultation of the underlying heart is often difficult.

Abnormalities of movement

Movement may be increased, as in dyspnoea, with accompanying use of the accessory muscles, notably the sternomastoid muscles, or diminished, as in the large, barrel-shaped chest of emphysema. Asymmetry of movement occurs in lobar pneumonia, pneumothorax, pulmonary collapse and pleural effusion. A pleural effusion, often unilateral, is not uncommon in cardiac failure.

The range of respiratory movement at nipple level should be measured with a tape measure.

Movements of the chest wall due to normal or abnormal activity of the heart may be significant, but vary considerably with the build of the patient and the presence or absence of emphysema. Very large hearts may produce abnormal movements at the apex of the heart or over the precordium, particularly in thinner individuals.

Inspection should also note:

- skin colour for cyanosis
- venous engorgement in the thoracic area
- the presence or absence of finger clubbing

Palpation

Palpation is used particularly for testing vocal fremitus, but is also valuable in determining the position of the trachea and apex beat. The trachea may be displaced by mediastinal movement. Causes include:

- pulmonary collapse
- pleural effusion
- pneumothorax

These may in turn affect the position of the cardiac apex and give a false impression of heart size. This apart, the hand is used to detect abnormal cardiac movement and thrills at the apex or over the precordium.

Very coarse rhonchi can often be felt and subcutaneous emphysema (as in some cases of pneumothorax or oesophageal rupture) can be recognized by a crackling sensation beneath the fingers. Areas of local tenderness over ribs, costochondral junctions or intercostal spaces may account for puzzling cases of chest pain.

Percussion

Percussion, although of little use in cardiology, is valuable in the diagnosis of respiratory disease. The combination of vocal fremitus, percussion and auscultation, for example, helps to differentiate pleural effusion, pulmonary collapse and pneumothorax from pulmonary congestion.

Auscultation

Auscultation will help to confirm the presence or absence of effusion, collapse, consolidation or pneumothorax by careful evaluation of the duration, intensity and tonal quality of the breath sounds. The presence or absence of adventitial sounds (rhonchi or crepitations), their pitch (low or high) and their quality (coarse, medium or fine) may help further with the diagnosis.

Rhonchi are almost exclusively the result of respiratory disease and are produced by reduction of air flow through narrowed bronchial tubes.

Fine crepitations can be associated with either cardiac or respiratory disease. Coarse crepitations are only found in respiratory disease.

Adventitial sounds in the upper lobes are rarely a sign of heart disease.

Crepitations due to cardiac failure

These may be fine or medium and are heard bilaterally in the mid and lower zones. They may be absent in the earliest stages of acute left ventricular failure.

Friction rubs

Auscultation may distinguish between pleural and pericardial friction.

Pleural friction is clearly associated with respiratory movements. It is heard over areas of the chest outwith the precordium and disappears when the breath is held.

Pericardial friction is best heard with the patient sitting up, leaning forward and in full expiration. It occurs in time with the heart beat and continues when the breath is held, although its intensity may vary with respiration.

A clicking pneumothorax is caused by air in the mediastinum. It is a crunching sound heard over the central chest area, occasionally without a stethoscope, and can cause confusion by being in time with heart beats. Subcutaneous emphysema may coexist.

Investigations

Further methods of examining the respiratory system include:

- radiology
- pulmonary function tests
- scanning procedures
- bronchoscopy
- sputum examination

Radiology

Normally this consists of a postero-anterior X-ray of the chest held in full inspiration at 2 metres. Lateral or oblique X-rays are also useful in some cases.

Other radiological techniques include fluoroscopy, by which cardiac and diaphragmatic movements can be detected, and tomography in which a series of X-rays, focussed at varying depths, may help with more accurate location of pulmonary shadows.

Principal features of the chest X-ray are:

- the cardiac shadow
- the rib cage and diaphragm
  In emphysema the ribs are horizontal and the diaphragm flattened.
- the lung fields
  These may show changes related to the degree of air filling or collapse, the pulmonary circulation and alterations in the pleura or pleural spaces, including the presence of fluid or air.

Other important radiological findings in cardiac disease are:

- hilar congestion in left ventricular failure
- fine linear streaks due to interstitial oedema at the costophrenic angles in longer-standing pulmonary oedema (Kerley's B lines)
- larger linear streaks due to past lung collapse or pulmonary infarction
- pleural effusion in cardiac failure
- evidence of pulmonary disease that might lead to cor pulmonale
- diminished or absent peripheral vascular shadows give the main pulmonary arteries a cut-off or pruned appearance in pulmonary hypertension

Pulmonary function tests

At a simple clinical level, the test most frequently used

is the assessment of expiratory flow and vital capacity using an instrument known as the vitalograph. This measures the forced expiratory volume in 1 second (FEV_1) and forced vital capacity (FVC). From these, it is possible to derive information identifying obstructive and restrictive forms of ventilation. More elaborate tests of gaseous exchange are available in specialized units to study possible diffusion defects.

Sputum examination

It is essential to collect and examine sputum in all cases of respiratory disease. The quantity, colour, appearance and viscosity are of importance, as is the presence of blood or pus. Samples can be sent for the identification of infecting organisms and their sensitivity to antibiotics. They can also be examined for neoplastic cells.

Lung scanning

Albumin labelled with technetium is used to examine the distribution of blood flow in the lungs, although the discriminatory value of the test is limited.

Bronchoscopy

Bronchoscopy is a valuable diagnostic technique in skilled hands and has been improved by the development of fibre optics. In addition to the more accurate location and identification of causes of bronchial obstruction, biopsies of lesions can be obtained for histology.

THE PERIPHERAL VASCULAR SYSTEM

The peripheral vascular system should not be examined in isolation but as an integral part of the cardiovascular system, after first noting the general physical and mental state of the patient.

Arterial system

Inspection of the limb

The affected limb should be observed for colour change, size, wasting, oedema and skin nutrition. It should be compared with the opposite limb.

Palpation of the limb

The temperature of the limb should be determined and areas of change from warm to cold noted. Again, the two sides should be compared.

Pulses – lower limb

The detection and evaluation of pulses is an important part of the examination of the peripheral vascular system. In the lower limb, the following should be noted:

- the femoral, at the mid-inguinal point
- the popliteal, behind the bent knee
- the posterior tibial, behind the medial malleolus
- the dorsalis pedis, lateral to the estensor hallucis tendon

These pulses are then compared with those on the opposite side.

Pulses – upper limb

In the upper limbs, the subclavian, brachial, radial and ulnar pulses should be examined. The blood pressure should be measured in both arms.

Auscultation of the limb

When pulses are diminished, a thrill may be felt or a murmur may be heard denoting proximal arterial stenosis, e.g. auscultation at the lower end of Hunter's canal may detect femoral stenosis.

Other tests

Further evidence of the degree of ischaemia may be obtained by elevating the lower limb and observing the sole of the foot for the onset of pallor in the pulps of the toes and the metatarsal pad. This may be emphasized by having the patient paddle the feet while they are supported behind the ankle.

After elevation, the foot is allowed to hang down and the time taken for the veins to fill is noted. This venous filling time, marked by the development of redness in the toes and foot, is normally about 10 seconds. A slow venous filling time, rubor on dependency and pallor on elevation, signify a marked degree of ischaemia.

Abdominal examination

The abdomen is now examined to feel the aortic, common iliac and external iliac pulses and for aneurysms. Auscultation may reveal a murmur suggestive of abdominal aortic stenosis, if it is central, or renal artery stenosis, if it is a little off centre. The renal murmur is likely to be localized. The aortic murmur may be transmitted down the iliacs.

The carotid pulses and the heart

The common carotid and bifurcation pulses should be felt for and auscultated. When listening for a murmur at the angle of the jaw, it is best to ask the patient to stop breathing for a few seconds. The presence of a thrill and murmur suggests internal carotid artery stenosis.

Finally, the heart should be examined.

Investigations

Arteriography

Arteriography is only carried out if the patient's complaint is severe enough to consider surgical treatment. For example, a claudication distance of as little as 200 metres would suggest the need for operation. Above that, it would be questionable and would depend upon age, occupation and pursuits. Arteriography reveals the anatomy of the arterial tree, but gives little idea of the physiological effects of obstruction. These must be determined in other ways (see below).

Blood flow

Using a pressure cuff, the pressure in the distal vessels can be obtained and related to normal arm blood pressure. An index of one to the other is also of value in the assessment of cases before and after operation.

Blood flow can be measured by techniques such as venous occlusion plethysmography, the clearance time of radioactive isotopes and Doppler ultrasound. These give a semiquantitative indication of the velocity of flow.

Treadmill

A patient's estimate of claudication distance is usually given approximately in yards or in minutes. Where quantitative analysis of the results of treatment is required, a treadmill that measures distance and incline is useful.

Venous system

Veins carrying the blood from the limbs back to the heart are of two types, the superficial veins and the deep veins.

The superficial veins

The superficial veins lie in the subcutaneous tissue. They are more muscular than the deep veins and also contain more sympathetic nerve fibres in their walls. They therefore respond readily to stimuli by contracting. This is often seen when a venipuncture needle has traversed a vein and is difficult to reinsert because of spasm.

The deep veins

The deep veins are less muscular, less well innervated and have less catecholamines in their walls than the superficial veins. They are therefore less responsive to stimuli.

The return of blood to the heart is encouraged by:

- muscular contraction of skeletal muscles massaging the blood upwards
- contraction of the muscle walls of superficial veins
- the arteriovenous gradient
- respiratory movement encouraging flow of blood into the chest
- gravity in the veins draining from head and neck

Inspection

On inspection, abnormalities of superficial veins such as varicosity, varicose dermatitis and varicose ulcer are obvious. Oedema, cellulitis and pigmentation along veins affected by thrombophlebitis are easily detected.

Palpation

Palpation may reveal thrombosis of the superficial veins, tender areas of thrombophlebitis and, if varicose veins are present, small defects in the deep fascia through which the perforating veins emerge.

In varicose veins, competence of the valves at the upper end of the veins should be tested. If the valves are incompetent, a cough impulse will pass down the veins in the thigh and tapping the upper end of the vein will produce a percussion wave.

Auscultation

Auscultation is rarely of use in the venous system unless there is an arteriovenous fistula, when a thrill may be felt in the dilated veins and a murmur heard on auscultation.

Investigations

The Trendelenburg test

This will demonstrate the competence of the saphenous valve. The patient lies down and elevates the leg to empty the veins. Pressure is applied proximally with the fingers over the saphenous opening to prevent the vein from refilling. The patient then stands with finger pressure still applied. The veins should remain empty, but when the fingers are removed immediate reflux of blood is seen to fill the varicose veins. This positive result indicates an incompetent valve. The same can be done using a number of tourniquets at various levels. Filling of the veins between tourniquets indicates presence of incompetent veins allowing the blood to pass from the deep into the superficial venous system.

Photography

This is rarely used except to record the collateral subcutaneous veins seen in the chest wall with superior vena caval thrombosis and in the abdominal wall with inferior vena caval thrombosis.

Thermography

It is possible, in the cooled limb, to detect the warmer blood from the deep veins refluxing back along the incompetent perforating veins to the superficial veins as hot spots on a Thermoscan. The equipment is expensive.

Fluorescein staining

A non-toxic dye, fluorescein, which fluoresces a brilliant yellow in ultraviolet light, may also be used to demonstrate the site of incompetent perforating veins.

Phlebography

This is the most commonly used technique for studying the anatomy of the deep venous system and is widely used to demonstrate the extent and position of venous thrombosis.

Contrast material is injected into the dorsal vein of the foot and forced into the deep veins by a tourniquet above the ankle. Various manoeuvres are used to ensure filling of the lower veins. The iliofemoral segment can best be demonstrated by direct injection into the femoral vein under X-ray control. Intra-osseous phlebography allows good opacification of the deep veins when injection into the femoral vein is not possible. The injection is made into the bone marrow with a special cannula.

Labelled fibrinogen

Fibrinogen labelled with radioactive iodine (^{125}I) is injected intravenously. If fresh thrombus is forming, the radioactive fibrinogen will be incorporated into the thrombus, giving a rise in radioactivity in that area. The level of radioactivity in the legs is expressed as a percentage of the precordial count. The difference in the counts between different areas in the legs can then be demonstrated on the same day or successive days.

Lymphatic system

Although disorders of the lymphatic system are much less common than those of the arterial or venous systems, they are nevertheless important.

The lymphatic system has two functions:
- to drain lymph from the tissues
- to assist in the control of infection by producing antibodies and lymphocytes

The lymphatics of the limbs remove large protein molecules from the interstitial fluid where their accumulation would cause increased tissue colloid osmotic pressure and fluid retention in the interstitial space, thus producing oedema.

Lymphatic disorders result in oedema – lymph-oedema. It is important to exclude other causes of oedema such as cardiac, renal, low plasma proteins and the oedema that follows venous thrombosis.

Early lymphoedema is soft and pitting. Later, skin changes such as thickening (elephantiasis) occur and fine warty excrescences may appear. Evidence of recurrent cellulitis may also be present.

Investigation

This is by lymphography. An injection of 0.5 ml of 10% Patent Blue Violet is made into a web space on the hand or foot. The dye diffuses into the lymphatics and outlines them. One lymph vessel is then exposed by incision and cannulated. Lipiodol, a radio-opaque medium, is injected and its passage up the lymphatics is visualized by X-ray.

THE PAEDIATRIC PATIENT

The methods and techniques used in the examination of paediatric patients differ fundamentally from those used in adults.

History

Babies and young children are unable to give a history. Older children are often reluctant to talk and may also be unreliable witnesses, either because they are anxious to please or because they fear the possible consequences of what they might say.

Commonly, both parents accompany a child on a first visit, which tends to be a major and somewhat worrying family experience. They are the main source of information about their children, but again their comments are much more likely to be influenced by emotions, such as pride and protectiveness, than they would be if they were telling the story about themselves.

As genuine cardiac symptoms are somewhat unusual in children with suspected heart disease, much of the history depends upon question and answer. Find out:

- about other children in the family and how the patient compares with them in growth and development. If the patient is an only child, ask how he compares with friends' and neighbours' children of the same age

- how he gets on at school

- if he plays games
  Does he play in a team and in what position on the field? Is he more tired and breathless than the other children during and after the match?

Remember that normal, healthy children vary greatly in their activities and in what gives them pleasure (ball kickers, tree climbers, chess players, bookworms etc.). So, what they do may depend more upon what they want to do than upon what they are able to do.

Breathlessness and chest pain on exertion are uncommon symptoms in children in the absence of cyanosis. Even when there are no physical signs to indicate the presence of a lesion, however, many doctors are reluctant to dismiss them in case they may be missing one of the intrinsic myocardial disorders. These conditions are nearly always accompanied by cardiac enlargement or ECG changes or both and, in their absence, such symptoms can confidently be ignored.

An infant's response to exertion is less obvious. In the main, exertion consists of eating, crying and, to a lesser extent, emptying the bowels, especially when constipated. Babies with serious heart disease are slow feeders and bad doers. They tend to be irritable because of fatigue. Their energy is used up by the heart to maintain a barely adequate circulation. They fall asleep during meals, not because they are satisfied, but because they become exhausted by the effort involved. Questions and answers about these matters give a good guide to the severity of the lesion and the adequacy of cardiac reserves.

Examination

Observation is a very important part of the examination in babies. Take a good long look at a baby before disturbing it. Watch it lying in its cot, watch it sleeping, watch it feeding, watch it crying. Note the state of nutrition, muscle tone, colour and general demeanour. There is usually nothing seriously wrong with the cardiovascular system if an infant looks well-nourished, happy and contented. Babies with serious heart disease are often pale, flabby, anxious and easily disturbed.

Look out for cyanosis at rest and on exertion. Note how long it takes for the colour to return to normal when the exertion stops.

When it comes to physical examination, the child must be handled with care and each case judged on its merits. By and large, one collects information as stealthily as possible while disturbing the patient as little as possible. Once an infant is upset or made to cry, satisfactory examination of the cardiovascular system is impossible and may not become possible again until the next visit.

The two most commonly made mistakes are:

- to treat little children like miniature adults

- to have them stripped to the waist

Never take infants away from their mothers and lay them on an examination couch, even if the mother comes and stands beside it. Always examine them sitting on their mother's lap and remember that they often cry if forced to lie down flat. Observation of crying and the response to it are important, but should be kept, if possible, until all other necessary information has been obtained.

Never insist on removing the last layer of clothing from small children before auscultation. It is nearly always resisted and causes loss of confidence. It is better to listen to the heart through a thin vest than through the sobbing that so often follows its forced removal.

Also, remember to auscultate before applying your hands. Keep things that may cause a scene, such as feeling for thrills, palpating the liver and estimating the femoral pulses, until the end of the examination.

Communication

Be careful what you say about the heart in front of parents or their children. Remember that even the suspicion of heart disease is a great worry for parents and that even very young patients have long ears. The seeds of a cardiac neurosis can be sown at a very early age.

More children are referred to exclude heart disease than to confirm it. If you hear a faint murmur and decide that it is an innocent noise, don't tell them about it and then, in the next breath, not to worry about it. Say nothing about the murmur or, if you have to say something because someone else already has, say 'I'm pleased to be able to tell you that I can find nothing wrong with your child's heart'.

Also, refrain from commenting or be wary when commenting on odd findings such as an unusual ECG or heart X-ray that are difficult to explain in the absence of abnormal physical signs. This is especially true in young children where the situation is likely to change rapidly with growth and development. If there is nothing you can do about it, such information is best kept to yourself and recorded only in the notes.

SECTION III

The Presentation of Cardiovascular Disease and the Diagnostic Possibilities

PRESENTING PROBLEMS IN CARDIOVASCULAR DISEASE

This section considers symptoms referrable to the cardiovascular system rather than diseases of the cardiovascular system, each with its own catalogue of symptoms and signs: a presentation-orientated approach that closely approximates the situation faced in clinical practice. Complaints do not, of course, always present singly, but in combinations that may themselves suggest the diagnosis. The recognition of such patterns is a function of experience. Here, for descriptive purposes, they are considered individually.

CHEST PAIN

When a patient complains of chest pain, the range of possible diagnoses is considerable. It is important to remember that chest pain and heart disease are not synonymous. Angina pectoris, 'a choking feeling in the chest', does not necessarily imply that a patient has atherosclerotic coronary heart disease.

When dealing with such a patient, the first priority is to take a careful history. If the pain is due to heart disease, this is likely to be more helpful in making a diagnosis than physical examination and further investigations because these often reveal no abnormality.

Causes of chest pain

Various diseases present with chest pain and may mimic angina. Those related to the structures listed in Table 9 are examples of conditions that must be considered in the differential diagnoses.

Angina pectoris

Angina pectoris is a symptom, not a diagnosis. Examination and investigation are required to establish the cause.

It is a tight or choking feeling in the chest brought on by effort and less often by excitement. It is often worse in cold or windy weather and after heavy meals. It does not last long when the precipitating factor is removed, being relieved by rest or nitrates.

Causes

Angina pectoris is due to transient myocardial is-

TABLE 9

Structure	Disease
Chest wall:	
skin	Herpes zoster
muscles	Myalgia
ribs	Fracture
Neck	Cervical spondylosis
Lungs and pleura	Pneumonia
	Pulmonary infarction
	Pleurisy
Mediastinum	
aorta	Dissection
oesophagus	Oesophagitis
Alimentary tract	Hiatus hernia
	Cholecystitis
	Peptic ulcer
	Pancreatitis

chaemia. It occurs when myocardial oxygen demand is greater than supply. The usual cause of angina (cardiac pain) is narrowing of the major coronary arteries due to atherosclerosis. This is present in 80% of patients. Other causes are possible and must be sought and excluded before making a diagnosis of coronary heart disease.

Among those to be considered are the following:

- systemic hypertension
- valvar heart disease
- disturbances of heart rhythm
- anaemia
- thyroid disease

Systemic hypertension

Both systolic and diastolic hypertension increase cardiac work and therefore increase myocardial oxygen demand. Atherosclerosis may also be accelerated by the raised pressure and cause further arterial damage. Angina may be greatly relieved if the hypertension is controlled.

Valvar heart disease

Anginal pain is common in the late stages of severe aortic stenosis, which may be either rheumatic or congenital and is commoner in men than in women. It is often unsuspected and the patients may have quite normal coronary arteries. With aortic stenosis, left ventricular pressure is increased to overcome the obstruction at the aortic valve. There is increased intramyocardial tension and diminished diastolic filling of the coronary arteries. The clinical signs are those of a forceful apex beat due to left ventricular hypertrophy, a systolic thrill and a rough aortic systolic murmur conducted upwards into the neck.

Prolapse of the mitral valve may occasionally be associated with chest pain that sometimes occurs on exertion. It is characterized by a late systolic murmur due to mitral incompetence and, in some cases, a midsystolic click. This rare syndrome is commonest in young women and may be confused with coronary disease, especially if the ECG is abnormal.

Disturbances of heart rhythm

Patients should be asked whether or not they have been aware of changes in heart rate (palpitation) and whether or not such changes are associated with pain or breathlessness.

Both tachycardia and bradycardia may lead to diminished cardiac output and diminished coronary filling. In rapid tachycardia, the heart is too rapid to allow adequate ventricular filling; in extreme bradycardia the heart rate is too slow to maintain an adequate output, even although stroke volume is satisfactory.

Anaemia

There are two main reasons why anaemic patients may have angina. The heart is being supplied with blood that is deficient in oxygen while at the same time being asked to increase its output to maintain peripheral tissue perfusion.

Conversely, polycythaemia (too many red cells) makes the blood more viscous, increases cardiac work and may also cause angina.

Thyroid gland disturbances

Both hyper- and hypothyroidism can be associated with angina. This may or may not be due to associated coronary disease. Weight loss, sweating, tachycardia etc. suggest increased thyroid activity; weight gain, dry skin, hoarse voice etc. suggest hypothyroidism.

Syphilis

Years ago, syphilis would have a prominent place in a list of causes of angina because it narrowed the ostia of the coronary arteries. Nowadays it is a rarity.

The approach to a patient presenting with chest pain

History

Information should be sought on the:

- site of pain
- type of pain
- radiation of pain
- factors producing pain
- factors relieving pain

The pain of angina pectoris is usually over the centre of the chest but can be felt anywhere from the epigastrium to the jaw and arms (see p. 72). It is usually brought on by exertion, less often by excitement or stress, and is relieved by rest.

Other types of chest pain have different features. Thus, well-localized chest wall pain, especially if it is in the left submammary area and is tender to the touch, is not due to cardiac disease and is unlikely to have any organic basis.

Cervical spondylosis often causes tingling in the arm and discomfort in the neck.

Pleural pain is usually experienced on one or other side of the chest and is made worse by deep breathing or coughing.

Abdominal pain due to gallbladder disease, hiatus hernia or peptic ulcer may also be mistaken for cardiac pain in some cases. A careful history and the signs associated with these conditions should avoid confusion.

Examination

No matter how clearcut the history, physical examination should never be skimped or omitted. Most often it excludes other causes of chest pain rather than revealing positive findings. What must be avoided at all costs is making a diagnosis of coronary heart disease when the patient has, for example, unsuspected aortic stenosis, anaemia or peptic ulceration.

In a review of 200 patients seen consecutively at a Chest Pain Clinic, the final diagnoses were as follows:

Coronary heart disease	50%
Non-specific chest pain	30%
Other	20%

The 'other' included previously unknown:

Paroxysmal tachycardia	6
Aortic valve disease	4
Cholecystitis	2
Hiatus hernia	1

Investigations

It is again emphasized that history is most important, often all-important, in the diagnosis of cardiac pain. Physical examination and further investigation, though also important, are often non-contributory to the diagnosis in patients with coronary heart disease.

DYSPNOEA

Breathlessness is a common symptom. Everyone can and frequently does become breathless, but dyspnoea is inappropriate breathlessness. It occurs when the degree of breathlessness is out of proportion to the amount of exertion that has caused it.

Dyspnoea is not exclusive to cardiac disease. It is also a common presenting feature in many respiratory disorders and in some types of anaemia. However, it does not always signify major disease. Psychogenic breathlessness is not uncommon. In this condition, the breathlessness is quite out of proportion to the clinical condition. The breathing is often sighing or jerky in character with a considerable range of depth. As a rule, no underlying disease can be found.

It is useful to grade dyspnoea according to its severity:

- Grade I
  No breathlessness on ordinary physical activity

- Grade II
  Breathlessness on strenuous exertion such as running for a bus or climbing a steep flight of stairs

- Grade III
  Breathlessness on ordinary exertion such as carrying a shopping bag, climbing a slight incline or keeping up a normal pace on the level

- Grade IV
  Breathlessness on the slightest exertion, perhaps even when confined to bed

Two other important types of breathlessness are:

- orthopnoea
  This describes dyspnoea occurring in the recumbent position: inability to breathe except in the upright position. It usually occurs during the night and can be relieved by sitting up in bed or by using more pillows.

- paroxysmal nocturnal dyspnoea
  This is a dramatic symptom: breathlessness that comes on suddenly during the night. Patients awake, usually after sleeping for an hour or two, with a sudden feeling of suffocation and may be extremely frightened. The need for fresh air is uppermost in their mind. They have to get up to find it, often by opening a window. In the most severe form, pulmonary oedema occurs, when a dry cough is followed by the copious production of bloodstained frothy fluid pouring from the mouth and nose; the patient is drowning in his own secretions. This condition, once seen or experienced, is never forgotten.

Mechanism

The mechanism of dyspnoea is uncertain. It is often associated with pulmonary congestion, increased stiffness of the lungs and with the sensation that an increased effort is required to breathe.

Causes

Diseases of the heart and lungs are the main causes of breathlessness. When only one system is involved, it is usually not difficult to decide which. When both are involved, the principal cause of the breathlessness is often difficult to determine.

When dyspnoea is due to heart disease, the cause is usually found to be on the left side of the heart, because there is obstruction to or impairment of left ventricular filling or emptying. The pressure rises first in the pulmonary veins and then in the pulmonary capillaries. A point is reached when the intracapillary and venous pressure exceed the pressure in the tissues. Fluid is forced from the capillaries into the interstitial tissues of the lungs, which become waterlogged. The lymphatics become engorged. If the capillary pressure continues to rise, the lymphatic drainage is overwhelmed and fluid passes across the alveolar capillary membrane. This causes pulmonary congestion or even pulmonary oedema. Common causes are:

- myocardial ischaemia (usually, but not always due to coronary heart disease)
- hypertension
- aortic and mitral valve disease
- disorders of heart muscle (cardiomyopathy)

The progression of dyspnoea differs according to

TABLE 10

Primary cause	Secondary cause
Airways obstruction	Chronic bronchitis Asthma
Restrictive defect	Fibrosis of the lung Deformities of the spine and thoracic cage (kyphoscoliosis)
Obstruction to pulmonary circulation	Pulmonary thromboembolism

the cause. For example, in mitral disease, symptoms develop insidiously over many years, whereas in aortic disease, they develop suddenly after many years without symptoms.

Pulmonary causes of dyspnoea include those listed in Table 10.

The patient

History

First assess the severity of the breathlessness and establish its duration and rate of progress. Longstanding breathlessness is likely to be due to longstanding disease of heart or lungs. Sudden onset of severe breathlessness suggests a major clinical event such as left ventricular failure due to myocardial infarction or to a respiratory problem such as pneumonia, pneumothorax or pulmonary embolism. Pulmonary tuberculosis may have produced marked lung destruction and fibrosis or possibly the patient has an industrial lung disease. Other important factors in the history that may help to pinpoint the system involved are:

- pain
- cough and sputum
- wheezing

Pain

Find out:

Is it increased on effort and relieved by rest, suggesting a cardiac cause.

Does it become worse on deep inspiration, suggesting pleural irritation.

About the site of the pain; central pain suggesting a cardiac origin, peripheral pain a pulmonary one.

Cough and sputum

Patients with chronic obstructive airways disease give a history of longstanding cough and excessive sputum production. In the winter, they are likely to have episodes of acute infection with purulent, yellow or green sputum. Patients with pneumonia or pulmonary infarction will frequently have a rusty blood-stained spit or frank haemoptysis. Patients with chronic left heart failure may also have a cough. This is usually an irritating, non-productive cough, occurring mainly after going to bed and due probably to lung stiffness caused by fluid accumulation.

Wheezing

A long history of episodic wheezing is usually a respiratory problem. Sudden episodes of nocturnal wheezing can be due to left heart failure and are known as cardiac asthma.

Examination

A general examination should be carried out before concentrating on the cardiorespiratory system. For example, pallor and pale mucous membranes suggest anaemia. Peripheral cyanosis, associated with a warm skin and bounding pulses, is more likely to be due to respiratory than cardiac disease. A vasoconstricted periphery is more likely to be cardiac in origin.

Examine the configuration of the chest. Severe skeletal deformity of the sternum, ribs or spine suggests a mechanical problem of lung function. The hyperinflated chest of emphysema is also a diagnostic clue.

Cardiovascular examination is most helpful in terms of congenital or valvar disease. Both mitral and aortic valve disease are associated with breathlessness: as previously stated, mitral valve disease causing a long history of gradually progressive dyspnoea, aortic valve disease remaining asymptomatic and unsuspected for many years before presenting abruptly with rapidly progressive symptoms.

Chest examination will give information about collapse, consolidation and effusion. Alterations in breath sounds can range from bronchospasm in asthmatics to basal crepitations in those with heart failure.

Finally, remember that it is often not possible to separate cardiac from respiratory causes of breathlessness without pulmonary function studies. Diseases of the heart can affect the lungs and diseases of the lungs can affect the heart. In certain situations, therefore, breathlessness may be due to a combination of effects.

FATIGUE

Fatigue is a non-specific symptom. Patients often complain about lack of energy; they realize that a task normally accomplished easily now takes much longer. Often, this is accompanied by a loss of initiative, with difficulty in starting as well as completing an undertaking.

There are many causes of fatigue. They include organic, psychosomatic and psychiatric disorders.

Disease of any system may cause fatigue. In cardiovascular disorders, it is thought that a chronically inadequate cardiac output both at rest and on exertion impairs cellular function. Other important symptoms, such as pain and breathlessness, should be sought. Both valvar and coronary heart disease may have fatigue as a prominent feature. This seems to be especially true in mitral valve disease where fatigue may be the patient's most prominent symptom.

A psychosomatic disorder should never be diagnosed without a careful history and physical examination. In these circumstances fatigue is often accompanied by sighing respiration, palpitation, precordial pain and faintness – these symptoms and the patient's demeanour often suggesting anxiety.

COUGH

Although a patient who complains about a cough is likely to be suffering from some type of respiratory disorder, cough is a moderately frequent accompaniment of cardiac failure.

History

Cough in cardiac disease

This is usually:

- short
- irritating
- unproductive of sputum
- worse on exertion and on lying down

In severe left ventricular failure with pulmonary oedema there may be copious frothy spit occasionally tinged with blood.

The cough in cardiac conditions is probably activated by compression of receptors in the walls of alveoli and smaller bronchioles because of excess interstitial fluid.

In an attack of acute dyspnoea, an accompanying cough may suggest that the breathlessness is due to a cardiac cause rather than to bronchial asthma. In the latter, cough and sputum production often appear only at the conclusion of the attack.

Cough in respiratory disease

In acute respiratory infections the cough is short, sharp and painful, either locally in the tracheobronchial area or more peripherally in a pleural distribution. At first the cough is unproductive, later sputum appears, frequently purulent and occasionally bloodstained.

In chronic respiratory disease, cough is more persistent, usually productive of sputum, sometimes clear, often sticky. It is worse:

- on rising
- on changing room temperature
- in dusty or smoky atmospheres
- with exacerbation of infection

Cough is also a feature of bronchial neoplasm.

Chronic cough

Smokers tend to have a chronic morning cough, probably due to varying degrees of pharyngitis and bronchitis.

Chronic bronchitis with or without emphysema is the commonest cause of a chronic cough. It is important to realise, however, that mitral valve disease and chronic bronchitis may coexist.

Pulmonary heart disease is also commonly associated with chronic bronchitis and emphysema and under these circumstances persistent cough is a dominating feature.

HAEMOPTYSIS

Haemoptysis is an important and not infrequent symptom of cardiovascular disease. It must always be investigated to discover the cause, which may be cardiac or an accompanying respiratory condition.

Causes

The following general cardiovascular conditions should be considered:

- pulmonary infarction
- pulmonary hypertension (e.g. in mitral stenosis)
- pulmonary oedema (e.g. left ventricular failure from any cause)
- arteriovenous fistula
- rupture of aortic aneurysm

Haemoptysis can be due to bleeding from a variety of vascular sources. These include:

- venous capillary bleeding

  This occurs in mitral stenosis and in left ventricular failure with or without pulmonary oedema. The bleed is usually small in amount, varying from a clear spit flecked with blood to copious pink, frothy sputum

- rupture of a bronchopulmonary venous anastomosis

  This occurs most often in mitral stenosis, but occasionally also in pulmonary infarction and may produce quite large volumes of blood

- arterial haemorrhage

  This can occur in pulmonary hypertension due to any cause. It is frequently brisk

Pulmonary infarction

This is usually caused by an embolus arising from thrombosis in deep leg or pelvic veins or less frequently in the right atrium. The embolus lodges in a pulmonary artery and depending upon its size and the local reaction to it, may or may not be accompanied by such symptoms as cough, breathlessness, pleural pain and haemoptysis.

Atrial fibrillation may contribute to pulmonary infarction in patients with mitral stenosis by causing stasis and encouraging thrombus formation. This may occur even in those with sinus rhythm.

Cardiac patients, with their congested lung bases, are particularly liable to develop pulmonary infarcts, sometimes as a consequence of local thrombosis.

Pulmonary hypertension may also cause pulmonary arterial thrombosis with the result that a peripheral pulmonary artery is obstructed by a thrombus rather than an embolus.

Bleeding from other sources

Rupture of an aortic or arteriovenous aneurysm is a rare cause of haemoptysis, but when it occurs frequently causes a large haemorrhage that may be fatal.

OEDEMA

Causes

Signs of severe generalized oedema in adults are usually due to cardiac, hepatic or renal disease.

A history of orthopnoea, effort dyspnoea or angina suggests cardiac failure. Alcohol abuse or previous jaundice suggests hepatocellular failure. Chronic kidney disease suggests renal failure.

In cardiac failure oedema affects the most dependent parts, i.e. the ankles of ambulatory patients or patients confined to a chair and the sacrum and thighs of patients confined to bed. By contrast, facial puffiness is prominent in renal oedema. A raised jugular venous pressure (JVP) supports a finding of heart failure, but it should be remembered that oedema and a raised JVP can also be caused by constrictive pericarditis and pericardial effusion without heart failure. In hepatic oedema, other signs of hepatic failure such as spider naevi, splenomegaly and palmar erythema are usually present.

In renal disease, the diagnosis is not so obvious on clinical examination but can be quickly substantiated by examination of the urine and blood.

In children, oedema may be due to acute glomerulonephritis.

In the absence of cardiac, hepatic or renal disease, other causes of oedema must be considered. Facial puffiness may be an allergic phenomenon and, in women, quite marked oedema may occur premenstrually in otherwise normal individuals. The possibility of pregnancy as a cause of oedema should also be kept in mind.

Inadequate ingestion of vitamin B_1 or protein may cause oedema in deprived or mentally disturbed patients and in those with the malabsorption syndrome.

Localized oedema

When oedema is confined to the ankles, certain specific diagnoses should be considered:

- varicose veins

  Patients with varicose veins are very susceptible to dependent oedema, notably towards the end of the day

- venous thrombosis in the deep calf veins

  When this is present, there may be tenderness and swelling of the calf although these signs are frequently absent

- venous or lymphatic obstruction

  This can be due to a pelvic tumour and may cause oedema that extends up to the thighs

- arthritis

  Here pain and tenderness are prominent

By a process of exclusion one may reach the conclusion that the ankle swelling is due either to immobility or to prolonged standing. Patients with cerebral vascular accidents often develop oedema due to immobility. Standing or sitting for long periods can cause oedema in normal individuals, particularly during warm weather.

PALPITATION

Palpitation is an abnormal awareness of the heart beat. Most people experience it from time to time and anxious persons may associate it with cardiac disease. It is often, but not always, an expression of an abnormal rhythm and the description may suggest the abnormal rhythm involved. Thus, patients often complain of 'fluttering in the chest' or 'missed beats' when they are having extrasystoles, or may describe 'racing of the heart' when they are having paroxysmal tachycardia.

The patient

Patients of any age and either sex can be affected. Anxiety is often prominent, but this is frequently a secondary feature caused by the symptoms rather than the primary problem. There may be evidence of underlying rheumatic or thyrotoxic heart disease, which are frequently associated with atrial fibrillation. In ischaemic heart disease, ventricular dysrhythmias are more likely.

Most often, however, the heart appears to be normal.

History

It is important to take a careful history in order to find out exactly what the patient means by 'palpitation'. In this way it is often possible to deduce with a fair degree of certainty what abnormal rhythm is causing the symptoms.

For example, when palpitation is due to ectopic beats, patients have often become aware of the compensatory pauses that follow them, rather than of the ectopic beats themselves; or they may notice the thumps of the postectopic contractions because of their increased stroke volume. Symptoms are often most marked at rest or in bed and tend to pass unnoticed when the patient is active, busy or preoccupied.

Patients with paroxysmal tachycardia often describe the onset of rapid regular beating, a racing of the heart, a fluttering in the chest or a throbbing in the neck. It usually begins suddenly and may end equally suddenly or pass off gradually. Sometimes vagal stimulation (carotid sinus pressure, gagging, Valsalva) will stop it and such a story is typical of supraventricular tachycardia.

When the paroxysm is irregular, this suggests atrial fibrillation or multiple ectopic beats.

Examination

This is often unhelpful. Few patients have symptoms at the time of examination, except for those with frequent ectopic beats. Likewise, an ECG is most unlikely to detect the abnormality unless it is recorded continuously on tape for 24 hours or more. Most patients have no clinical evidence of underlying heart disease.

SYNCOPE

Syncope, or sudden loss of consciousness due to cerebral hypoxia, is a common symptom affecting people of all ages.

Causes

It has a wide differential diagnosis that includes the following:

- vasovagal attack
- postural hypotension
- epilepsy
- vertebrobasilar insufficiency
- Adams–Stokes attacks
- drug induced hypotension
- cardiac syncope of aortic stenosis or pulmonary hypertension
- cough syncope
- micturition syncope

- minor strokes
- transient attacks of cerebral ischaemia
- subclavian steal syndrome

Single episodes of syncope may occur with acute myocardial infarction or pulmonary embolism.

The patient

The age of the patient is of some diagnostic value. Vasovagal attacks, for example tend to occur in young people, Adams–Stokes attacks and vertebro-basilar insufficiency in older patients.

History

An accurate account of the syncopal attack is essential. Often, the patient's own account is limited. In these circumstances an eyewitness account is invaluable and should always be sought. The eyewitness may describe the striking pallor and subsequent flushing sometimes seen in an Adams–Stokes attack or the cyanosed, rigid appearance seen in epilepsy. They may also be able to say whether the patient had convulsions.

Details of premonitory symptoms or precipitating factors and what drugs are being taken may positively identify the cause of syncope.

Examination

Physical examination often gives no clue to the cause of the syncopal attack. When it has a cardiac cause, this may be obvious, as in severe aortic stenosis or complete heart block, or it may leave no clues, as in a paroxysm of very rapid tachycardia.

As with palpitation, a routine ECG is unlikely to be helpful, except when the heart rate is slow, unless it is recorded for 24 hours or more.

FEVER

Fever and febrile symptoms are not common in patients with cardiovascular disease.

Causes

Fever and febrile symptoms are usually prominent in acute pericarditis and myocarditis, but may not occur in endocarditis until the condition is well established. In febrile patients with myocarditis, the heart rate is often disproportionately fast.

A little fever is quite common for a day or two after myocardial infarction, although the patients are seldom aware of it. On the other hand, sweating and lassitude are common following myocardial infarction even in patients whose temperature is not elevated.

Mild pyrexia is also present in other destructive lesions such as dissection of the aorta, pulmonary embolism and pulmonary infarction, so it has little value in the differential diagnosis in patients with precordial pain.

HEADACHE

Headache is a very common symptom. Its cause is often difficult or impossible to determine and although many patients with cardiovascular disease complain of headaches, a cardiovascular cause is seldom found to explain them.

Causes

Most extracranial structures are supplied with pain fibres, particularly arteries and muscles in the scalp. Inside the skull, pain fibres are confined to the arteries and dura around the base, the venous sinuses and their tributaries, and cranial nerves V, VII, IX and X. The mechanisms and examples of headache are shown in Table 11.

TABLE 11   Organic causes of headache

Causes	Examples
Vascular	Migraine, glyceryl trinitrate
Muscle contraction	Tension headache
Traction on intracranial structures	Intracranial space occupying lesions, lumbar puncture
Inflammation:	
intracranial	Meningitis, subarachnoid haemorrhage
extracranial	Giant cell arteritis
From neighbouring structures	Nose and paranasal sinuses Eyes (glaucoma) Ear Teeth Skull or neck
Cranial nerves	Trigeminal neuralgia

The patient

Headache is so common that the age and sex of the patient can give only the broadest indication of probable causes. For example, migraine commonly starts in adolescence. Tension headache is often seen in young adults, particularly females in whom it may persist into later life. Hypertensive headache is more a feature of middle age. Trigeminal neuralgia and giant cell arteritis are diseases of later life.

History

For history taking see p. 76.

Examination

Particular features to look out for on examination include:

- level of consciousness
  Consciousness may be clouded with vascular or space-occupying neurological lesions, sub-arachnoid haemorrhage, meningitis and hypertensive encephalopathy
- neurological signs
  Full neurological examination is essential to exclude a neurological cause for the headache
- optic fundi
  Papilloedema and haemorrhages may be due to raised intracranial pressure from cerebral tumour, but in these circumstances associated neurological signs are usually present. Their absence suggests malignant phase hypertension as the probable cause
- hypertension
  A grossly elevated blood pressure will support this cause, but single readings can be misleading and it is of great assistance to have previous records
- proteinuria
  This is a feature of malignant phase hypertension
- other features
  A tense patient suggests tension headaches. A check should also be made for such things as neck stiffness or inflamed temporal arteries. The nose, eyes, ears, teeth and neck should also be examined

Rarely, a patient may be seen with paroxysmal hypertension caused by a pheochromocytoma. In such a case, severe headache, tachycardia, sweating and pallor may be observed when the blood pressure rises abruptly.

Headache and hypertension

Severe (malignant phase) hypertension may produce early morning headache, gradually easing during the day. It is particularly troublesome if the patient stays late in bed. A similar headache may be experienced during paroxysmal hypertension.

On the other hand, many patients with hypertension are symptom free so that their headaches are usually due to other causes. Because of the supposed association, blood pressure is usually measured in patients with headache. In some it is raised and the 'association' continues. Studies have shown, however, that blood pressure is no more likely to be raised in patients with headache than in those without. The headache may be due to anxiety on learning about raised blood pressure in which case it responds to reassurance or even a placebo. Nevertheless, the significance of hypertension is such that routine measurement of blood pressure is recommended.

CYANOSIS

Cyanosis is the blue or purplish colour seen in the skin or mucous membranes when the oxygen content of the blood in the superficial vessels is abnormally low.

It becomes apparent when more than 5 g per cent of the circulating haemoglobin is reduced. It is therefore fairly common in patients with polycythaemia and rare in those who are grossly anaemic.

It is more often detected by the doctor during clinical examination than complained of by the patient during interrogation.

When detected it must be differentiated into one of two types:

- peripheral cyanosis
- central cyanosis

Causes

Peripheral cyanosis

This results when there is increased extraction of oxygen from blood that has left the heart fully saturated. It is the outcome of reduced peripheral circulation and may be due either to vasoconstriction of the peripheral vessels or to a low cardiac output.

Cold is the most common cause of peripheral vasoconstriction and in cold climates, peripheral cyanosis is commonly seen in the hands and faces of normal healthy people. Warm mucous surfaces, such as the inside of the mouth, are usually not affected.

Peripheral cyanosis is also seen when the peripheral circulation is slow because of a low cardiac output. In serious heart disease this may be enhanced by differential vasoconstriction diverting blood from the skin to more vital organs.

Central cyanosis

This results when the arterial blood leaving the heart is less than fully saturated. As a rule, it does not become clinically obvious until the saturation has fallen below about 80%. If affects both warm and cold surfaces, and may originate in either the heart or the lungs.

Some congenital cardiac malformations allow part of the systemic venous return to escape into the arterial side of the circulation without passing through the lungs. This is called a 'right to left shunt' and the resulting central cyanosis is caused by mixing of venous and arterial blood.

Central cyanosis of respiratory origin is due to inadequate oxygenation of blood as it passes through the lungs. It is seen in destructive diseases that produce airways obstruction and in infiltrative conditions that create diffusion defects, particularly when they are sufficiently advanced to cause pulmonary heart disease.

Differential diagnosis

It is usually fairy easy to differentiate between peripheral and central cyanosis.

When possible, the patient should be examined in a good natural light. The skin temperatures should be assessed and the mucous membranes inspected.

If in doubt, remember that peripheral cyanosis should lessen when the skin is warmed. Central cyanosis is little influenced by changes in temperature, but is increased by exercise. It can always be confirmed by measuring the arterial oxygen saturation.

Severe central cyanosis caused by congenital cardiac malformations is accompanied by clubbing of the fingers and toes, and injection of the conjunctivae. Severe central cyanosis caused by chronic respiratory disease is often accompanied by peripheral vasodilation and warm blue hands.

In both types of cyanosis, polycythaemia leads to increased viscosity of the blood and slows its circulation through the skin capillaries with the result that peripheral and central cyanosis may coexist.

Abnormal blood pigments

Abnormal pigments, such as sulphaemoglobin and methaemoglobin, are rare causes of cyanosis and can be detected by spectroscopy.

HYPERTENSION

Patients with high blood pressure often have no symptoms. They are discovered either during routine medical examination for such things as life assurance or when they are examined because of an unrelated complaint.

Under conditions of physical or emotional stress a normal person's blood pressure can be considerably elevated for short periods. To identify hypertension as a problem, the blood pressure must either be so high that it is clearly abnormal or a more modest rise must be shown to persist over several readings, preferably on different occasions.

Because of the Gaussian distribution of blood pressure, it is not possible to give an exact figure above which the blood pressure can be said to be too high (see p. 147). To some extent, this must be an arbitrary decision.

The patient

Patients of any age may have high blood pressure. It is most common in middle age when an underlying cause is rarely found. It is less common in young patients, when it is more likely to be secondary to underlying disease. It is also frequently found in the elderly, when its significance is less certain.

History

Patients with severe hypertension may complain of headache. Otherwise, relevant symptoms will be due to complications of hypertension or its underlying cause and are shown in Table 12.

Nocturia and polyuria

These may signify underlying renal disease, either the cause or the result of the hypertension. They are also occasionally seen with gross hypokalaemia from aldosterone excess. Recurrent frequency and dysuria may signify recurrent urinary tract infection associated with chronic pyelonephritis. A past history of nephritis or proteinuria may be elicited in patients with chronic glomerulonephritis.

TABLE 12 Important features in the assessment of hypertension

	For aetiology	For prognosis
History	Urinary symptoms	Angina pectoris
	Polyuria	Breathlessness
	Palpitations	Oedema
	Pregnancy	Claudication
	Renal disease	Stroke
	Family history	Failing vision
	Drug therapy	Urinary symptoms
Examination	Cushing's syndrome	Blood pressure
	Renal size	Arcus senilis
	Renal bruit	Xanthelasmata
	Femoral pulses	Fundal changes
		Cardiac impulse
		Urine
		Cardiac failure
		Peripheral pulses

Paroxysms of palpitations

These, if accompanied by sweating, pallor or headache, suggest the possibility of pheochromocytoma.

Angina pectoris

This will signify coexisting myocardial ischaemia, as will a past history of myocardial infarction.

Breathlessness and oedema

These may be due to cardiac failure, usually the result of coronary artery disease but to which uncontrolled hypertension contributes.

Claudication

Atheroma in peripheral vessels may produce claudication and progress to cause rest pain or even gangrene.

Cerebrovascular disease

Cerebrovascular disease usually presents as a sudden hemiplegia or dysphasia. Multiple micro-infarcts may produce a less dramatic neurological loss. Sudden onset of headache, usually with clouded consciousness or neurological signs, suggests subarachnoid haemorrhage. Atheroma (often of the carotid or vertebral arteries) may compromise cerebral circulation without producing infarction and cause transient neurological symptoms – the transient cerebral ischaemic attack.

Retinal changes

The retinal changes in malignant hypertension can produce visual deterioration.

Joint pains

Collagen diseases may be suspected if there are joint pains or recurrent pleurisy.

Pregnancy

Hypertension may be preceded by pre-eclampsia in pregnancy.

Family history

A family history may be given in some cases of essential hypertension and also in some patients with secondary hypertension, e.g. polycystic renal disease.

Drug history

It is important to exclude such drugs as corticosteroids and the contraceptive pill as possible contributory causes.

Examination

The blood pressure

The most important physical sign is the blood pressure itself. It is important to reduce the natural variations by using standard conditions. Adequate warmth will avoid the pressor effect of cold; lying for 5 minutes on the couch will help to achieve mental and physical relaxation; and careful support of the extended arm will avoid significant isometric exercise. A significant postural fall in blood pressure is especially likely in the presence of atheroma or sympathetic blocking drugs, so, it is good practice to measure the pressure routinely with the patient standing up as well as lying or sitting.

Retinopathy

In the normal optic fundus, the disc is a distinct round white-to-pink area at the optic nerve head. From it radiate arteries and veins branching into subdivisions. The arteries usually appear narrower than the corresponding veins (with a ratio of 3:4) and cross in front of them without reducing the venous calibre.

The retinal changes of hypertension are classified into four grades.

- Grade I
  Thickening of the arterial wall causes an increased light reflex and narrowing of the column of blood within the arteries, but only minimal depression of the veins at the arteriovenous crossings
- Grade II
  Focal arterial spasm may reduce the arteriovenous ratio to 1:3. The arteriolar light reflex is broader and largely hides the column of blood (copper wire appearance). The veins are compressed at the arteriovenous crossings, and appear interrupted and to change direction
- Grade III
  The arteriovenous ratio is further reduced and the light reflex broader and lighter (silver wire appearance). The important feature is the appearance of bilateral retinal haemorrhages, usually flame shaped, and soft 'cotton wool' exudates
- Grade IV
  The changes of Grade III are seen together with papilloedema, a pink swollen disc with loss of its margin

Cardiovascular system

The pulse is usually regular. The cardiac impulse may suggest left ventricular hypertrophy.

The second heart sound in the aortic area is often accentuated and may show reverse splitting. A fourth sound indicates a failing heart. A systolic murmur caused by aortic sclerosis is not uncommon.

Absent peripheral pulses may confirm peripheral vascular disease. Femoral pulses are delayed or absent in coarctation of the aorta. An epigastric bruit or a bruit in the flank is occasionally heard with renal artery stenosis. Atheroma of the major vessels in the neck may lead to reduced carotid pulsation or a bruit in the neck

Respiratory system

Persistent basal crepitations indicate left heart failure.

Renal system

Proteinuria is present in severe hypertension or with underlying renal disease. Urine microscopy may show casts and cells in glomerulonephritis or pus cells in pyelonephritis. Large kidneys are usually palpable in polycystic renal disease. Renal tenderness may signify active infection in a patient with pyelonephritis.

Central nervous system

Cerebrovascular disease produces focal neurological signs, particularly hemiplegia. Neck stiffness and a positive Kernig's sign suggest subarachnoid haemorrhage or sometimes cerebral haemorrhage. Consciousness may be clouded.

Other signs

Cushing's syndrome can usually be detected by the characteristic facial and body appearance. Collagen disease may produce pallor, joint signs and pleural friction. The presence of an arcus senilis or xanthelasmata suggest coincidental hyperlipoproteinaemia or diabetes mellitus, which, like obesity, may need treatment.

HYPOTENSION

Acute hypotension may lead to syncope (see p. 104).

Chronic hypotension is due to loss of the vasomotor reflex. Patients have a normal or low blood pressure when reclining, but it falls when they stand up and causes symptoms of weakness, blurred vision, dizziness and syncope that disappear rapidly when they lie down again. In milder cases the blood pressure only falls low enough to produce symptoms when they exercise in the upright posture.

Causes

The commonest cause of postural or exertional hypotension is drug therapy, particularly sympathetic neuron blocking drugs or vasodilator drugs given for the treatment of hypertension. Other causes include:

- diabetic autonomic neuropathy
- tabes dorsalis
- prolonged bed rest (or weightlessness)
- idiopathic postural hypotension

It is important to recognize the symptoms and then measure the blood pressure with the patient lying, standing and exercising. A reading taken lying down may be normal or even raised and on occasion this has resulted in the dose of an offending drug being increased instead of reduced, with resulting dangerous aggravation of the hypotension.

When caused by drugs, the hypotension can usually be relieved by reducing the dose or changing the drug. If the syndrome is idiopathic or due to neuropathy, treatment is more difficult. It sometimes responds to fludrocortisone or the wearing of elastic tights.

HEART MURMURS

Heart murmurs are common at all ages, particularly in the young and the elderly.

Nearly all children and adolescents have auscultatory abnormalities associated with a hyperdynamic circulation. Many of them have innocent systolic murmurs that often originate outside the heart itself in such places as the great vessels, the fascial planes of the neck, the pleuropericardial spaces, or the pulmonary arteries. In many, no cause can be found despite extensive investigation. Whatever their cause, most of them will disappear as the patient matures.

Many old people develop murmurs as degenerative changes take place in the heart and great vessels that are also of little or no importance.

Heart murmurs are of many different types (see p. 85). By their very nature, some are more likely to be significant than others. Systolic murmurs may or may not be significant. Diastolic murmurs are nearly always significant. In general, loudness correlates quite well with significance, although there are important exceptions to this rule as, for example, in small ventricular septal defects, where a little hole may make a disproportionately loud noise.

Presentation

Patients with heart disease may present with characteristic symptoms and examination will reveal a murmur that confirms the diagnosis, e.g. breathlessness and fatigue in mitral stenosis or angina and syncope in aortic stenosis.

Patients with heart disease, but without symptoms, may present because a murmur has been detected at a routine medical examination. They are without symptoms either because the lesion is not serious enough to cause symptoms or because it has been detected early in the course of its natural history before it has started to cause symptoms, e.g., a modest degree of mitral valve disease in a young married

woman or an atrial septal defect in a teenage girl.

Patients with heart disease may present because a murmur has developed during the course of their illness, e.g., mitral incompetence following myocardial infarction or aortic incompetence following endocarditis.

Patients with or without heart disease may present because a murmur has been detected during the course of an illness that does not involve the cardiovascular system, e.g., a recurrent chest infection.

Patients without heart disease may present because a murmur has been heard during a routine medical examination, e.g., at a well-baby clinic, at school, for employment, for life assurance, in the antenatal clinic or before a surgical operation.

Assessment of significance

Most heart murmurs are of no significance. When assessing their significance it is important to remember that most people associate heart murmurs with heart disease and heart disease with the fear of death. Patients vary a lot in this regard and often quite unpredictably, but, once told of a heart murmur, a significant number will soon develop appropriate symptoms or, if parents of the patient, observe appropriate symptoms.

Innocent murmurs

Once it has been decided that a murmur is of no consequence, it should be labelled an innocent noise, a description that begs the question of aetiology. The adjectives 'functional' and 'organic', so often applied to such murmurs, are meaningless terms and should be abandoned.

If the patient already knows about the murmur, strong reassurance should be given that there is nothing wrong with the heart and that the murmur will affect neither the way of life nor life expectancy. It is often helpful to liken the cardiovascular system to a central heating system. This too may make noises as the water flows through it, but they do not necessarily mean that there is anything wrong with the system.

If the patient does not know about the murmur, it is best to say nothing about it.

Heart disease

If a diagnosis of heart disease is made, its significance

can be determined from the patient's history, physical signs, heart size, ECG, echoes, X-rays etc.; to which should be added the physician's knowledge of the natural history of the disease concerned. So far as the patient's history is concerned, it is well to remember that patients with seemingly identical lesions may react differently to them because of differing attitudes towards illness.

In the absence of cyanosis, genuine cardiac symptoms are uncommon in children unless they have very severe lesions, so the presence or absence of symptoms is of little or no help in assessing the significance of murmurs. Parents often maintain that the affected child is the most active member of the family and are often reluctant to accept a diagnosis of heart disease. Sometimes they admit to a little fatigue on prolonged exertion but say that after a short rest, the child is off again lively as ever. A few children take advantage of their condition and produce symptoms to make sure that they are spoiled by their parents.

IMAGINARY HEART DISEASE

When considering imaginary heart disease, or 'cardiac neurosis' as it is often called, it is important to appreciate that in the lay mind, the heart is the vital organ, the very font of life itself. This has been so since ancient times. Most gestures and expressions of emotion are related to it. The breast is beaten in anguish. The heart is said to be broken, to have its strings torn, to jump for joy and to have its cockles warmed by a good dram on a cold day. Nice people are said to be warm-hearted and nasty people are said to be stony-hearted.

Because of this deep-seated emotional response, the fear of heart disease is widespread in all communities. Most patients will tolerate considerable suffering and disability with remarkable fortitude, yet strong men blanch when they overhear the words 'heart disease' whispered at the foot of the bed. It is associated not with suffering or disability, but with dropping down dead.

The panic-like reaction of many people with apparently healthy hearts to the thought that they might have heart disease is in striking contrast to the matter-of-fact attitude shown by so many of those who know that they do; and is often helpful when taking the history and making a differential diagnosis.

Worry about heart disease and its consequences may cause a variety of symptoms under different circumstances.

Patients with asymptomatic heart disease, and who are unaware of it, often develop symptoms soon after they are told about it. These may be either typical cardiac symptoms, such as breathlessness on exertion or fatigue, often quite out of keeping with the severity of the lesion; or they may be typical neurotic symptoms, such as stabbing apical chest pain and the sort of breathlessness that is sighing in character or described as the inability to take a really deep breath.

Patients with symptomatic heart disease often have symptoms that are not caused by their cardiac lesion. For example, much of the chest pain felt by some of those with coronary heart disease is not true angina. Such symptoms are often referred to as an 'overlay'.

Patients without heart disease, but who think that they may have heart disease, present in many ways, varying from those with occasional neurotic symptoms to those with a full-blown anxiety state that is really a disease in its own right and which has been given a variety of names such as 'soldier's heart', 'effort syndrome' and 'neurocirculatory asthenia'.

Diagnosis and treatment

Diagnosis seldom presents much difficulty in patients with imaginary heart disease, either because the symptoms themselves do not ring true or because they do not match up with the physical findings. Sometimes they are clearly caused by the effects of the autonomic nervous system or the cerebrum on the heart rather than by the heart itself. If neurotic symptoms overlie genuine cardiac symptoms, it is often much more difficult to disentangle one from the other.

When talking to such patients it must be constantly kept in mind that although the heart disease is imagined, the symptoms are real. Nothing is more irritating to those who feel genuinely unwell than to be labelled neurotic and given the impression that their symptoms are imaginary. They require sympathy, understanding and an explanation of how such symptoms can be produced. For example, a witness to a particularly gory accident may feel sick and even vomit. These gastrointestinal symptoms are not imagined, they are real, as testified by the vomit. Most patients will take the point that they are not caused by gastrointestinal disease. So it can be explained that worry about heart disease causes anxiety; anxiety causes tachycardia; tachycardia causes the patient to become aware of the heart's action and feel the pulse (such patients are often secret pulse-takers); it misses beats, this causes further anxiety and the resulting release of adrenaline causes a sensation of constriction in the chest accompanied by throbbing in the neck, a chokiness in the throat and light, shallow breathlessness. Now, genuinely agitated, the patient feels faint, weak, dry-lipped and light-headed, then breaks into a cold sweat with the worry about what may happen next.

Not everyone has such serious symptoms or goes through this full sequence of events, but, if the way in which one thing can lead to another is explained in simple language, most people can be persuaded that the heart is the victim rather than the culprit.

Treatment is often difficult unless the symptoms are of recent onset and the patient merely wishes to be reassured that there is nothing wrong with the heart.

Those with established disease are a mixed bag, many of whom have suffered for years and have been seen by many doctors. Some have reached a stage where, even if they wished to, they would be incapable of shaking off the invalid status. Some continue to be worried about it; some are prepared to accept it; some use it for their own ends and some appear almost to enjoy it. By and large, the longer it has been present, the more refractory it is to treatment and attempts at cure may be either consciously or subconsciously resisted.

It is essential to adopt a positive and unambiguous attitude right from the start when dealing with such patients, especially in those who are being seen for the first time, because there is little doubt that many patients with imaginary heart disease, if not doctor-produced, are doctor-perpetuated.

THE SWOLLEN LIMB

Swelling of the lower limbs is a common complaint. Swelling of the upper limbs is much less common. Before considering possible diagnoses it is important to find out:

- if the swelling is bilateral or unilateral and if bilateral, if the limbs are equally affected
- if the limbs are swollen all the time or only at certain times
- if anything makes the swelling worse or better
- if it is associated with pain, tenderness, colour or temperature changes

- if it started suddenly or gradually

Causes

A limb becomes swollen because its fluid content is increased. Although sometimes this is with blood, as in the vascular congestion of venous thrombosis, the main component is usually tissue fluid, which may be increased for a variety of causes:

- venous
- cardiac
- renal
- lymphatic
- allergic

Factors affecting fluid exchange

Fluid normally flows across the capillary walls because the pressure at the arterial end is greater than the pressure in the interstitial tissues. At the venous end, the reverse is true (see LD-35).

Factors are summarized in Table 13.

TABLE 13

Factors	Cause
Increased filtration pressure	High venous pressure Low serum albumin
Increased interstitial pressure	Lymphatic blockage
Capillary leakage	Allergy

A rise in the blood pressure at the venous end of the capillaries is the most common cause of oedema. This is seen at its greatest when the venous system becomes blocked, as in iliofemoral venous thrombosis or to a lesser extent in localized blockage, as in calf vein thrombosis. A high venous pressure also causes oedema in severe varicose vein disease. Bilateral oedema suggests a general cause such as raised central venous pressure due to cardiac failure.

In lymphatic oedema, the capability of the lymphatics to remove fluid from the interstitial tissues is impaired. This may be due to such conditions as congenital hypoplasia, neoplastic infiltration or, rarely in Britain, filariasis. Surgical excision of lymph glands, especially if it is followed by radiotherapy that results in further damage to the lymphatics, is a common cause of oedema, as when cancer of the breast is treated by radical mastectomy followed by radiotherapy.

ACUTE PERIPHERAL CIRCULATORY DEFICIENCY

When the peripheral circulation is suddenly interrupted, immediate recognition of the following features is vital if the affected limb (usually the leg) is to be saved by medical or surgical measures:

- pain
- paralysis
- pallor
- pulselessness

It is also important to recognize the stages through which these features progress so that the severity of the condition and prognosis can be assessed at the time the limb is examined. The three important stages are:

- early: the ideal time for treatment
- intermediate: the stage of apparent recovery, although time is really running out
- late: the limb cannot now be saved

Symptoms are summarized in Table 14, below.

The early stage

Characteristically, the first symptom is sudden, severe pain in the leg and almost immediately there is total loss of function. The limb feels numb, heavy and cold. Examination shows a waxy pallor that progresses rapidly upwards from the toes. The pulses are absent below the site of obstruction, but the pulse immediately above the block may feel stronger than normal. This is the stage at which the condition must be recognized and treatment started to have a good chance of saving the limb.

The intermediate stage

Within a few hours the foot becomes oedematous. Paradoxically, at this stage there may be a slight recovery of voluntary movements in the more proximal joints and the area of pallor may recede slightly.

These signs may cause understandable, but inadvisable, optimism. They must not be allowed to delay active treatment or the condition will inevitably progress to necrosis and gangrene.

The (too) late stage

Later, the leg becomes progressively more oedematous, the toes become darkly cyanosed and there is a mottled cyanosis more proximally. By this time, the limb is very cold, the foot moves into plantar flexion and the leg is completely anaesthetic and powerless.

About 8–12 hours after the onset of acute ischaemia, progressive small vessel thrombosis and tissue necrosis occur and it becomes impossible to save the leg. Early diagnosis and urgent treatment are vital if this disaster is to be avoided.

TABLE 14 Symptoms in acute peripheral circulatory deficiency

The early stage	The intermediate stage	The (too) late stage
Sudden, severe pain	Pain is less severe	Anaesthetic
Total loss of function	Some functional recovery	Completely powerless
Progressive pallor	Pallor recedes	Mottled cyanosis
Coldness	Coldness	Coldness
Pulses absent below the obstruction	Distal oedema develops	Marked oedema Plantar flexion of the foot

Causes

The causes of acute arterial obstruction are:

- thrombosis
- embolus
- trauma

Thrombosis

Acute thrombosis is the commonest cause, occurring in a previously diseased and narrowed atheromatous vessel. Thrombosis may be precipitated by a sudden fall in cardiac output.

Embolus

Emboli may arise from blood clots, vegetations on

heart valves or atheromatous plaques. Emboli originate mainly from the heart. In the past, they usually occurred in patients with mitral stenosis and atrial fibrillation: now they most frequently follow recent myocardial infarction. Less often, emboli originate from atheromatous plaques in the proximal arterial tree or in aortic aneurysms.

One way and another, therefore, atheroma plays the major role in the aetiology of acute arterial obstruction.

Sites of emboli

Emboli most often lodge in the lower limb vessels, at or just beyond the bifurcation of a major artery. The commonest sites are at the bifurcation of the:

- common femoral artery
- common iliac artery
- aorta

Acute obstruction of upper limb vessels is much less common.

Thrombosis or embolus

Embolism is commonly followed by local thrombotic extension and so the differentiation between thrombosis and embolus may be difficult.

Atrial fibrillation or a recent myocardial infarction suggests an embolus. The absence of a cardiac abnormality or the presence of peripheral vascular disease, such as a history of intermittent claudication, suggest thrombosis.

Trauma

Traumatic injuries may also cause acute circulatory deficiency. Such injuries may be

- open, and therefore obvious
- closed, and much less obvious

An open wound with a damaged artery is obvious, but internal arterial damage may have occurred even when the external surface of the vessel looks intact.

Closed injuries with distal ischaemia should always suggest the possibility of arterial damage. Injuries, especially those close to joints, may cause occlusion of vessels by pressure from a fractured or dislocated bone or from an expanding haematoma. Those around the elbow and dislocated shoulders are particularly dangerous.

Arterial injuries must be recognized quickly, because urgent surgical exploration is essential if severe ischaemic damage is to be avoided.

Dissecting aneurysm

Dissecting aneurysms may cause sudden peripheral circulatory deficiency. The dissection usually begins in the thoracic aorta and symptoms start with pain in the chest, abdomen or back. Signs of limb ischaemia may present later, but may improve spontaneously as the dissection passes the origin of the involved artery.

CHRONIC PERIPHERAL CIRCULATORY DEFICIENCY

Chronic peripheral circulatory deficiency most commonly presents with signs and symptoms in the lower limbs. The underlying pathology in most cases is atherosclerosis causing progressive arterial occlusion.

When assessing a patient with chronic circulatory deficiency, remember that the disease process seen in the limbs is only one manifestation of generalized arterial disease. Such patients usually have coronary and cerebral arterial disease as well and this may be more important and potentially more life-threatening than the peripheral arterial disease.

The plan of management must always be decided with this in mind, after a full assessment of the whole cardiovascular system.

The patient

Patients with chronic peripheral circulatory deficiency usually complain of:

- pain
- skin changes

The severity and distribution of these symptoms are important, because they can indicate the probable site and potential danger of the disease process.

Limb pain

This is of two types depending upon the severity of the condition:

- pain that comes only on exertion (intermittent claudication)
- pain that is present at rest

Intermittent claudication

This is pain felt in active muscles. It indicates that their blood supply, which is adequate at rest or on slight exertion, becomes inadequate as effort increases. Such pain is usually the first symptom of peripheral circulatory deficiency in younger patients (45–55 years).

The pain of intermittent claudication comes on after walking a specific distance – the claudication distance – and is fairly constant for the individual. It is a dull, cramp-like pain that is related to the distance walked and the effort expended. Thus, the claudication distance is less when the patient walks quickly. The pain increases in severity until the patient has to stop. This relieves the pain in a few minutes. He then walks on and the pain returns after a similar or slightly shorter distance. There is often an associated loss of sensation and a feeling of coldness in the foot. Because of the regular need to stop to relieve the pain, patients with claudication, like those with untreated angina, often become expert window-shoppers.

The site of arterial narrowing can be predicted because it is always proximal to the area of claudication. Thus:

- buttock claudication indicates an aorto-iliac occlusion
- calf claudication indicates a femoral occlusion
- foot claudication indicates an occlusion below the knee

Claudication is felt in the muscles of propulsion, most often in the calf, less often in the buttock and only rarely in the foot. The natural history is variable and difficult to predict. The symptoms tend to improve as collateral vessels open up, but may remain static or deteriorate quite quickly if the disease progresses.

Rest pain

This occurs in an older group of patients (over 55 years) with chronic peripheral circulatory deficiency.

At first, pain is felt in the forefoot when lying in bed at night, but may progress to become. constant throughout the day. It is usually described as a severe burning pain that dominates the patient's life. It is only controlled by powerful analgesics and the patient will often plead to have the painful foot amputated.

Although the patient feels that the foot is hot, it is cold to the touch.

In an attempt to gain relief from the pain, which comes on whenever the leg is raised to the horizontal position, the patient characteristically sits in bed with the knee bent, holding on to the forefoot. He may hang the leg out from under the bedclothes or put it down onto a cold floor. In severe cases, he may sit up in a chair all night rather than go to bed.

Rest pain is of much more serious prognostic importance than claudication because it indicates that the blood supply has become inadequate, even at rest. In severe cases, urgent treatment is needed if the limb is to be saved.

Skin changes

These vary with the severity of the condition. The patient may first notice cold feet, numbness or paraesthesia and, as the blood supply decreases, he may notice his foot has become pale and wasted. In more advanced cases ischaemic ulcers appear over pressure points or between the toes and these hardly ever heal spontaneously. Finally, frank gangrene supervenes.

Impotence

Male patients may sometimes complain of impotence, because they cannot achieve or sustain an erection. This can be caused by bilateral occlusion of the internal iliac arteries, either in isolation or in association with an aortic occlusion. The triad of:

- impotence
- absent femoral pulses
- intermittent claudication of buttock muscles

is called the Leriche syndrome after the surgeon who described it.

When examining and assessing patients with chronic peripheral circulatory deficiency, it is important to assess not only the local circulation but also the patient's physical status and life style. For example, serious coronary or cerebral arterial disease may be more important than the claudication and preclude surgical treatment. A sedentary, retired, car owner with a claudication distance of 200 metres is unlikely to need an operation, whereas a postman would be significantly disabled and unable to earn a living in such circumstances.

VARICOSE VEINS

Varicosity of the lower limb veins is a common

complaint, especially amongst women after they reach middle age, and is a cause of considerable physical and mental discomfort.

The normal direction of blood flow in the lower limb veins is from the superficial veins through the deep fascia to the deep veins and thence to the iliac veins. Because of the upright posture, this one-way flow relies upon:

- the pumping action of the lower limb muscles to drive blood upwards under pressure
- competent one-way valves to prevent reflux (LD-104, LD-105)

Veins become varicose when a valve becomes incompetent. This allows blood at a higher than normal pressure to reflux into the superficial veins, which lie unsupported in loose subcutaneous tissues and dilate. In an adult, the pressure when standing is that of a column of blood about 115 cm (45 inches) long from the ankle to the level of the heart. This high pressure acts on the next valve along the system, which eventually also becomes incompetent, and so the condition tends to progress.

Varicose veins are dilated and elongated superficial veins, visible through the skin when the patient stands. As the condition progresses, the veins become more and more tortuous, and their walls become thickened and fixed to the surrounding superficial tissues.

Causes

Varicose veins can be classified as

- primary
- secondary

Primary (or idiopathic)

Most cases fall into this category. No predisposing cause can be found, though there seems to be a familial tendency.

Secondary

Predisposing causes include

- deep venous thrombosis
  This destroys the valves between the deep and superficial systems and allows blood at high pressure to enter the superficial veins.

- pelvic tumours
  These may obstruct flow through the large pelvic veins and increase venous pressure in the legs. This applies also to the pregnant uterus and may be one reason why varicose veins are more common in women.

- constipation
  pressure from an overloaded colon is suggested as a cause for the higher incidence of varicose veins in left leg.

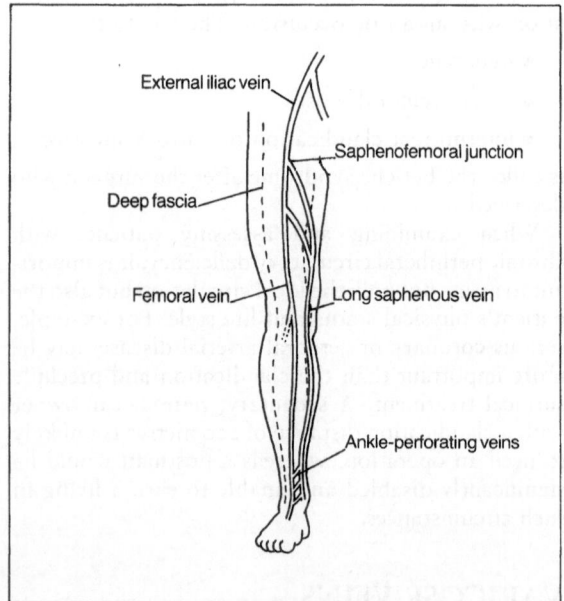

LD-104. *Front of leg showing the superficial veins and the positions of the more important one-way valves*

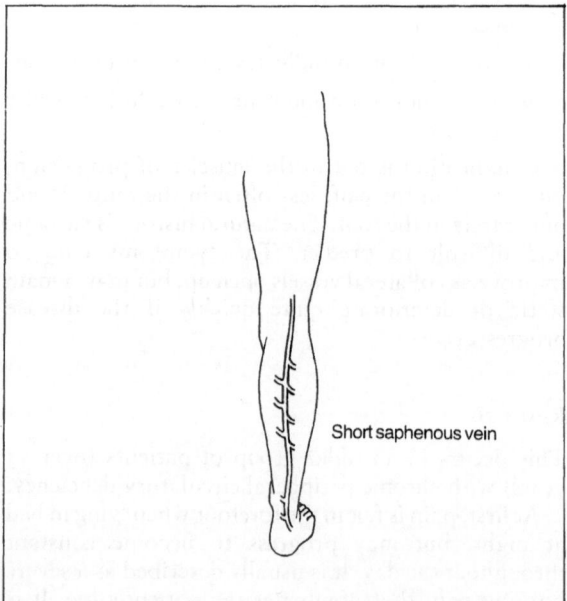

LD-105. *Back of leg showing the superficial veins and the positions of the more important one-way valves*

The patient

History

Patients may present for various reasons:

- prominent veins
  These are easily seen when the patient stands and treatment may be sought for cosmetic reasons
- discomfort and fatigue
  Many patients describe an aching discomfort and a heavy dragging sensation, worst after prolonged standing or walking. It is relieved by elevating the legs and reduced by wearing compression stockings. Pain may be localized to particular varicosities if they are affected by thrombophlebitis. Localized pain may also be a feature of infected varicose ulcers
- ankle oedema
  This is due to poor venous return
- microvarices
  These are prominent subcutaneous venules seen as a flare, especially over the medial side of the ankle. This is a danger signal; varicose eczema and subsequently varicose (gravitational) ulceration may develop if the veins are left untreated
- blow-outs
  These are swellings that occur at the site of incompetent valves. They are non-pulsatile and easily compressible. A fluid thrill can be felt when the vein below is gently tapped. They disappear when the limb is elevated and the veins emptied. At the saphenous opening such a blow-out, called a saphena varix, can be confused with a femoral hernia

Complications

These include:

- phlebitis
- ulceration
- haemorrhage

Phlebitis

Superficial thrombophlebitis causes localized pain and signs of inflammation. In severe cases, the leg is swollen and the pain more diffuse and throbbing.

Ulceration

Chronic venous insufficiency causes nutritional changes in the skin, particularly over the medial malleolus, that may eventually lead to ulceration. Ulcers may become infected and, in longstanding cases, malignant changes may occur.

Haemorrhage

Bleeding from varicose veins caused by trauma can be considerable and very alarming. It is however, easily treated by elevating the limb and applying pressure to the bleeding point.

Management

Management includes:

- compression stockings
- compression sclerotherapy
- surgical ligation of incompetent veins and stripping of superficial varicosities

Treatment is described in more detail on pp. 233 and depends on the careful localization of the sites of incompetence by the Trendelenburg test (see p. 94). The present trend is to deal surgically with varicosities above the knee and to treat those below the knee by compression sclerotherapy. The use of compression stockings is reserved for mild cases and for those unwilling or unfit to have definitive treatment.

THROMBOSIS AND EMBOLISM

Occlusions of blood vessels may occur anywhere in the body. They are caused either by thrombosis *in situ* or by embolism from a distant source.

Thrombosis

Thrombosis results from many factors including:

- damage to the vessel wall
- stasis or sluggishness of blood flow
- alterations in the clotting mechanism

Certain conditions appear to predispose:

- age

- bed rest and immobility
- the postoperative state
- the female sex
- oral contraceptives
- pregnancy
- obesity
- neoplastic disease

Age

Thromboembolism is most common after the age of 50. The reasons for this are not certain. Many associated diseases such as cancer and heart failure are then also more common, as are immobility and venous stasis.

Bed rest and immobility

Changes may occur in the clotting mechanism as a result of immobility. In bedfast patients, the weight of the lower limb compresses the veins and this, along with reduction in normal muscle pumping, leads to venous stasis. These factors encourage clotting, but the underlying disease causing the immobility may be an equally important factor.

The postoperative state

This seems to be a particularly vulnerable period, especially for patients in the older age groups. Those having major abdominal surgery or suffering major injuries are at greater risk.

Sex specificity and oral contraceptives

Females are more prone than males to thrombotic events. This was recognized long before the advent of the contraceptive pill, which itself increases the risk of thrombosis. The increased thrombotic tendency is probably related to oestrogen, because oral contraceptives that contain large amounts of oestrogen are most likely to cause thrombosis. It appears that during the follicular phase of the menstrual cycle and in those using oral contraceptives, there is increased activity of many of the natural clotting factors.

Pregnancy

Various factors operate in pregnancy, especially during the puerperium. These include a degree of venous stasis in the lower limbs and immobility due to bed rest. The suppression of lactation by oestrogens is a further predisposing factor.

Obesity

Obese patients are often relatively immobile and suffer from associated conditions such as varicose veins, but the real reasons for their acknowledged increased risk of thrombosis is not known.

Neoplastic disease

The reasons for the increased clotting tendency in patients with carcinoma, particularly of the bronchus, stomach and pancreas, are not understood but probably relate to changes in levels of several clotting factors and platelets.

Site

Thrombosis occurs in veins and arteries.

Veins

It is more common in veins than in arteries and those most commonly affected include the:

- deep veins of the calf and thigh
- veins of the pelvis

Thrombosis may also occur within the heart. Causes for this include:

- mitral stenosis
  Clots form in the atria, usually but not always in the left atrium and especially in the presence of atrial fibrillation
- myocardial infarction
  Thrombosis may occur over the infarcted area of myocardium usually in the left ventricle
- infective endocarditis
  Thrombus forms at the site of infection, usually on valves or occasionally in association with a congenital malformation.

Arteries

Thrombosis commonly occurs in:

- coronary arteries
- pulmonary arteries
- carotid and cerebral arteries
- retinal arteries

Less commonly the arteries supplying the kidneys, spleen or mesentery may be involved.

The symptoms and signs of thrombosis are due to:

- obstruction of the blood supply to the affected organ
- detachment of a clot that causes embolism in a distant organ

Embolism

Although usually due to blood clot, it may also be caused by:

- fat
- air
- tumour cells

The source of emboli may be either venous or arterial (systemic).

Venous emboli

These most commonly originate in the deep veins of the lower limb or pelvis; occasionally in the right atrium.

Systemic emboli

These often originate in the heart from the sources detailed above; occasionally from atheromatous lesions in the aorta and its major branches.

The target organ depends on the origin of the embolus.

Venous emboli end up in a branch of the pulmonary artery. They may occlude a large branch or break up and occlude one or more smaller branches. The result is pulmonary infarction.

Systemic emboli from the heart commonly find their way to the limbs or the brain. They may also obstruct arteries supplying internal organs, notably those of the kidney, spleen or mesentery and, occasionally, the coronary arteries. Emboli from the aorta usually find their way to the lower limbs; those from the carotid arteries into the vertebrobasilar system. Organs most seriously affected by embolism are those supplied by end arteries where the result is infarction.

Fat and air emboli cause their greatest damage in the brain.

TEST-YOURSELF QUESTIONS
Sections I, II and III

1. Match the statement on the left with the most appropriate condition on the right.

1) Commonest cause of death in males
2) Commonest cause of death in females
3) Highest consultation rate in males in general practice
4) Highest consultation rate in females in general practice
5) Commonest cause of death in Japan

a) Chronic rheumatic heart disease
b) Coronary heart disease
c) Hypertensive disease
d) Cerebrovascular disease
e) Other forms of heart disease

2. Which of the following statements is/are true concerning the heart?

a) About 85% of the blood is contained within the systemic circulation
b) The resistance to flow in the pulmonary circuit is greater than in the systemic circuit
c) As the heart rate increases the duration of diastole is reduced to a lesser extent than the duration of systole
d) The parasympathetic control of the heart is mainly concerned with ventricular contractility
e) An increase in sympathetic activity has a positive chronotropic effect by acting on the SA node

3. In relation to electrical excitation of the heart put the following in sequence order.

a) AV node
b) Ventricular muscle
c) Bundle of His
d) Sinoatrial node

4. a) What does Poiseuille's law tell us about blood vessel resistance and flow rate?
   b) What happens to flow rate when you halve the radius of the vessel?

5. Match the conditions on the left with the most appropriate item in the list on the right.

1) Pericarditis
2) Myocarditis
3) Rheumatic heart disease
4) Brown atrophy
5) Cardiomyopathy

a) Abnormal immune response to group A β-haemolytic streptococci
b) Uraemia
c) Alcoholism
d) Coxsackie B infection
e) Increase in pigment lipofuscin

6. Which of the following findings are abnormal on an ECG?

a) P wave of 0.16 s
b) PR interval of 0.24 s
c) Isoelectric S T segment
d) Presence of U wave
e) Inverted T wave in V1

7. What are the typical ECG changes of a myocardial infarction?

8. Match the ECG changes on the left with the site of the infarction on the right.

a) 11, 111 + aVF
b) V1-3
c) Precordial leads, I and aVL
d) V4-6

1) Anterior infarction
2) Anterolateral infarction
3) Inferior infarction
4) Anteroseptal infarction

9. Which of the following statements is/are true of radiological examination of the heart?

a) Increased pulmonary blood flow is usually more obvious in the left side
b) Evidence of pulmonary venous hypertension is usually more readily detected in the upper lobes
c) Kerley's B lines are a feature of chronic interstitial pulmonary oedema
d) Films should be taken with the breath held in full expiration

10. Which of the following make up the left border of the heart on postero-anterior X-ray.
a) The aortic arch
b) The left ventricle
c) The superior vena cava
d) The pulmonary trunk
e) The right atrium

11. For each of the features on the left select the most appropriate diagnosis on the right.
a) Orthopnoea
b) Pulmonary crepitations
c) Jugular venous disternum
d) A third heart sound
e) Hepatic congestion

1) Left heart failure
2) Right heart failure
3) Neither

12. If a patient complains of a pain in the chest, what seven items of information should you establish about the pain?

13. A patient complains of palpitations. What further questions should be asked relating to the palpitations?

14. A patient complains of syncope. What further questions should you ask?

15. What is the name for each of these findings on examination of the pulse?
a) Rate quickening towards the end of inspiration and slowing during expiration
b) Pulse rate at wrist less than rate measured on cardiac auscultation
c) Beats are 'coupled'
d) Regular rhythm with regular changes in pulse pressure
e) An abnormally rapid upstroke

16. Match the murmurs on the left with the conditions on the right.
a) Early systolic murmurs at apex
b) Ejection murmur at base
c) Pansystolic murmur at mitral area
d) Early diastolic murmur down left sternal border
e) Mid diastolic murmur at apex

1) Aortic stenosis
2) Mitral incompetence
3) Aortic incompetence
4 Mitral stenosis
5) Of no pathological significance

17. List five causes of angina.

18. List four cardiac causes of dyspnoea and three respiratory causes.

19. What five cardiovascular conditions should be considered in a patient with haemoptysis?

20. What causes would you consider in a patient who complains of oedema of the ankle?

21. In a patient with severe generalised oedema what features in the history suggest a cardiac cause?

22. List ten causes of syncope.

23. For each of the features below indicate whether you think it is typical of
1) central cyanosis
2) peripheral cyanosis
3) central and peripheral cyanosis
a) More than 5 g per cent of the circulating haemoglobin is reduced
b) Lessens when the skin is warmer
c) Increased by exercise
d) Associated with clubbing
e) Found in polycythaemia

24. List the important features to be ascertained from the history in the assessment of hypertension.

25. List five symptoms of acute peripheral circulatory deficiency.

26. In relation to acute peripheral circulatory deficiency
a) what is the commonest embolic cause
b) what is the commonest site for emboli?

27. List three conditions that predispose to varicose veins.

28. List six conditions which predispose to thrombosis.

The answers to these questions can be found on p.277.

SECTION IV

Description of Specific Diseases

CORONARY HEART DISEASE

People are living longer in the Western world largely because infectious disease has been controlled. As a result, coronary heart disease (CHD) has become the leading cause of disability and death. In CHD, the coronary arteries become narrowed and blood flow to the heart is impaired. The usual cause is atherosclerosis, fibrofatty plaques that form in the arterial wall. These plaques are vulnerable to further pathological changes such as haemorrhage, ulceration and thrombosis that may result in abrupt clinical deterioration.

During the past 20 years, a great deal has been learned about CHD but, although many of those at risk can now be identified, and theories abound, its cause remains a mystery.

Prevalence

A total of 200 000 Americans under 65 years of age dies each year from the consequences of CHD. By the age of 65, 50% of Americans have significant stenosis of at least one coronary artery. An autopsy study of American soldiers (average age 22) killed in action in Korea showed that 75% of them already had some gross evidence of coronary artery disease. Similar findings were noted during the Vietnam war.

In the United Kingdom, CHD is the major cause of death in middle and old age. In men aged 45–54, 52% of all deaths in 1973 were due to cardiovascular disease and more than 75% of these deaths were due to CHD. This compares with 26% of deaths due to cancer. The death rate in younger men has increased more than it has in older men. It is higher in Scotland and Northern Ireland than in England and Wales. Age specific incidence and mortality rates rise more or less logarithmically throughout life, approximately doubling every 10 years.

The male:female ratio diminishes progressively from a maximum of 6:1 below 40 years of age to about equality in later life.

The picture is not completely bleak. In the United States the death rate from CHD – although still unacceptably high – has fallen by around 25% in the past few years. Similar trends may be developing in the Netherlands, Finland and Belgium. In the United Kingdom, the death rate seems to be on a plateau. The reasons for this change remain obscure, although some claim that it is related to less cigarette smoking, better diet, more exercise and improved treatment.

CHD in the community

Hospital admissions give only a limited view of the problem. Community studies are more informative, as can be seen in Table 14.

TABLE 14

	Oxford Region	Edinburgh
Total population	325 000	500 000
Cases registered	373	1858
Attack rates per 1000 men per annum aged 40–69	6	16
28-day fatality rate	59%	33%
Deaths in hospital as a fraction of the total	28%	27%

More than half of all deaths from CHD occur within 2 hours, many of them suddenly, so that most of those who do not survive heart attacks die outside hospital without medical treatment. The long term aim in the management of CHD must therefore be prevention rather than cure.

Pathology

Experimental myocardial infarction has been shown not to be an instantaneous process. It progresses over several hours with increasing cell death that starts in the core of the ischaemic area and, in time, involves more and more of the periphery. In the dog, 3 hours after ligation of the circumflex coronary artery, one third of the ultimate infarct area remains viable. This agrees with the clinical impression that myocardial infarction can progress over several hours and has led to a concentrated effort to lessen infarct size in the human. Oxygen, drugs and surgery have all been used. Disappointingly, no definite benefit has yet been shown.

In the early stages of infarction, little may be apparent either to the naked eye or with conventional staining methods. Special staining for enzyme activity can indicate areas of damage and potential or established necrosis (Table 15).

Atheroma

The cause of myocardial infarction is usually atheroma, fibrofatty deposits in the arterial intima.

There is a lack of good experimental models because man is almost unique in suffering from spontaneous occlusive vascular disease.

By the time atheroma presents as a clinical prob-

TABLE 15

Time since infarction	Pathological change
12–18 h	Cytoplasmic clumping, cellular infiltration
24 h	Infarct identifiable as a yellow or pale area
48–72 h	Loss of muscle striation
3–4 d	Necrosis maximal
5–6 d	Development of connective tissue and new blood vessels at periphery
3rd week–6th month	Fibrosis and scar formation

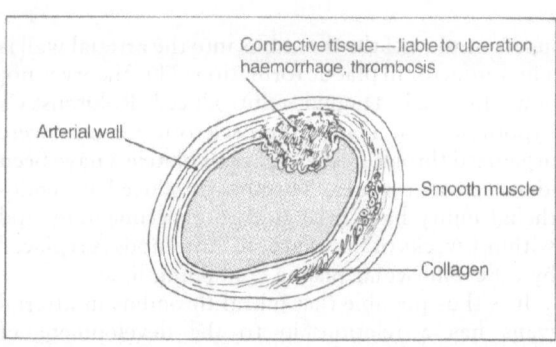

LD-106. *Fibrolipid plaque*

lem, it is usually far advanced. Its development is a lifelong process. The target organs (heart, brain etc.) may be so severely affected that symptomatic treatment is all that can be offered.

Mechanism

Although the precise mechanisms of atherosclerosis remain uncertain, there is considerable clinical and experimental evidence to suggest that the initiating factor is endothelial injury. Normal endothelium allows only minimal entrance of lipid into the arterial wall, but, when local damage occurs, lipids and other plasma constituents can and do infiltrate the wall.

Clinically the process develops in stages:

- damage to the arterial wall
- thrombus formation on plaques leading to narrowing or occlusion
- reduction in target organ blood flow

The obstruction may be either gradual or sudden.

Cause

The aetiology of atherosclerosis remains obscure despite large scale clinical, epidemiological, biochemical and pathological studies. It has been defined as a common process affecting the large elastic and muscular arteries and characterized by areas of intimal thickening. These thickened areas consist partly of proliferated connective tissue, partly of lipid and other material from the plasma and partly of cell debris. The process is, therefore, a combination of proliferation and degeneration.

The classical lesion is the fibrolipid plaque. This is raised above the arterial lining and has a rich lipid base (LD-106).

There have been many theories concerning atherosclerosis and its cause. The current view is that under normal circumstances the arterial endothelial cells protect the intima and media by acting as a filtration

barrier. These cells may be damaged by turbulent blood flow or other adverse factors such as catecholamines, high blood pressure, cigarette smoking and anoxia. Once endothelial change occurs, platelets aggregate, blood fats enter the intimal space and smooth muscle cells migrate into the area. Fibrinogen from the plasma may also infiltrate the lesion, collagen fibres are laid down and a fibrofatty plaque is formed that reduces the lumen of the vessel.

Cholesterol is a major constituent of atherosclerotic plaques. It constitutes 65–85% of the total lipid present. Turnover studies suggest that it is mostly derived from plasma lipoproteins. Recent immunofluorescence studies suggest that lipoproteins can cross the intact intimal wall and that more passes across when the blood pressure is elevated. Either an increase in permeability of the arterial barrier or a decline in clearing mechanisms seems probable. Among the causes could be:

- mechanical injury
  high blood pressure, shearing stress at certain parts of the wall due to turbulent blood flow etc.
- chemical injury
  anoxia, catecholamines etc.

Injury to the arterial wall is followed by an attempt at repair. Platelets adhere to the damaged area. Smooth muscle cells proliferate in response to the secretion of a low molecular weight protein by the platelets. Such proliferation of smooth muscle cells can also be induced by low density lipoprotein (LDL). It is possible that the smooth muscle proliferation also acts as a non-specific repair process.

Deposition of lipid in the wall, the development of atherosclerotic plaques and the complications of haemorrhage, thrombosis and calcification represent one theory of atherosclerosis.

An alternative theory has also been proposed. This suggests that mural thrombosis with subsequent incorporation of the thrombus into the arterial wall is a major factor in plaque formation. This theory is not new. In 1946, Duguid reintroduced Rokitansky's hypothesis that many atherosclerotic plaques were organized thrombi. Aggregates of platelets have been identified in plaques. Thrombi produced by endothelial injury have been studied experimentally and within 3 weeks of the injury, the thrombus is replaced by a fibromuscular plaque containing lipid.

It is thus possible that mural thrombus in arterial walls has a relationship to the development of atherosclerotic plaques and it seems likely that the presence of thrombus can bring about a prompt proliferative response.

Risk factors

Risk factors are characteristics found in healthy or apparently healthy individuals that relate to the subsequent appearance of CHD. There are considerable gaps in our knowledge of risk factors and what they contribute to the occurrence of CHD. Many individuals who would appear to be at high risk do not develop CHD. Others, who have no apparent risk factors, do develop CHD.

In general, the risk of CHD is determined by the aggregate of individual risk factors, perhaps better regarded as risk indicators. Some factors that help to identify individuals at high risk cannot be modified. These include age, sex, diabetes and family history. Other risk factors such as physical inactivity, cigarette smoking and obesity can be modified.

The risk factors to be considered are:

- plasma lipids
- cigarette smoking
- blood pressure
- diabetes mellitus
- obesity
- lack of physical activity
- stress
- oral contraceptives

Plasma lipids

Plasma lipids have for long occupied an important place in thoughts about the cause of CHD. It is possible, although not yet certain, that their importance has been overemphasized.

Plasma cholesterol

Population studies throughout the world have consistently shown a relationship between the mean level of cholesterol and the prevalence of CHD.

Lipoproteins

It is usual to measure both cholesterol and triglyceride levels. These are markers for underlying disorders of lipoproteins. The combination of lipid and protein is the method whereby water-insoluble lipids can be transported in blood.

Prevention

There is no doubt that plasma lipid levels can be lowered by diet, by drugs or by their combination.

The results, in terms of reducing CHD, are disappointing. The Los Angeles Veterans study has faults in design and is a mixed study of primary and secondary prevention. One group was given a diet low in unsaturated fat and high in polyunsaturated fat. There were fewer CHD events in the treated group, but this did not reach clinical significance and there was no difference in total mortality. The study conducted in Finnish mental hospitals (1958–71) also had faults in design. There was a tendency overall for the treated group to have a lower incidence of CHD but no definite conclusions could be made. The large scale study conducted in three European cities under the auspices of the World Health Organization has produced many important results. The effect of clofibrate on cholesterol levels and CHD was investigated. Overall, the results suggested that clofibrate could reduce cholesterol by 7–10% and that the incidence of CHD was lower in the high risk group. However, there was also an increase in gallstone formation and in deaths from other causes such as alimentary cancer that did not occur in the corresponding control group. Overall, so many more deaths from other causes occurred in the treated group that they outweighed the reduction in deaths from CHD. On balance, clofibrate appeared to do more harm than good and cannot be recommended as a lipid-lowering agent for the prevention of CHD in the general population. It should be reserved for those with the appropriate lipoprotein disorders.

It is not surprising that attempts to lower plasma lipids by relatively small amounts in middle-aged men have not had a dramatic effect in the incidence of CHD. Theoretically at least, such therapy would need to be started early in life and continued on a lifelong basis.

Good general advice is to reduce the amount of fat

in the diet from 40% to 30% by eating less animal (saturated) fat. There is no evidence, however, that taking extra polyunsaturated fat is beneficial.

Cigarette smoking

The relationship between lung cancer and cigarette smoking is well known. What is less well known and requires emphasis is that the risk of a cigarette smoker dying from CHD is about twice that of a non-smoker. Pipe and cigar smokers, though at less risk, are not immune from the consequences, if they inhale.

The reason for the increased mortality among smokers is not clear. Cigarette smokers have increased atheroma. It may be that nicotine releases catecholamines that damage the endothelium. Smokers also have increased carboxyhaemoglobin levels that may damage endothelium and impair myocardial function.

Prevention

Stopping smoking is worth while. There is evidence that stopping reduces the chance of developing infarction. Those who stop smoking after a myocardial infarct have a lower incidence of reinfarction than those who continue to smoke.

Blood pressure

Raised blood pressure is a major risk factor in CHD. A single casual blood pressure reading is a powerful indicator of the extent of the risk. Both systolic and diastolic levels provide such indications. For middle-aged men, CHD increases by nearly 20% for each 10 mmHg increase in systolic pressure. Mild hypertension should not be ignored. Because of its prevalence, it contributes considerably to the occurrence of CHD.

It is uncertain how hypertension increases CHD. It may be because the vessel wall is damaged with a consequent increase in atheroma. In addition, left ventricular hypertrophy increases myocardial oxygen demands and aggravates ischaemia.

Prevention

The treatment of high blood pressure lowers the incidence of strokes and renal failure. It has not been shown convincingly that it lowers the incidence of CHD. Several studies currently in progress suggest that it does.

Diabetes mellitus

Atherosclerosis is common in patients with disorders of carbohydrate metabolism. It is almost invariably present in those who have had diabetes for more than 5 years and there is a high incidence of preclinical diabetes in those with premature or unexplained coronary heart disease.

Acceleration of coronary atherosclerosis is especially striking in women, even in those with normal blood lipids who are premenopausal and normotensive. As a result, angina and myocardial infarction occur as commonly in diabetic women over the age of 40 as they do in men – the risk of these conditions being twice as high for men and three times as high for women as it is in the general population.

The risks associated with coronary heart disease are also considerably increased. About 40% of those receiving medical care do not survive their first infarct and fewer of those who survive are alive at the end of 5 years than in non-diabetics.

Obesity

Obesity is thought of by the public as a major contributor to CHD. There is no doubt that fat people tend to have high blood pressure, raised lipids and sedentary habits, but obesity alone, unless gross, is probably not such an important risk factor as it was once thought to be. None the less, there are good physical and psychological reasons why weight should be reduced. Not least is that people feel better when they get their weight down.

Lack of physical activity

Physical activity is also in the public eye, as evidenced by jogging, which many believe will prevent heart attacks. This may well be true, although there is no hard evidence that it does. Active exercise lowers lipids, improves myocardial oxygen consumption and may promote coronary collateral circulation. Care should be taken by those who are overweight, are over 40, have had a previous infarct or have not exercised for some years. Such people should have a physical examination before starting on an exercise programme and should start off gradually under medical supervision.

Stress

Many lay people link heart disease with stress. Stress is difficult to define, however, and its role as a risk factor is not clearly established. Obviously, it must be considered along with other factors, but many people enjoy the stimulus of a challenging situation and appear to thrive on it.

Oral contraceptives

Oral contraceptives, especially those with a high oestrogen content, have recently received publicity as a possible cause of myocardial infarction in young women. The risk appears to rise considerably in those with a family history of CHD, a raised blood pressure, obesity, in those who smoke cigarettes, and who are over 40.

Clinical features

Coronary atheroma is so common in the adult population that it is now regarded almost as a normal finding. Many postmortem studies have shown extensive coronary atheroma at all ages in people who have no cardiac symptoms and who have died from non-cardiac causes.

Thus, those with coronary atheroma will not necessarily develop symptoms and it is important to distinguish between coronary artery disease and coronary heart disease (CHD). The natural history of CHD is notoriously variable. Some with extensive atheroma in their coronary arteries have no symptoms, some are crippled by angina, some have recurrent episodes of myocardial infarction and some drop down dead. Those affected may be in their early twenties or late eighties and it is now becoming increasingly common in women of child-bearing age.

Even after the disease has become clinically obvious, its effects on those who survive are unpredictable. Many who recover from major infarcts lead apparently normal lives for many years; others survive for only a short period before succumbing to another attack.

Although the outcome clearly depends to some extent upon the severity of the arterial disease and the number of major vessels involved, this is by no means the whole story, because patients with what appear to be identical lesions may follow a vastly different clinical course.

Angina pectoris

Definition

Angina pectoris is a feeling of tightness or discomfort in the chest (and also in other areas) brought on by effort or excitement or both. It is usually of short duration and is relieved by resting or by taking sublingual nitrates.

The symptoms are due to myocardial ischaemia and occur when the myocardium demands more oxygen than the coronary circulation can supply.

The major determinants of myocardial oxygen consumption are:

- the magnitude of systolic wall stress (pressure/volume)
- the fraction of time during which stress is exerted
- the contractile state of the heart

When a patient has typical angina pectoris relieved by rest or glyceryl trinitrate there is an 80–90% chance that coronary atherosclerosis is the cause. The extent of the coronary atherosclerosis varies. Usually more than 50% narrowing of two major coronary arteries has occurred before angina develops, but this is not always the case. Coronary angiography has demonstrated that fairly severe angina may be present in patients who have only single vessel coronary artery disease.

Remember too that the presence of coronary atheroma does not necessarily cause angina. Many patients without angina, who die from unrelated causes, are found to have extensive coronary heart disease. Studies in both Korea and Vietnam have shown fairly extensive coronary atheroma in many apparently healthy young men killed in battle.

Causes

Although the usual cause of angina is atherosclerotic narrowing of the major coronary arteries, many other factors may contribute to myocardial oxygen imbalance:

- non-atherosclerotic disease of coronary arteries
  Disease of small intramyocardial vessels such as is reputed to occur in collagen diseases and perhaps in diabetes
- hypertension
  Increased cardiac work is required because of the increased afterload
- anaemia
  Increased cardiac work takes place in the presence of diminished oxygen supply
- polycythaemia
  Increased cardiac work is caused by the increased viscosity of the blood
- valvar disease of the heart
  Increased left ventricular pressure, increased intramyocardial tension and diminished diastolic coronary artery filling are caused by aortic stenosis. Other valve lesions associated

with angina are aortic incompetence and mitral stenosis. Patients with prolapse of the mitral valve sometimes present with somewhat atypical chest pain

- paroxysmal disorders of cardiac rhythm
  These may be either tachycardias or bradycardias
- cardiomyopathies
  These may affect the myocardium and its blood supply
- thyroid dysfunction
  Both hypothyroidism and hyperthyroidism can cause myocardial ischaemia
- syphilis
  Some years ago late syphilis would have been regarded as a major cause of anginal pain, but it is seldom seen nowadays in Britain

History

When evaluating chest pain to decide whether or not a patient has angina pectoris, the following points should be considered:

- the nature of the pain
- its site and radiation
- precipitating factors
- relieving factors

Nature

The patient often describes heaviness, gripping, crushing or tightness. The sensation is not always thought of as pain and pain may be denied. It is deep rather than superficial and, when present in the arms, they are often said to feel heavy, numb or weak.

When describing the pain, patients often clench a fist and place it over the precordium.

Site and radiation

Anginal pain caused by myocardial ischaemia is referred to a superficial somatic segment. The usual site is over the centre of the precordium but it may occur anywhere from the epigastrium to the jaw or even in the back between the shoulder blades. In one typical series:

- 96% had pain in the chest and in 62% it radiated.
  Of the latter:
    33% had radiation to the left arm
    10% had radiation to the right arm
    16% had radiation to the back
     9% had radiation to the lower jaw

Pain localized to the apex of the heart is unlikely to be due to coronary heart disease. This type of pain is often classified as innocent left submammary pain for which no organic cause can be found. It is important not to label such a pain as cardiac pain because this often sows the seed of a cardiac neurosis.

Precipitating factors

Anything that increases the heart's oxygen requirement can cause pain. Exertion is by far and away the commonest cause, hence the term 'angina of effort'. Most patients with genuine cardiac pain soon learn about precipitating factors and take steps to avoid them whenever possible. These include:

- overexertion
- cold (weather or rooms, especially bedrooms)
- strong winds
- heavy meals
- emotion

Walking into the wind on a cold morning after breakfast is a classical example.

Excitement and anger are also well known precipitating factors – the increased sympathetic activity leading to increased demand for oxygen that cannot be supplied. John Hunter recognized his own frailty when he said 'my life is at the mercy of any rascal that chooses to annoy or tease me'.

Relieving factors

The duration of angina is usually short. It is nearly always relieved by standing still. If not, and especially when precipitated by emotion, sublingual glyceryl trinitrate is of great help. In more than 75% of patients, pain will be relieved in 3 minutes or less. If the pain is not rapidly relieved in either of these ways, the diagnosis is in doubt.

Although angina is nearly always precipitated by exercise, it can occur at rest. This is usually associated with serious coronary artery disease and, if it is severe and lasts for more than 20 minutes, it is difficult to differentiate from the pain of myocardial infarction.

Nocturnal angina

This is not common, but is distressing. It awakens the patient from sleep and may be a consequence of dreaming.

Prinzmetal's angina

This is an atypical variant of angina in which the pain

often occurs at rest. It is related to coronary artery spasm and may occur in both normal and atherosclerotic vessels.

Onset

Angina characteristically develops after exercise or emotional upset but can occur spontaneously at rest. It is usually associated with a rise in heart rate and blood pressure and is, in effect, a short-lived episode of left ventricular failure. This accounts for the breathlessness that is often a feature of an anginal attack.

Stable and unstable angina

Angina is frequently described as being stable or unstable.

Stable angina is a pattern of symptoms that has been present for some time and shows little change in either frequency or severity.

Unstable angina refers to a situation where the angina has occurred for the first time or to stable angina that is either becoming increasingly severe or developing on less and less effort, possibly even at rest. Such patients have an increased risk of myocardial infarction and require urgent investigation and treatment.

Significance

Angina pectoris is a frightening symptom. It is associated in the lay mind with heart disease and the fear of dropping down dead. The truth is, however, that it is difficult to predict the course of patients who present with angina. Some develop stable angina that may persist for many years and be kept almost symptom-free with medical therapy. Some have myocardial infarcts and after recovery become pain-free. Some improve spontaneously; some become so disabled, despite intensive treatment, that surgery is required.

The symptoms may lessen or disappear in 10–20% of patients. This is probably due to the development of a collateral circulation to the ischaemic area. Hypoxia is the most potent stimulus to vasodilatation and revascularization. Medical treatment can contribute considerably to management. Individuals with angina should not be given a gloomy prognosis and regarded as invalids. They should be encouraged to make every effort to keep active and lead a normal life.

Approach to the patient

This can be summarized in the flow chart, LD-107.

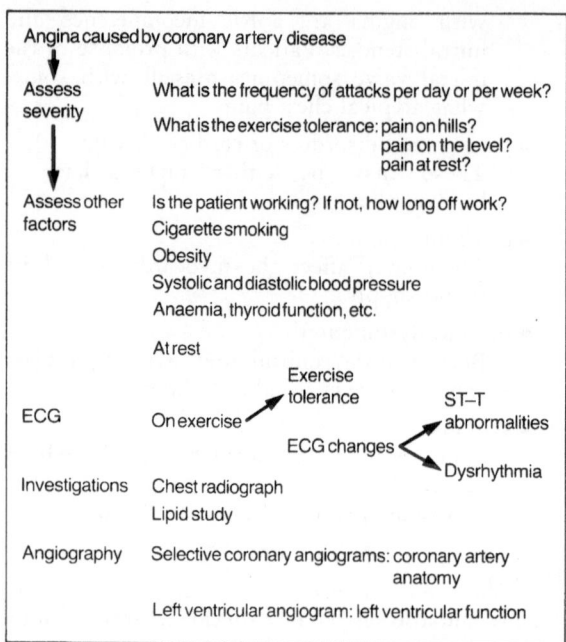

LD-107. *Flow chart of approach to patient*

The ECG

The resting ECG is normal in 50% of patients with angina. This should be no surprise. Their complaint is of chest pain on effort and the pain is due to transient myocardial ischaemia. When the patient rests, the myocardial ischaemia resolves and the symptoms subside. An abnormal ECG at rest means that the myocardium has already suffered permanent ischaemic damage. Such abnormalities may be those of previous myocardial infarction or ST segment depression, T wave flattening or inversion, or any combination of these (LD-108).

The ECG configuration gives only a rough guide to the site of ischaemia.

Changes in the inferior leads (III, AVF) are often associated with disease of the right coronary artery or the left circumflex coronary artery.

Changes in the anterior and lateral leads (I, AVL,

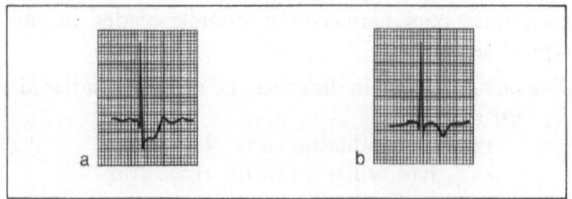

LD-108. *a, ST depression; b, T-wave inversion*

V_1–V_6) are usually associated with left coronary artery disease, especially the left anterior descending.

However, the relationship is not sufficiently close for an anatomical diagnosis of vessel disease to be made accurately on the basis of the ECG alone.

Exercise testing

If a patient complains of angina and the resting ECG is normal, an exercise test may be indicated. This is done using a treadmill or a bicycle ergometer. The slope and speed of the treadmill or the load on the bicycle are progressively increased every few minutes.

A normal exercise test demonstrates the patient's ability to increase the heart rate without causing angina or ECG abnormality. The target heart rate to be achieved is usually taken as 200 minus the age in years. Thus, a normal response in a man of 50 would be an exercise heart rate of 150 without either chest pain or an abnormal ECG.

A test may be positive in several ways. Angina can develop without ECG abnormality. This should cause suspicion, but is not diagnostic of myocardial ischaemia.

Conversely, the ECG may change without the development of chest pain. When this happens, the ECG changes should be studied carefully. Slight changes may occur normally with an increased heart rate. It is easy to overinterpret them and make a diagnosis of myocardial ischaemia where none exists. A positive exercise test shows ST segment depression of at least 1 mm, usually of 'square-wave' or 'plateau type' appearance (LD-109). In some cases the T wave also shows transient changes.

A further positive endpoint is the development of ectopic beats.

Exercise testing should never be done without careful supervision. A physician should either be present or immediately available and the ECG should be monitored continuously throughout the test. It is not sufficient to rely on symptoms; significant ECG changes may develop before pain.

Although exercise testing is usually a safe pro-

cedure, it should not be done unless resuscitation equipment is immediately available because major complications such as ventricular fibrillation, ventricular tachycardia or myocardial infarction are always possible.

Value of exercise testing

As noted above, the resting ECG is normal in 50% of patients with angina due to coronary heart disease. The combination of a resting ECG and an exercise test increases the yield of abnormalities from 50% to about 85% of those with angina who have demonstrable coronary disease.

In addition, the exercise test provides valuable information about the exercise tolerance and overall physical fitness of the individual being investigated.

Coronary angiography

Coronary angiography is a specialized and now widely used method of studying the coronary circulation. Radio-opaque contrast material is injected to outline the coronary arteries and cine films are taken in several planes to study the vessels. Each coronary artery is injected in turn, using pre-shaped catheters. The catheter can be inserted through the brachial artery or the femoral artery.

Coronary angiography is always accompanied by measurement of left ventricular pressure and left ventricular angiography. Cine films are taken during several cardiac cycles to assess left ventricular contraction and to detect areas of diminished or absent contraction and paradoxical pulsation.

Coronary angiography and left ventriculography complement each other, the aim being to assess both the state of the coronary arteries and the function of the left ventricle.

Indications

There are several indications for coronary angiography, but it is an investigation that causes both mortality and morbidity and should never be carried out without good reason.

The main indications are:

● assessment of patients with angina in the selection of those suitable for coronary bypass surgery

It is accepted that lesions occluding more than 70% of the external diameter of the vessel are likely to diminish coronary flow to a critical level

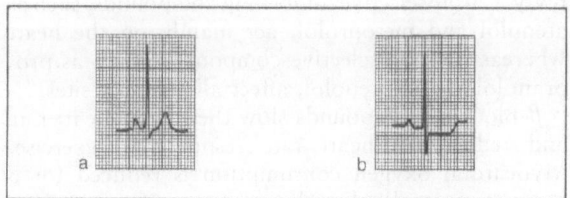

LD-109. *a, normal resting record; b, ST depression after exercise*

- assessment of the coronary circulation in patients with valvar disease to ensure that additional pathology is not present

  This is especially important in patients with aortic valve disease who are being considered for surgery

- diagnostic angiography to assess the coronary circulation in patients with recurrent episodes of chest pain of undetermined cause

  This may be necessary in those whose occupations involve the safety of others, e.g. drivers of public service vehicles and airline pilots

Prognostic value

It was realized long ago that knowledge about the extent of coronary disease might give valuable information about prognosis. As experience has accumulated, however, it has become clear that some patients with extensive coronary disease may have a better prognosis than had been initially reported. Patients with angina and significant disease of all three major coronary arteries, for example, are now known to have a 3 year survival rate of around 85%. For those with two-vessel disease, it is around 90%.

Patients with disease of the left main coronary artery before it divides into the left anterior and circumflex branches have a particularly bad prognosis and mortality probably reaches 40–50% over a 5 year period.

Who should have coronary angiography?

This causes considerable controversy. One point of view is that all patients with angina should have angiograms with a view to possible coronary bypass surgery. The alternative is that angiography should be reserved for those who fail to respond to medical treatment.

Medical management

New drugs have been developed for the treatment of angina and symptoms can be considerably relieved in most cases.

The first step in management is to give advice on the patient's life style. Risk factors, if present, should be corrected, for example:

- reduce obesity
- stop cigarette smoking
- advise about the level of activity
- avoid stress that is likely to produce pain

If pain persists, drug therapy should be considered.

Nitrates

These have been used for many years. Amyl nitrate was introduced by Lauder Brunton in Edinburgh more than 100 years ago.

Glyceryl trinitrate is at present the most widely used compound. It is taken sublingually and absorbed from the buccal mucosa. The standard dose is 0.5 mg. It is useful when taken prophylactically before effort that is known from experience to bring on pain. It is also useful in the treatment of the acute attack. Tolerance does not develop and tablets can be taken as required. The main side-effect is a pounding headache, probably due to dilatation of the cerebral vessels. This is most troublesome when glyceryl trinitrate is first used. Thereafter, it becomes less pronounced, although the beneficial actions persist. Often the dose can be reduced and pain relieved without causing a headache.

It acts not by dilating the diseased coronary arteries but by dilating the venous side of the circulation, the capacitance vessels. This reduces the venous return to the heart and the cardiac output so that less oxygen is required by the myocardium.

Intermediate and long-acting nitrates have been developed and, although these have been disappointing, there is now good evidence that a prolonged effect may be obtained.

β-Adrenoreceptor blocking compounds

Ahlquist developed the theory of the α- and β-adrenoreceptor system to explain the differing responses in various organs to catecholamines released from sympathetic nerve endings and the adrenal medulla. Black, in the early 1960s, used the theory to develop β-adrenoreceptor blocking compounds that would be useful in the management of angina. Propranolol was the first to be used successfully in long term management and remains the standard against which all the numerous newer β-blocking agents are judged.

A further development has been the recognition of β_1- and β_2-receptors. β_1-receptors are found mainly in the heart, β_2-receptors are found throughout the body. Cardioselective β-blocking compounds, such as atenolol and metoprolol, act mainly on the heart whereas the non-selective compounds, such as propranolol and oxprenolol, affect all receptor sites.

β-Blocking compounds slow the resting heart rate and reduce the heart rate response to exercise. Myocardial oxygen consumption is reduced for a given exercise level and symptoms of angina are relieved. The starting dose should be small and increased progressively until the symptoms are relieved or until symptoms occur because of bradycardia, which should not in itself be used as an indication to reduce the dose. Therapy should be discontinued slowly, never suddenly, because abrupt withdrawal of β-blockade can lead to worsening of angina or even myocardial infarction. β-Blockers should not be given in the presence of heart failure or bronchial asthma as both can be made worse.

Recent developments

Interest in longer acting nitrates has been revived with nitroglycerine ointments, pastes and patches, the concept of first pass metabolism in the liver and preparations that are slowly released and absorbed through the buccal mucosa.

A different approach to therapy has been the introduction of compounds that reduce calcium influx into the myocardial cell. This leads to diminished myocardial cell contractility and a reduced need for oxygen.

Results with drugs like nifedipine are promising and, when given in combination with β-blocking compounds, are effective in many patients who are difficult to treat. In some cases, however, calcium antagonists increase the severity and frequency of pain and have to be stopped.

The medical management of angina can, therefore, be summarized as follows:

- correct underlying and associated risk factors, e.g. weight, smoking, blood pressure
- use β-adrenoreceptor blockade, where suitable, as maintenance therapy and combine this when necessary with nifedipine
- use nitrates for immediate prophylactic purposes or in the treatment of an acute attack of pain and longer acting preparations where indicated

It is important to encourage optimism in patients with angina. They should be reassured and, short of sudden or obvious overexertion, encouraged to lead as normal a life as possible.

Surgical management

Coronary bypass surgery can be done with a mortality of as little as 2% in an experienced centre. Angina is relieved in about 80% of patients. Some evidence also suggests that in suitably selected cases, long term survival may also be improved. Because of this, a suggested policy is shown on the flow chart, LD-110.

Unstable angina

This is a term used to describe patients with stable

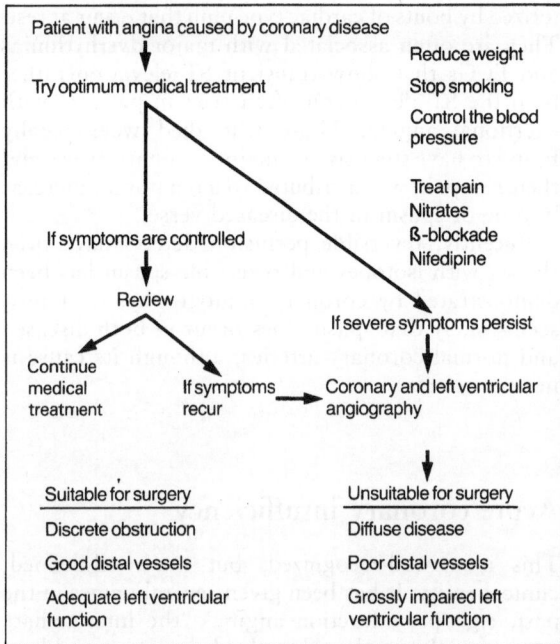

LD-110. *Flow chart of suggested policy for coronary bypass surgery*

angina or recent onset angina whose symptoms are rapidly becoming worse. It encompasses a wide clinical spectrum from those with occasional exertional pain that has become much less occasional, to those who have rapidly become incapacitated even at rest.

It was once thought to indicate that myocardial infarction was imminent, but, although serious, it is now known that, of patients whose symptoms are not severe enough to warrant admission to hospital, only about 5% will die and 10–15% will have infarcts during the following 6 months. Also, that by the end of this time 30% will no longer have symptoms.

Of those requiring admission to hospital, 20% will be dead at the end of 1 year and 25% at the end of 2 years. Most of them have extensive three-vessels disease, but 10% have obstruction in the left main coronary artery that may be relieved surgically.

Coronary spasm

The concept of coronary spasm is not new. Osler speculated on its presence in 1910. It again came to the forefront in 1960 with the work of Prinzmetal and his colleagues. They described what has become known as Prinzmetal's or 'variant' angina. This is characterized by bouts of cardiac type pain that occur at rest. They are often associated with major dysrhythmias and ECGs that show transient ST elevation rather than the ST depression often seen in patients with exertional angina. Those who died were usually found to have stenosis of a major coronary artery and their rest pain was attributed to a temporary increase in tone or spasm of the diseased vessel.

Recently, reversible perfusion defects have been shown with isotopes and reversible spasm has been demonstrated by coronary angiography, so it now seems likely that spasm does occur in both diseased and normal coronary arteries, although its cause is not yet certain.

Acute coronary insufficiency

This is a well-recognized, but not well-defined, clinical entity. It has been given several names in the past, e.g. 'pre-infarction angina', 'the intermediate syndrome'. It was thought to lead almost inevitably to infarction, but this is now known not to be so. The ECG shows changes in the ST segments and T waves. The ST segments may be elevated or depressed and the T waves flattened or inverted. These changes may develop rapidly and regress rapidly. Although infarction may be suspected on the basis of the prolonged pain and ECG changes, the enzymes do not rise. The management of this condition remains controversial and varies from those who treat it as no more than a prolonged attack of angina to those who advise emergency coronary artery surgery. Be that as it may, it is a good general rule to treat such patients as though they have had infarcts until it is proved otherwise.

Acute myocardial infarction

Onset

Myocardial infarction presents in many ways; from severe crushing chest pain to mild discomfort, from a little unexplained breathlessness to acute left ventricular failure, from transient lightheadedness to sudden death. It may even be silent, unsuspected and detected only on ECG. In the Framingham study, around 20% of all infarcts diagnosed by ECG were not suspected clinically.

There is thus a spectrum – ranging from the classical 'heart attack' that can be readily recognized,

through infarction that is only detected by ECG, to the unsuspected infarct that is only discovered at autopsy.

Prodromal symptoms

It has to be re-emphasized that many coronary deaths are sudden and unexpected. However, both prospective and retrospective studies have suggested that some who develop infarction have premonitory or prodromal symptoms before the real attack.

Unfortunately, vague cardiac symptoms are not uncommon in the general population. If prodromal symptoms could be accurately identified, early preventive measures might become feasible.

Several series have documented the types of prodromal symptoms that occur (Table 16).

TABLE 16

Prodromal symptoms	New York (%)	Edinburgh (%)	Aberdeen (%)
None	35	44[*]	32
Pain	59	44	55
Other symptoms such as: fatigue weakness dyspnoea	6	5	12

[*] In this series 16% had chronic 'stable' angina of effort that had not become worse during the preceding 3 months

Angina

Prodromal symptoms can last from hours to more than 3 weeks. Patients who complain of new, worsening angina or who find their angina rapidly becoming more severe and more limiting have what is termed 'unstable angina'. Although only a few will go on to acute infarction, it is currently impossible to select those at most risk and all should have urgent medical attention.

Sudden death

Myocardial infarction often presents as sudden death because ventricular fibrillation occurs soon after the attack begins. Many of those who 'die suddenly' survive long enough to be saved if prompt medical attention is readily available.

It used to be thought that all patients who died in this way following a 'heart attack' had not survived long enough for the pathological changes of infarction to develop. It is now known that some of those who are successfully resuscitated do not subsequently develop such changes and that ventricular fibrillation may occur as a complication of coronary heart disease without myocardial infarction.

Pain

Pain is the commonest symptom. It is usually intense, starts retrosternally and may spread across the chest and up into the neck, shoulders and arms. At times it passes through to the back. The arms, especially the left, can feel heavy and useless. The pain may come on at any time and is, as often as not, unrelated to exertion. It is usually prolonged and is not relieved by rest or sublingual glyceryl trinitrate (GTN). It is often accompanied by 'angor animi' (a feeling of impending death) and by systemic effects such as profuse sweating, pallor and nausea or vomiting due to the profound autonomic disturbance.

Breathlessness and heart failure

Occasionally, and quite frequently in the elderly, myocardial infarction presents with sudden breathlessness due to acute left ventricular failure. Pain is not a prominent feature in such cases, although a recollection of a prior episode of chest discomfort can sometimes be elicited on close questioning.

Syncope

Acute myocardial infarction can cause loss of consciousness for several reasons. Disturbances of rhythm such as a short period of asystole, bradycardia or tachycardia may all cause low cardiac output with impaired cerebral blood flow and consequent loss of consciousness. This mode of presentation is again common in the elderly.

Other presentations

The clinical presentation may not be of infarction itself but of a complication of infarction. This includes embolism from a mural thrombus, pain from pericarditis, breathlessness from mitral incompetence following damage to a papillary muscle and rupture of the ventricular septum.

Differential diagnosis

Conditions to be considered include:

- dissecting aortic aneurysm
  Check peripheral pulses. They may be absent or delayed. The blood pressure in the arms may be different. X-ray of the chest may show widening of the mediastinum

- pulmonary thromboembolism
  The circumstances often suggest the possibility. Examine the legs for deep venous thrombosis and the chest for signs of friction and consolidation. X-rays may be helpful

- pneumothorax and pneumonia
  Clinical examination of chest and an X-ray should exclude these possibilities

- others are:
  Oesophageal emergencies (reflux, rupture), upper abdominal emergencies (acute gallbladder disease, perforations etc.) and cervical disc problems

The important clinical decision is whether or not the pain is due to myocardial ischaemia. If it is, the differential diagnosis includes various types of acute cardiac pain:

- acute myocardial infarction

- acute coronary insufficiency

- a severe anginal episode without measurable myocardial damage, often referred to as an ischaemic attack

Examination

Clinical examination may not contribute a great deal to the diagnosis, but can at times be helpful and should never be skimped or overlooked. It usually reveals an anxious, pale, sweating and vasoconstricted patient who is distressed and suffering pain that demands immediate relief.

Pulse

The pulse gives information about the heart rate and and rhythm:

- rate > 150 and regular
  Consider dysrhythmias such as supraventricular or ventricular tachycardia

- rate > 150 and irregular
  Consider atrial fibrillation

- rate > 100 and regular
  Sinus tachycardia. This may be appropriate or inappropriate. It is appropriate if it reflects a response to myocardial damage and the need to maintain cardiac output. It is inappropriate if due to excess catecholamine release. If allowed to persist, it increases myocardial oxygen demand and may cause extension of the infarct.

● rate < 60

Sinus bradycardia is often associated with parasympathetic overactivity soon after infarction. It is often a temporary phenomenon, but may be associated with a reduced cardiac output and a low blood pressure

● rate < 40

Consider atrioventricular block – especially complete heart block

Irregularities of the pulse give an indication of the presence and number of ectopic beats but no indication of their origin.

Blood pressure

The response varies. Initially, about 20% of patients whose blood pressure was previously normal have a slight transitory increase in pressure because of sympathetic overactivity. More common is a slight fall in blood pressure. This may be associated with sinus bradycardia due to parasympathetic overactivity. Profound hypotension, progressive heart failure and cardiogenic shock can occur in those who have had a massive infarct that involves much of the left ventricle and severely disturbs its function.

Patients who were previously hypertensive may have an apparently normal blood pressure when first seen. This, for them, is a low pressure. It may indicate a precarious situation and that they are in danger of developing cardiogenic shock or heart failure.

Heart failure

Signs of heart failure are usually a consequence of a failing left ventricle. The patient may be dyspnoeic and moist sounds are heard in the chest. These may be basal or more widespread and accompanied by bronchospasm if the failure is severe. The venous pressure is usually normal but may be raised if significant failure persists. Occasionally, the infarct involves the right ventricle predominantly and, in this situation, the jugular venous pressure is raised because of right ventricular failure and the signs of left ventricular failure are minimal or absent.

Auscultation

There are no diagnostic features about the heart sounds, but they are often soft and of poor quality. The presence of a fourth (atrial) sound is associated with impaired left ventricular relaxation during atrial systole and can be an early sign of failure. A third heart sound, occurring early in diastole, is a more definite sign of impaired left ventricular function. A

rapid heart rate with an added sound is known as triple rhythm and indicates a labouring ventricle.

Pericardial friction develops in 15–20% of cases but is an evanescent sign and, to be sure of hearing it, repeated auscultation is necessary.

New systolic murmurs indicate complications such as mitral incompetence due to papillary muscle dysfunction or rupture of the ventricular septum.

Investigations

The most important investigations in a case of suspected myocardial infarction are the:

● ECG

● serum enzymes

● chest X-ray

ECG

The ECG is important, but remember that the first ECG (if recorded soon after the onset of symptoms) may not be diagnostic in up to 50% of patients subsequently shown to have had an infarct. Many such records are within normal limits.

The ECG gives the following main types of information:

● presence or absence of infarction

● site and nature of the infarct

● disorders of rhythm and conduction

Transmural infarction involves the whole thickness of the ventricular wall. The earliest sign is the presence of ST segment elevation, closely followed by the development of significant Q waves (usually more than 0.04s in duration and more than 25% of the depth of the following R wave, if one is present). Serial tracings, in uncomplicated infarction, usually show persistence of Q waves, return of the ST segments to the isoelectric level and inversion of T waves over the infarcted area. These are known as the sequential changes of infarction (LD-111). They occur over varying periods of time. The sequence can evolve over the course of a few days or may take 10–14 days to develop.

The site of infarction can be identified from the ECG pattern. Leads I and aVL usually reflect what is happening on the anterior surface of the heart; leads III and aVF, the inferior surface.

Chest leads:

● V_1–V_3 are anteroseptal

● V_3–V_5 are anterior

● V_5–V_6 are anterolateral

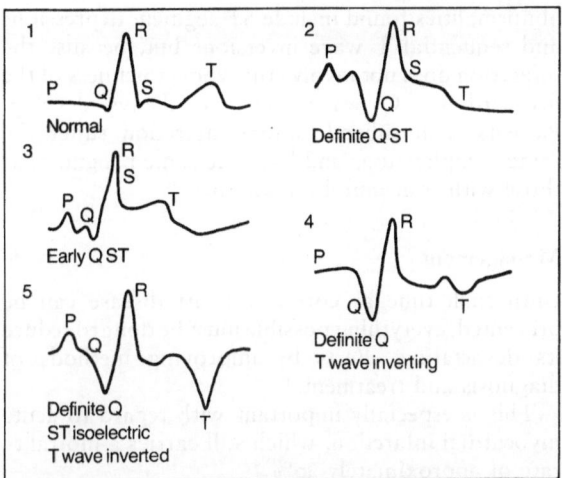

LD-111. *ECG changes on infarction*

Leads III and aVF should be examined with care. Q waves in these leads are not necessarily abnormal unless the tracing is recorded in full inspiration. True posterior infarction can be suspected from the presence of dominant R waves in the right chest leads (V_1-V_3) when they are associated with a clinical history suggesting infarction and abnormal enzyme values. A tracing taken with an oesophageal electrode may provide more detailed information in this situation.

It may be necessary to use additional electrode positions. For example, high lateral infarction may be found only by moving the exploring electrode further round the chest and moving one or two interspaces higher.

There is a rough correlation, but no more than that, between the site of infarction and the coronary artery involved. Thus, anterior infarction is usually associated with left anterior descending coronary artery disease and inferior infarction is associated with right coronary artery disease. The right coronary artery usually supplies the SA and AV nodes.

Serum enzymes

Myocardial ischaemia can cause pain and may alter the ECG. Myocardial infarction causes death of myocardial cells and the enzymes they contain leak into the blood stream. Five enzymes are commonly measured in patients with suspected infarction:

- creatinine phosphokinase (CPK)
  This enzyme is the first to be released. The blood level rises about 6 h after infarction,

peaks at 18–36 h and then falls slowly over 2–3 d. The normal level is less than 100 U/ml. With infarction, a wide range of maximum values occur. In massive infarction, the levels may rise to 1000 U or more and such levels imply a poor prognosis. Lesser values are consistent with infarction, but small increases to around 200 U/ml may be harder to evaluate. Intramuscular injections can cause an increase of 70–100 U and so can pulmonary infarction. Where the cause of the raised CPK is in doubt, it is possible to measure the specific cardiac isoenzyme CPK (MB). This will usually resolve the dilemma.

- SGOT and SGPT
  Serum aspartate transferase (previously glutamic oxaloacetic transaminase, SGOT) and serum alanine transferase (previously glutamic pyruvic transaminase, SGPT) are standard investigations. These enzymes are found predominantly in the heart and liver but are released in different proportions depending on the organ involved. The concentration of SGOT is higher in heart muscle. Thus, in myocardial infarction, the increase in SGOT levels is at least two to three times higher than the rise in SGPT levels. In liver damage, both rise to similar values. Normal values for each are around 50 U/ml but vary between laboratories. An increase in SGOT to above 100 U/ml is suspicious of infarction. Levels rise a little later than CPK values. They are raised by 12–24 h, peak at 34–48 h and slowly decline over 3–4 d.

- lactic acid dehydrogenase (LDH) and P-hydroxybutyric dehydrogenase (HDB)
  These enzymes are not of value in the early diagnosis of myocardial infarction but can be helpful when patients present a few days after the suspected infarction has occurred at a time when other enzyme values are returning or have returned to normal. They may give good evidence on which to base a retrospective diagnosis. Values begin to rise after 2–3 d and remain raised for up to a week. LDH may also be raised in liver disease. If there is any doubt about the LDH increase being a 'false positive' for infarction, the isoenzyme values may again be helpful. There are several isoenzymes for LDH. When the rise is due to cardiac damage, the isoenzyme LDH 5 is raised to a greater extent than is isoenzyme LDH 4.

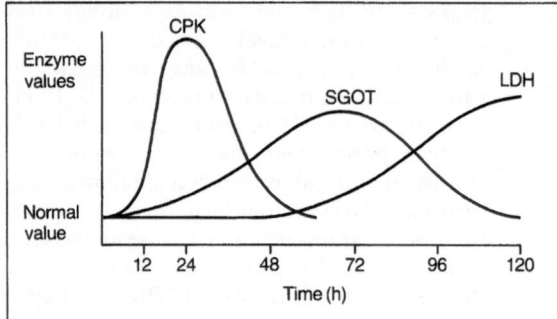

LD-112. *Enzyme changes after infarction*

Chest X-ray

This can give helpful information, especially about left ventricular failure. Radiological signs of pulmonary congestion often appear before symptoms or clinical signs and indicate the need for treatment. The chest X-ray is also a convenient way of assessing heart size. Cardiomegaly is associated with a poor prognosis but care is needed when interpreting portable X-ray films because they may give a false impression of increased heart size.

Conclusion

The combination of history, ECG and enzyme values usually allows the diagnosis of myocardial infarction to be confirmed or refuted. The investigations are complementary. For instance, the patient may give a history that suggests acute infarction but, though the ECG changes are not diagnostic, raised enzymes confirm the clinical diagnosis.

Each enzyme has its own use. The CPK is especially valuable in coronary care units. It rises early and allows prompt diagnosis and management decisions.

Other systemic manifestations of infarction occur and were once widely used for diagnosis. Some 24–48 hours after infarction, there is a slight pyrexia, a raised erythrocyte sedimentation rate (ESR) and an increasing polymorphonuclear leukocytosis. These changes are non-specific, but can help to confirm the diagnosis. A raised temperature occurring 4–5 d after infarction usually has a different cause and should prompt a search for such conditions as thrombophlebitis, chest infection or urinary tract infection.

Subendocardial infarction

Clinically, this is similar in all respects to transmural infarction. The enzyme rise is consistent with cell necrosis but the ECG changes may be different. The abnormalities found include ST segment depressions and sequential T wave inversions but, because the infarction does not involve the whole thickness of the myocardium, Q waves do not always develop. Patients with subendocardial infarction suffer the same complications and have the same prognosis as those with transmural infarction.

Management

Until such time as coronary heart disease can be prevented, everything possible must be done to reduce its devastating effects by improving methods of diagnosis and treatment.

.This is especially important with regard to acute myocardial infarction, which still carries a mortality rate of approximately 40%.

Recent advances include the:

- demonstration that external cardiac massage can maintain blood flow to essential organs
- application of electrical current to restore normal cardiac rhythm
- development of cardiac pacemakers
- concept of acute coronary care units in hospitals and mobile coronary care units in the community

These, along with advances in drug therapy, have greatly increased the chances of successful cardiac resuscitation.

Attempts at resuscitation are not new. In 1809, Allan Burns of Glasgow wrote: 'Where, however, the cessation of vital action is very complete and continues long, we ought to inflate the lungs and pass electric shocks through the chest'.

Home or hospital

There is considerable discussion and controversy over which is better. There is no doubt that the impact and benefit of treatment depends upon the time lapse between the onset of infarction and help reaching the patient. The decision on whether the patient remains at home or is taken to hospital should be based mainly on how long it has been since the symptoms began. Thus, if more than 6 hours have passed and the patient's condition appears stable so far as rhythm and blood pressure are concerned, transfer to hospital may be of no great benefit, especially if the home circumstances are good and the hospital has no coronary care unit.

The decision may also be influenced by the distance to the nearest suitable hospital and the method of transport available. Long journeys in ambulances without staff and equipment for resuscitation may do more harm than good at a crucial phase of the illness.

The decision whether or not to send a patient with suspected myocardial infarction to hospital is an important one. Once it has been made, monitoring and resuscitation facilities should be available as soon as possible. Depending on circumstances, these may be:

- in the ambulance
- in the hospital emergency room
- in the coronary care unit (CCU)
- wherever the patient happens to be (mobile CCU)

The basic requirements are ECG monitoring, an intravenous cannula so that there is immediate access to the circulation and a defibrillator.

If such facilities can be made available at home and maintained throughout the journey, there is no great urgency about movement and the patient's condition should be stabilized before transport to hospital.

If no such facilities exist outside hospital, no time should be wasted once the decision to send the patient to hospital has been made.

Coronary care units

A coronary care unit (CCU) provides a means whereby the minimum number of trained staff can look after the maximum number of patients at most risk following myocardial infarction. Immediate action can be taken, not only to treat life-threatening emergencies, but also to prevent them arising. CCUs have an invaluable but limited role. Invaluable, because they reduce mortality in those admitted to hospital soon after infarction. Limited, because at least 50% of those who do not survive are dead within 2 hours of the onset of symptoms and, at present, relatively few patients reach hospital within this time.

There are several reasons why patients die before medical care becomes available:

- death may be instantaneous or occur before help could arrive
- patients fail to recognize the significance of their symptoms
  Many think, or hope, that they are due to indigestion and do not summon immediate aid. This is especially true of first infarcts. Those having a recurrence are usually quick to suspect the diagnosis
- inability to contact the family doctor
- inability of the family doctor or the ambulance to come at once when sent for

- delay may occur in the emergency department before the patient is transferred to CCU

Mobile coronary care units

Recognition of the importance of early medical treatment has led to the development of mobile coronary care units that take aid to the patient, the aim being to provide coronary care facilities as quickly as possible.

Such mobile units need not be staffed by doctors and nurses. Good results have been obtained using specially trained ambulance drivers and firemen.

Mobile coronary care is not without its critics. The overall impression, however, is that these units can be useful but require a considerable team effort by motivated staff with adequate back-up facilities in hospital. Also, that the public must be made more aware of the importance of early treatment if the units are to realize their full potential.

Relief of pain

After myocardial infarction, patients usually have severe pain and are intensely anxious. Continuing pain not only causes distress but can have adverse effects upon the heart rate and blood pressure, possibly increasing the size of the infarct. Its relief takes priority.

Cyclimorph 10–15 mg (morphine plus cyclizine) or 5 mg diamorphine with 50 mg cyclizine depending on the size of the patient, should be given by intramuscular injection. It is seldom necessary to give these drugs intravenously unless there is profound hypotension or peripheral circulatory failure that would delay absorption. The dose may be repeated within 1 hour if necessary. Morphine should not be given alone because of its liability to cause vomiting.

For less severe pain, weaker analgesics such as dihydrocodeine can be used.

Anxiety

Anxiety following myocardial infarction is usually maximal during the first 48 hours. Diazepam, 2–5 mg three times a day, is given during this period, and for a longer period if the patient remains anxious. In addition, diazepam 5–10 mg can be given at night as a hypnotic.

Oxygen

Arterial hypoxia may cause acidosis, reduce myocardial contractility and predispose to dysrhythmias.

There is controversy about its use after myocardial infarction. On balance, it is probably of some value, but care must be taken to keep the concentration low in those who also have chronic respiratory disease.

Anticoagulants

Anticoagulant therapy has no confirmed place in the treatment of myocardial infarction, but is still used to prevent venous thrombosis and its possible sequelae (e.g. pulmonary embolism). Calcium heparin 5000 U is given subcutaneously every 12 hours while the patient is confined to bed.

Those sustaining pulmonary or systemic emboli during the course of the acute illness require carefully controlled treatment with heparin and warfarin.

General

Patients are kept under continuous observation in the coronary care unit until their condition is stable and any complications that may have arisen are under control. Uncomplicated cases are usually discharged to the wards after 2 or 3 days.

Nowdays, mobilization begins towards the end of the first week and most patients are ready for discharge after about 14 days. Progress depends upon the severity of the infarct and possible complications.

Complications

Immediate complications include:

- cardiac arrest – sudden death due to ventricular fibrillation or asystole
- conduction defects (heart block)
- dysrhythmias
- cardiogenic shock
- heart failure

Complications occurring 1 or more days after infarction include:

- pulmonary embolism
- systemic embolus from mural thrombus
- cardiac rupture
- papillary muscle dysfunction or rupture causing mitral incompetence
- rupture of the ventricular septum
- any of the *immediate* complications listed above

Complications occurring later include:

- postmyocardial infarction syndrome, with fever pericarditis and possibly pleural effusion
- shoulder–hand syndrome and frozen shoulder
- ventricular aneurysm
- depression

  Depression is an important and often un-recognized complication. The patient believes that his active life is over, his job is threatened and he may become an invalid. Active rehabilitation and reassurance are needed to dispel such fears.

Cardiac arrest

Cardiac arrest may occur after warning dysrhythmias or it may develop unexpectedly in a previously uncomplicated illness. The usual cause is ventricular fibrillation.

Ventricular fibrillation (VF)

Ventricular fibrillation occurring soon after infarction usually reverts to normal rhythm when promptly treated by electrical cardioversion (see p. 266).

Ventricular fibrillation occurring later in the illness or in patients with other complications such as cardiogenic shock or heart failure has a poorer prognosis and often leads to asystole.

Cardiogenic shock

This indicates massive myocardial damage. The blood pressure is low, the cardiac output is low, the urine output falls and the patient is cold and clammy.

The prognosis is poor despite intensive medical treatment. Many therapeutic regimes have been tried without much success. Catecholamines (dobutamine, dopamine) are used to improve cardiac output by increasing myocardial contractility. Vasodilators (nitroprusside, isosorbide, prazosin) can be tried, to reduce the amount of work required of the left ventricle. These are powerful agents, however, and must be used with great care if they are not to do more harm than good.

Intra-aortic balloon pumping has been used to reduce left ventricular work and improve coronary, cerebral and renal blood flow. The results have been disappointing because it has proved difficult to wean patients off the pump.

Heart failure

Acute left ventricular failure requires immediate and intensive treatment with oxygen, i.v. frusemide (80 mg), morphine and digoxin (if the latter has not already been prescribed). Vasodilators may also be required.

Lesser degrees of heart failure are common after myocardial infarction and are manifest clinically by breathlessness, pulmonary crepitations and possibly a gallop rhythm. Evidence of pulmonary congestion is also present on the chest X-ray.

Initially, treatment consists of potent diuretics such as frusemide (40 mg) or bumetamide (1 mg). If this does not control failure, digoxin should be added and the dose of diuretic increased.

Cardiac rupture

It has been suggested that 5–10% of deaths following myocardial infarction are due to cardiac rupture. Rupture may also occur as a consequence of over-enthusiastic cardiac massage, especially in the elderly.

The blood pressure falls dramatically, cardiac output diminishes rapidly and asystole or ventricular fibrillation develop. Death is the usual outcome, although occasionally some patients survive small ruptures.

Ventricular septal defect

Myocardial infarction may be complicated by the development of a ventricular septal defect (VSD) caused by rupture of an infarcted septum.

On examination, a rough blowing pansystolic murmur can be heard over the lower part of the precordium, being maximal at the left sternal edge. Pulmonary blood flow is increased and may cause heart failure if there is a large left to right shunt.

If vigorous medical treatment does not result in rapid clinical improvement, emergency surgical treatment should be considered.

Papillary muscle dysfunction

Ischaemia of the papillary muscles often results in minor mitral valve dysfunction. Increasingly severe damage can lead to major mitral incompetence. The systolic murmur that develops often suggests the diagnosis but may not reflect the severity of the regurgitation, which is often worse than the signs suggest. Minor degrees of incompetence need no action. If failure develops and continues despite intensive medical therapy, it may be necessary to consider mitral valve replacement.

Ventricular dysfunction and aneurysm formation

Infarction heals by fibrosis. Myocardial contraction in the fibrosed area is impaired and may compromise ventricular function.

There are various grades of malfunction:

- hypokinesis (impaired contraction)
- akinesis (absent contraction)
- dyskinesis (paradoxical movement when, instead of contracting during systole, the damaged segment bulges outwards)

In most cases, ventricular function remains adequate for normal demands. Patients with grossly impaired ventricular function may remain breathless and some may remain in chronic heart failure. If they do not respond to medical treatment, surgical treatment should be considered. In general, those with widespread dysfunction do badly, but some with localized areas of malfunction may be greatly improved by resection.

Dysrhythmias

There is a high incidence of dysrhythmias in patients seen shortly after infarction (Table 17).

TABLE 17

Dysrhythmia	Incidence %
Bradydysrhythmias	20
Ventricular extrasystoles (VES)	90
Ventricular tachycardia (VT)	5
Ventricular fibrillation (VF)	10
Supraventricular dysrhythmias	20
Second or third degree heart block	10

Both parasympathetic and sympathetic overactivity may occur, although parasympathetic overactivity is more frequent. Both predispose to ventricular dysrhythmias and increase infarct size.

The early management of infarction is based on:

- relief of pain
- prevention or correction of dysrhythmias
- correction of autonomic imbalance

Dysrhythmias after infarction are important because they may:

- be life-threatening in themselves
- be precursors of more significant and life-threatening dysrhythmias
- increase morbidity, for example by precipitating heart failure
- predispose to increased infarct size

Remember that ventricular fibrillation can occur without warning – even in those receiving apparently adequate antidysrhythmic treatment.

Mechanisms

These include:

- predisposing conditions:
    previous infarction
    large heart
    previous or current heart failure

- cardiogenic shock

- catecholamine excess

- local myocardial changes, including accumulation of potassium and free fatty acid

- increased automaticity of damaged cells

- injury potential leading to localized depolarization

- re-entry due to slowed conduction

There are two major causes of dysrhythmias:

- focal automaticity

- re-entry

Focal automaticity occurs when an abnormal focus, perhaps an ischaemic area of ventricle, regularly initiates an action potential independent of the underlying basic sinus rhythm.

With myocardial infarction or ischaemia, areas of ventricular muscle are being depolarized and repolarized at different rates and times. Impulses conducted across the Purkinje–myocardial junction pass in various directions. For example, if one pathway is refractory and the impulse is blocked, impulses can arise from distant cells and re-enter the circuit when the refractory period ends (see p. 195).

The object of therapy is to control the abnormal process by:

- controlling or abolishing focal automaticity

- interrupting re-entry pathways

The requirements for the effective treatment of cardiac dysrhythmias are:

- accurate diagnosis

- identification and treatment of initiating factors

- appropriate drug therapy

Management has improved because of enhanced detection, better understanding of the electrophysiology and the introduction of new antidysrhythmic drugs.

The drugs' mechanisms of action are mainly to:

- increase the threshold potential

- slow the rate of rise of diastolic depolarization

- lengthen the refractory period

- slow the re-entry circuit

Incidence

Nearly all patients have some abnormality of rhythm after a myocardial infarct (Table 17). The incidence is highest soon after the acute episode. It decreases rapidly within 6 hours of the infarct, but serious dysrhythmias can still develop with startling rapidity, give no warning and cause death.

Autonomic disturbances are common immediately after infarction. Parasympathetic overactivity is indicated by sinus bradycardia and a low blood pressure; sympathetic overactivity by sinus tachycardia and transient hypertension.

The highest incidence of autonomic disturbance is recorded before analgesia and most settle once pain and anxiety are adequately relieved.

Significance

Many dysrhythmias are of little or no significance; some are precursors of more serious dysrhythmias; a few are life-threatening and may cause sudden death. The details of their recognition and treatment are given on pp. 195–210, 266. Over the years it has become appreciated that they should not be treated for their own sake, but only when they either warn of trouble ahead or become haemodynamically significant.

Prognostic value

There is little doubt that, as a group, those who have serious abnormalities of rhythm soon after the onset of myocardial infarction are less likely to survive and leave hospital than those who do not.

Postinfarction dysrhythmias can be controlled by such drugs as mexiletine, disopyramide or quinidine, but no convincing evidence has as yet emerged that this improves long term survival.

Ventricular ectopic beats (VES)

Most ventricular ectopic beats after myocardial infarction are of little significance. Some people still treat multiple ectopics and multifocal ectopics, but this is probably unnecessary.

Ventricular ectopic beats that start before the end of the preceding T wave, the so-called 'R on T ectopics', are liable to be followed by ventricular fibrillation and should be treated.

It is important to remember, however, that in at least 50% of cases in which ventricular fibrillation complicates myocardial infarction, there is no warning dysrhythmia. So, a good case can be made for prophylactic therapy in all patients, provided the treatment is effective and not harmful.

Ventricular tachycardia (VT)

This is liable to be followed by ventricular fibrillation and should normally be treated with suppressive drugs, such as lignocaine, disopyramide or mexiletine. In those with shock or heart failure, immediate d.c. cardioversion is indicated.

Recurrent episodes of VT that are resistant to drug therapy occasionally require overdrive ventricular pacing.

Ventricular fibrillation (VF)

When this occurs in the early phase of the illness (primary VF), it nearly always responds readily to a d.c. shock and the prognosis is good after successful resuscitation (see p. 266).

When ventricular fibrillation occurs later in the course of an illness complicated by recurrent dysrhythmias, cardiogenic shock or heart failure (secondary VF), the prognosis is poor. Cardioversion under these circumstances often induces asystole and resuscitation is frequently unsuccessful.

Ventricular asystole

This is a common terminal event in those who have been seriously ill with complications following massive myocardial infarction. Although it seldom responds to treatment, cardiac resuscitation and the insertion of a pacemaker is occasionally successful.

Supraventricular tachycardias

Sinus tachycardia is common, especially after large infarcts. It indicates severity and requires no specific treatment.

Atrial fibrillation, atrial flutter and paroxysms of atrial tachycardia are not uncommon, but should only be treated if they are causing haemodynamic upset or if the ventricular rate is so fast that it might cause extension of the infarct by greatly increasing the myocardial demand for oxygen.

Sinus bradycardia

A slow heart rate is common, especially after inferior infarction. It often responds to the relief of pain and the associated autonomic upset.

If accompanied by shock, heart failure or dangerous ventricular ectopic beats, it should be treated with atropine. If it does not respond, cardiac pacing may be necessary.

Heart block

First, second or third (complete) degree heart block is fairly common and occurs in 10–15% of patients after myocardial infarction. It does not always require treatment, but should always alert those in charge to the possibility that treatment may be required.

The insertion of a cardiac pacemaker is effective in most cases where an adequate circulation cannot be maintained because of a slow heart rate. The indications for emergency prophylactic pacing vary a little in different centres.

Some patients do not develop complete heart block, but conduction defects of the right bundle and one fascicle of the left bundle (hemiblock), usually the anterior fascicle. This combination of right bundle branch block and left anterior hemiblock is not an absolute indication for immediate cardiac pacing, though if it persists, pacing may well be required before long. If the PR interval is also prolonged, considerable interference with conduction is obviously present and pacing should be commenced at once because of the risk of asystole.

Second degree heart block of the Wenckebach type, where there is progressive lengthening of the PR interval followed by a dropped beat, may be left untreated. Second degree heart block of the Mobitz type, where the PR interval is usually normal and unexpected drop beats occur due to failure of AV conduction, is a sinister dysrhythmia. Pacing is justified in these circumstances because sudden asystole can occur.

Complete heart block may or may not be associated with poor cardiac output and falling blood pressure. If it is, pacing is indicated.

The type and prognosis of heart block in inferior and anterior infarction differs. Heart block develops more commonly with inferior infarction but is usually of relatively short duration and is often a consequence of ischaemia rather than infarction of the AV node. Treatment is only required if shock or heart failure results or is exacerbated by the slow ventricular rate.

By contrast, the occurrence of heart block after anterior infarction is an ominous development. It usually indicates massive myocardial damage and carries a grave prognosis. If either second or third degree block develops, emergency pacing should be carried out without regard to the patient's haemodynamic state.

The differences can be summarized as shown in Table 18.

The use of temporary on-demand pacing has been of great value in the treatment of heart block following acute myocardial infarction and can often

TABLE 18

	Inferior infarction	Anterior infarction
Size of infarction	May be small	Usually large
Subsidiary pace-maker site	Low junctional	Idioventricular
QRS complex	Narrow	Wide
Mortality	< 20%	> 80%

be life-saving. The technique of insertion is relatively simple and easily learned.

Pacemakers should be left *in situ* for a few days after a return to sinus rhythm because many patients who need them have recurrent short episodes of heart block.

Prognosis

The high immediate mortality rate in acute myocardial infarction has already been discussed.

What does the future hold for those who survive to leave hospital? Overall, the mortality is around 10% in the first year and about 5% each year thereafter. Those who have already had an infarct more often die of a further infarct and have a greater chance of dying suddenly than those who have not. However, the overall picture is not a good predictor so far as the individual is concerned.

Various indices have been calculated to assess prognosis. They can be used to separate patients into high risk and low risk groups. Those in the low risk group have an 85–90% chance of surviving for 5 years; those in the high risk group have only a 30–35% chance of doing so. Adverse features include:

● age
● hypertension
● previous infarction or angina
● atrial dysrhythmias following infarction
● heart failure
● cardiomegaly

When dealing with such an unpredictable disease, a prognostic index can have only a limited value in the management of individual patients. It can, however, provide rough guidelines for deciding where prolonged follow-up and treatment may be necessary and in setting targets for rehabilitation.

Attempts are being made, by continuous monitoring of cardiac rhythm, to predict those at greatest risk, in the hope that the risk can be lessened by the long term administration of antidysrhythmic drugs. Other

drugs, such as those that affect platelets, are also under test.

Rehabilitation

A positive and encouraging attitude is essential if chronic invalidism is to be avoided. Patients should be encouraged to take the heart attack in their stride and get back to normal as quickly as possible. To achieve this, education of both the patient and the spouse is important. Both are afraid that exertion may cause a further attack and the fear or dropping down dead constantly lurks in the background.

Rehabilitation should begin at the start of the illness and should continue until return to a normal or near normal life. In some cases, it may even be to a better life.

Early mobilization and discharge from hospital have been shown to have no adverse affects. In uncomplicated cases the patients should be:

● out of bed sitting in a chair on the third or fourth day
● walking about by the seventh day
● ready for home (or a convalescent home) on the fourteenth day

After a transfer from the CCU to the ward, physical activity should be gradually and progressively increased so that on returning home they will not be confronted by activities that are more physically demanding than those performed in hospital.

Patients should be educated about the nature of a 'heart attack' and should be counselled about such things as smoking, drinking, dieting, exercise, sex, driving and returning to work.

Smoking

Cigarette smoking should be prohibited because stopping is beneficial and improves prognosis even if the patient has smoked for many years. Smoking an occasional pipe or cigar is less harmful provided the patient does not inhale.

Alcohol

In moderation, alcohol does no harm and may be beneficial especially at night before retiring.

Diet

Patients should modify their diet if they are above ideal weight and should avoid all types of dietary excess.

Exercise

Exercise should be encouraged as it promotes physical and mental well-being. Competitive sports such as squash, and isometric exertion such as weight-lifting, should be avoided.

Those who have taken no exercise for years should start gradually on a planned programme, as should those suffering from breathlessness. Angina is no contraindication, but should be treated to allow physical activity to continue.

Sex

Normal sexual activity is moderate exercise with emotional overtones. Its resumption is a source of anxiety to many patients and their spouses. Many do not ask about it, fearing that it may be forbidden, and many doctors are reluctant to discuss it unless pressed to do so.

Intercourse may be resumed gradually in most cases about 1 month after discharge from hospital. Modifications in sexual practices may be required for those who become unduly breathless or develop angina during the act.

Driving

Although the prevalence of sudden death is increased in postinfarction patients, there is little evidence that it causes an increase in road accidents. Most patients appear to have sufficient warning to pull into the side of the road and stop before they lose consciousness.

Driving should be discouraged for a month or two until patients are fully mobile and their confidence in themselves has been restored. At first, long journeys, motorways and heavy traffic should be avoided.

Those with known coronary heart disease may not again drive heavy transport or public service vehicles.

Employment

The longer a person is off work the harder it is to return to it. Prolonged invalidism following myocardial infarction is often in no way justified by the patient's medical condition.

Most of those who survive have little or no disability and should be encouraged to return to their previous employment within 2 or 3 months. Some with breathlessness or angina may require lighter work but, with proper medical care and encouragement, they should be the exception rather than the rule.

Patients who have had several infarcts may find their exercise tolerance becomes progressively de-creased and may eventually develop chronic heart failure requiring digoxin and diuretic therapy. In these circumstances, early retirement is probably the best course of action.

Hyperlipoproteinaemia

Primary and secondary prevention of atherosclerosis and its consequences should logically begin with the detection and treatment of risk factors. One of the risk factors is hyperlipoproteinaemia. In general, the results of correcting abnormal lipid levels have been disappointing. The reduction in lipid levels and in coronary disease have been less than had been hoped and there seems to have been little effect on the overall mortality. Dietary control of abnormal lipid values remains the cornerstone of treatment. Drug treatment is reserved for those with a major metabolic problem when dietary management is not sufficient, but is not without its complications.

Clinical features

Differential diagnosis

Every care should be taken to ensure that the diagnosis of hyperlipoproteinaemia is based on adequate evidence. Single, random samples of venous blood are insufficient and can be completely misleading. The basic investigations are measurement of cholesterol and triglyceride. It may also be necessary to quantify the concentration of the various lipoprotein fractions – namely low density lipoprotein, very low density lipoprotein and high density lipoprotein. This is usually done by ultracentrifugation and precipitation techniques. The cholesterol content of each isolated fraction can then be measured.

Usually a minimum of three adequate samples is required before making a firm diagnosis and before starting treatment.

For adequate sampling, subjects should:

• fast for 12 hours
• be on their usual diet
• have a stable weight
  Those who are on a weight reducing diet can considerably alter their lipid levels and this makes diagnosis difficult

Patients who have had a myocardial infarction are often referred for lipoprotein typing. There is an understandable wish on the part of clinician and patient to 'get things started'. There should be no rush. Cholesterol usually falls considerably immediately after infarction – possibly a stress response – and triglyceride levels can rise. Thus, patients after myocardial infarction should not have lipid measurements taken until at least 8–12 weeks after the acute episode.

Classification

In the past 20 years new techniques and new methods of classification have helped considerably to define the various types of metabolic problems. It should be remembered, however, that simple methods can still provide a great deal of information. Measurement of cholesterol and triglyceride, and inspection of a serum sample will allow diagnosis in many instances. Upper levels of normal are arbitrary and vary from population to population. However, cholesterol levels of above 250 mg per cent (6.5 mmol/l) and triglyceride levels of more than 200 mg per cent (2.3 mmol/l) can be used to define hyperlipoproteinaemia. In general, such patients can be divided into three main groups. Those with:

- raised cholesterol alone
- raised triglyceride alone
- raised cholesterol and triglyceride

Considerable information can be gained by looking at the serum sample kept overnight in the refrigerator at 4 °C (*not* frozen). If the plasma is clear, then triglyceride is probably normal. When the triglyceride value is above 300 mg per cent, the plasma sample is hazy and turbid and this becomes increasingly so as the triglyceride level rises. If chylomicrons are present, a creamy layer is present floating on the surface. The usual cause of this is the patient's failure to fast.

With the use of additional techniques, such as lipoprotein electrophoresis, preparative ultracentrifugation and precipitation of lipoproteins, six major types of lipoprotein disorders can be defined. Further advances are being made in this field. Instead of relying on measurements of cholesterol and triglyceride, it is likely that more specific markers, probably genetic, will become available and the current views may well be altered considerably.

Although at least six types of disorders are described, from the cardiological point of view Type II (both IIA and IIB) and type IV are by far the most important. The others are rare although of considerable metabolic interest.

Overview of management of lipid control

It should be remembered that cholesterol and triglyceride (as markers of lipoprotein abnormality) are only a facet of management of atherosclerosis. It would be facile to expect major reductions in cardiovascular mortality by controlling lipid levels in those with coronary disease established over the years. Primary prevention studies have been difficult to carry out and those published have stirred considerable controversy. It seems likely that, for the majority of adults, a prudent diet is all that can be achieved and weight should be kept as near to the ideal as possible. Dairy produce and animal fat cannot be avoided but should be taken in reasonable amounts. So far there is little evidence that the substitution of vegetable fat makes any difference and it is better to concentrate upon reducing the total intake of fat rather than to worry about its nature. Drug therapy should only be considered in those who have persistently abnormal lipids and especially in those who have a family history of premature vascular disease.

High density lipoprotein (HDL)

Most reports have concentrated on the adverse effect of raised lipids on coronary mortality. Somewhat belatedly, it is being suggested that not all lipoproteins are bad. High levels of HDL have been shown to correlate with low levels of vascular disease and, conversely, low levels of HDL seem related to increased vascular disease. HDL possibly acts as a scavenger, retrieving cholesterol from cells and returning it to the liver for further metabolism and perhaps removal. Attention is thus being directed to raising HDL levels. Adequate physical exercise at present seems the most sensible way of achieving this.

SYSTEMIC ARTERIAL HYPERTENSION

Definition

The term hypertension refers to pathological elevation of the systemic arterial blood pressure. Its exact definition is difficult, because an individual's blood pressure varies markedly from moment to moment and from day to day. Also the blood pressure measurement of a population shows a slightly skewed normal distribution. This is shown for the diastolic pressure in LD-113. From this it can be seen that to define hypertension by selecting a cut-off point is somewhat artificial. The proportion of hypertensive

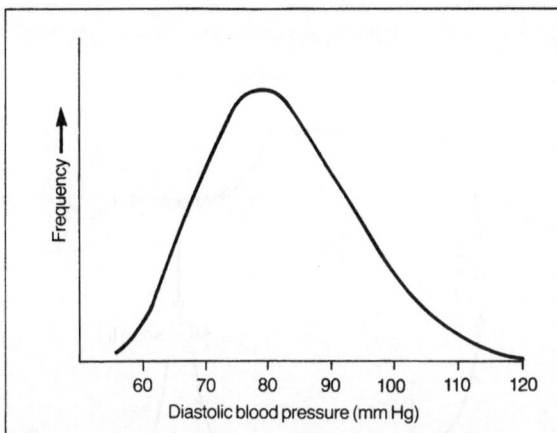

LD-113. The distribution of diastolic blood pressure in a
population

patients will be considerably increased if 90 mm
rather than 100 mm is used in the definition.

Nevertheless, hypertension is an important finding
because patients with a high blood pressure have a
reduced life expectancy that can be improved by
treatment.

Aetiology of raised blood pressure

Hypertension may be classified as (1) essential or
idiopathic hypertension, which is by far the commonest cause, and (2) secondary hypertension. Causes
of secondary hypertension include:

- renal artery stenosis
- chronic pyelonephritis
- acute glomerulonephritis
- chronic glomerulonephritis
- polycystic renal disease
- connective tissue diseases
- coarctation of aorta
- Cushing's syndrome
- Conn's syndrome
- pheochromocytoma
- drugs

Essential hypertension

In the majority of patients with raised blood pressure,
particularly those in the older age groups, no under-

lying cause can be found. This is usually known as
'essential' hypertension.

Essential hypertension could be either an inherited
disease or the result of environmental influences.
Blood pressure in a population cannot be neatly
divided into a normal group and a hypertensive
group. This makes it unlikely that inheritance is by a
single gene, but relatives of patients with hypertension have a higher than normal blood pressure and
twin studies suggest that about half the variation in
blood pressure between individuals is inherited, probably by several genes.

Environmental factors also appear to be important.
Normal subjects and patients with essential hypertension show an increase in blood pressure with age,
except in communities with a very low sodium intake
(e.g. Solomon Islands or Highlands of New Guinea)
where blood pressure remains stable. Also, severe salt
restriction causes a fall of blood pressure; lesser
degrees of restriction having a lesser effect. Obesity
leads to a rise in blood pressure that can be reversed by
weight reduction (probably even if sodium intake
remains constant). There is a tendency for those under
stress or who do not display their emotions, to have a
higher than normal blood pressure, but this correlation is not good.

Extensive research has so far failed to find a
mechanism for the raised blood pressure in essential
hypertension. There is no evidence of an abnormal
pressor substance. Some studies have shown an
increase in plasma catecholamines with an exaggerated response to stress, but the changes are very
slight and could be the result, rather than the cause, of
the hypertension. There is no consistent abnormality
of plasma renin, angiotensin or aldosterone and
cortisol levels are also normal. Some borderline
hypertensives have a hyperdynamic circulation with
an increase in cardiac output. In more longstanding
hypertension, the cardiac output falls and peripheral
resistance is increased. There is evidence that the
aortic arch baroceptors are less responsive in hypertensive patients, but the significance of this is uncertain; as is the significance of the finding of reduced
venous compliance. A consistent finding in hypertension is a fall in the renal blood flow, possibly due to
vasoconstriction in afferent arterioles. Recent work
in hypertensive patients has shown interesting changes in sodium and potassium transport across cell
membranes, possibly due to a humeral factor.

Clinical features

The history and findings on examination are given on
p. 109. The absence of features of secondary hypertension (see below) is of paramount importance.

Management

For details of management, see pp. 154–155.

Renovascular hypertension

Wilson and Byrom first showed that hypertension may be produced by clamping a renal artery and causing renal ischaemia. This ischaemia stimulates the secretion of the renal hormone renin from the juxtaglomerular apparatus. Renin splits renin substrate in the plasma to angiotensin I, which in turn is converted into angiotensin II, an active octapeptide that causes intense vasoconstriction and a rise in blood pressure. Angiotensin II in turn stimulates the zona glomerulosa of the adrenal cortex to produce aldosterone, which causes sodium retention in the distal convoluted tubules of the kidneys (LD-114). The sodium retention adds to the rise in blood pressure.

This humoral sequence may be interrupted by adrenergic β-blocking drugs, which reduce renin release from the juxtaglomerular apparatus, by the converting enzyme inhibitor captopril, which prevents the formation of angiotensin II, and by saralasin, which is a competitive inhibitor of angiotensin II.

Fibromuscular hyperplasia of renal artery

In this condition, which is most common in women in the third and fourth decades of life, hypertrophy of the media of one or both renal arteries produces stenosis usually with post-stenotic dilatation. The affected artery may have several stenosed segments giving a beaded appearance. The cause is uncertain; an association with unusually mobile kidneys has been suggested.

Clinical features

The patient presents with hypertension that may be severe. The only abnormal physical sign (present in 10% of cases) is a bruit heard over the affected renal artery.

Investigations

Intravenous urography (IVP) shows the affected kidney to be smaller than the one on the other side. The excretion of contrast is delayed and its concentration may appear increased. The diagnosis can be confirmed by renal arteriography.

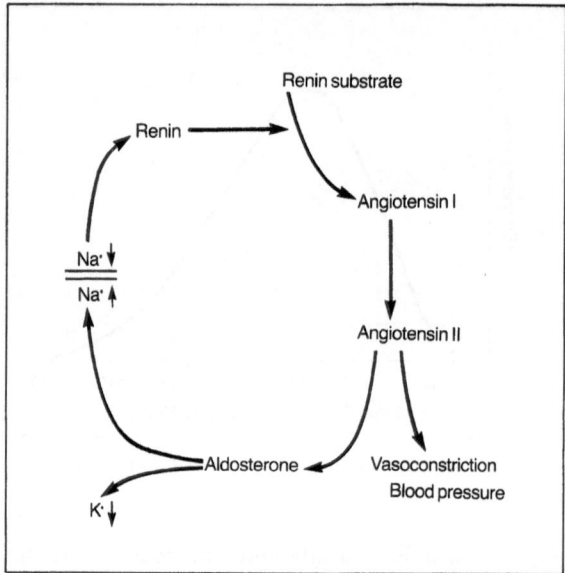

LD-114. *The renin–angiotensin–aldosterone system*

It is important to demonstrate that the stenosis is the cause of the raised blood pressure before considering surgery. The renal veins are catheterized to demonstrate a high secretion rate of renin from the affected kidney. Another useful test is reversal of the hypertension with oral captopril.

Management

Definitive treatment is surgical; it may be possible to bypass the stenosis but at times nephrectomy is necessary. If the patient is not fit for surgery or if the hypertension persists after the surgery, conventional drug therapy will be required.

Atheromatous stenosis of the renal artery

This is commoner than fibromuscular hyperplasia. It occurs in older patients, often in males with evidence of atheroma elsewhere. Usually, the mouth of the renal artery is stenosed by an atheromatous plaque. Again, post-stenotic dilatation is common.

Clinical features

The patient may have evidence of coronary, peripheral or cerebrovascular disease and then develop hypertension that is sometimes severe.

Investigations

The signs and investigations are similar to those

described under fibromuscular hyperplasia. The arteriogram will usually show extensive atheroma of the aorta with partial occlusion of the origin of the renal artery. Often an anatomically demonstrated atheromatous stenosis is not the cause of the hypertension but simply a feature of associated atheroma. And, even when increased renin secretion is demonstrated on the affected side, the results of surgery are not so good as in fibromuscular hyperplasia.

Management

Most cases are treated medically. Surgery is sometimes indicated. In certain cases it is possible to dilate the stenosed artery with a balloon catheter.

Parenchymal renal disease

Virtually any parenchymal renal disease may cause raised blood pressure by the renin–angiotensin mechanism. In the early stages this may be reversible, but as the renal disease becomes chronic, the hypertension becomes fixed despite a fall of renin secretion to normal.

Chronic pyelonephritis

Acute pyelonephritis is not associated with hypertension. Most cases heal with no sequelae, but some progress to chronic pyelonephritis, although it is not yet clear if all chronic cases result from continuing infection. The histological changes may be indistinguishable from those seen with persistent hypokalaemia or analgesic abuse. Chronic pyelonephritis is characterized by cortical scarring, shrinkage of the kidney and adhesion of the capsule. There is usually inflammation in the medulla and pelvis. Progressive scarring may lead to chronic renal failure. Sometimes it is unilateral with hypertrophy of the other kidney.

Chronic pyelonephritis is often associated with hypertension.

Clinical features

Patients with hypertension due to chronic pyelonephritis may have a history of recurrent acute pyelonephritis and loin pain or, if presenting late, may have symptoms of chronic renal failure and anaemia. The hypertension may be mild or severe.

Investigations

The urine may contain pus cells and may be infected.

Proteinuria will be present even with mild hypertension. The diagnosis is confirmed by demonstrating small scarred kidneys on intravenous urography.

Management

Conventional drug therapy is usually needed to control the hypertension. Occasionally there is a place for unilateral nephrectomy in a younger patient if the other kidney appears entirely normal. Antibiotics are indicated to treat infection and long term antibiotic suppression may be needed for persistent or recurrent infection.

Acute glomerulonephritis

Hypertension is a frequent feature of acute post-streptococcal glomerulonephritis. Patients present with malaise and smoky haematuria. Continuing streptococcal infection requires treatment and hypertension responds to the usual drugs. The condition is self-limiting and the drugs can usually be withdrawn after a few weeks.

Occasional patients may develop malignant hypertension and hypertensive encephalopathy requiring urgent treatment of the raised blood pressure.

Chronic glomerulonephritis

Hypertension and renal failure are common features in chronic glomerulonephritis of all types. The hypertension may be mild or severe. It is accompanied by heavy proteinuria and other stigmata of renal disease such as cells and casts in the urine. The diagnosis can be confirmed by renal biopsy.

Management

Treatment of the hypertension may help to slow the progression of renal failure, but as renal failure progresses the hypertension may be increasingly difficult to control. Haemodialysis sometimes helps and bilateral nephrectomy has been carried out to allow control of severe hypertension in the presence of advanced renal failure. Use of the converting enzyme inhibitor captopril usually makes this unnecessary.

Polycystic disease of the kidneys

This is a congenital abnormality. The distal nephrons fail to link with the proximal parts and the resulting cysts are usually multiple and bilateral. Severe cases present with abdominal distension at birth or rapidly progressive renal failure in infancy. Less severe cases lead to hypertension in early adult life and progressive renal failure. The hypertension may be mild or severe and its treatment may help to slow the progress of the renal failure.

Clinical features

Patients may present with hypertension, renal failure or abdominal pain and haematuria. The characteristic physical sign is marked bilateral renal enlargement together with haematuria.

Management

The hypertension requires therapy along the usual lines.

Surgical puncture of cysts has no place except in isolated cysts that can be punctured under ultrasound control. Cytology of the cyst fluid helps to exclude a cyst in a hypernephroma. There is an increased incidence of renal carcinoma in polycystic disease.

Connective tissue disease

Polyarteritis nodosa

Polyarteritis nodosa affects small and medium arteries throughout the body. It is characterized by fibrinoid necrosis leading to thrombosis, stenosis, haemorrhage or aneurysm formation. In some patients, the kidneys are involved with resulting hypertension. This may present as rapidly progressive hypertension associated with otherwise unexplained disease. Steroid therapy helps to slow the progression of renal disease and treatment of the hypertension is an essential part of the management.

Other connective tissue diseases

Systemic lupus erythematosis and other connective tissue diseases may cause hypertension. Treatment includes steroid and antihypertensive therapy.

Diabetes mellitus

Diabetic renal disease produces sclerosis of the afferent arterioles leading to destruction of the glomeruli and progressive renal failure with proteinuria. Hypertension is often a feature and its treatment may help to slow the progress of the renal failure.

Less common causes of renal hypertension

These include:

- analgesic abuse
- radiation damage to the kidneys
- amyloidosis

Coarctation of the aorta

Coarctation of the aorta is a congenital malformation that causes hypertension in the upper half of the body. The usual site of constriction is between the origin of the left subclavian artery and the insertion of the ductus arteriosus. Coarctation is often associated with berry aneurysms in the circle of Willis and abnormalities of the aortic valve.

Clinical features

An extensive collateral circulation develops to bypass the coarcted area. The most characteristic clinical signs are absent or weak and delayed femoral pulses, suprasternal pulsation in the root of the neck and palpable collateral arteries around the scapulae.

Management

Recognition of coarctation of the aorta is important because it can cause severe hypertension in childhood and early adult life with the risk of subarachnoid haemorrhage and malignant hypertension. The condition should be treated surgically by excision of the coarcted area. Some patients remain hypertensive after surgery but can usually be easily controlled with drugs.

Endocrine causes of hypertension

Cushing's syndrome

Cushing's syndrome is caused by excessive production of corticosteroids in the adrenal cortex. It may be due to excess production of ACTH by the pituitary because of a basophil adenoma – Cushing's disease. This leads to bilateral adrenal cortical hyperplasia and excess cortisol production. Alternatively, a primary adrenal abnormality, either an adenoma or, uncommonly, a carcinoma may produce cortisol autonomously. Rarely, ectopic production of ACTH, usually from a bronchial carcinoma, leads to increased adrenocortical function.

Clinical features

Patients may present because of hypertension or the characteristic appearance and features of Cushing's syndrome: a plethoric appearance, moonface, obesity of the trunk with a buffalo hump and wasting of the limb muscles, hirsutism, osteoporosis and diabetes.

Investigations

The diagnosis rests on demonstrating autonomous cortisol production. Adrenal adenomas can be localized by computerized axial tomography or adrenal venography.

Management

An adrenal adenoma is treated by unilateral adrenalectomy. Patients with pituitary tumours are best treated by bilateral adrenalectomy that may be followed by pituitary radiotherapy. Surgery is carried out under hydrocortisone cover and patients subjected to bilateral adrenalectomy require lifelong steroid replacement therapy.

Conn's syndrome

Conn's syndrome or primary hyperaldosteronism is due to excess production of aldosterone by the zona glomerulosa of the adrenal cortex. This may be because of a unilateral adenoma or bilateral hyperplasia.

Excess aldosterone production leads to sodium retention and hypertension. In addition, excessive loss of potassium in the urine leads to hypokalaemia.

Clinical features

Patients often present with mild symptomless hypertension. The malignant phase is rare. The hypokalaemia may occasionally cause polyuria.

Investigations

The diagnosis is often first suspected when hypokalaemia is discovered on routine blood testing. It is confirmed by demonstrating that plasma renin is suppressed and that plasma aldosterone is elevated. An adenoma can be visualized by computerized axial tomography or adrenal venography. Adrenal venous blood samples can be obtained to estimate aldosterone concentration.

Management

An adenoma can be removed surgically. Treatment with the competitive aldosterone antagonist spironolactone will reverse, in most cases, the biochemical changes and the hypertension.

Pheochromocytoma

Pheochromocytoma is a rare tumour of the adrenal medulla that produces adrenaline, noradrenaline or other catecholamines. It is usually found in one or other adrenal but is occasionally ectopic in the posterior abdomen or thorax. A proportion are malignant.

Clinical features

The catecholamine production leads to vasoconstriction, tachycardia and hypertension that is often severe. The secretion is often paroxysmal, producing bouts of headache, palpitation, pallor, sweating, chest pain, thyroid swelling and hypertension.

Investigations

The diagnosis depends on demonstrating excess excretion of catecholamines or their metabolites in the urine. The site of the adenoma may be established by computerized axial tomography, arteriography or retroperitoneal air studies.

Management

Surgical removal of the tumour is curative. The risk of profound hypotension during surgery can now be avoided by adequate premedication with adrenergic α- and β-blocking drugs.

Drug induced hypertension

Corticosteroid therapy

Corticosteroid therapy may cause hypertension and changes similar to those found in Cushing's syndrome. The blood pressure usually falls when the drug is discontinued. So, remember to check the blood pressure of patients receiving steroid therapy.

Contraceptive pill

Oestrogen therapy tends to produce a small rise in blood pressure. In some, it causes hypertension. Withdrawal of therapy usually leads to a fall in blood pressure, although this can take as long as 4 months. A few remain hypertensive, but it is difficult to attribute this to the drug. Because of this complication, however, it is important to measure blood pressure before women start to take the contraceptive pill and at regular intervals during therapy.

Significance of hypertension

Malignant phase hypertension

Severe hypertension is characterized by fibrinoid necrosis in the arterioles. This is responsible for the characteristic retinal signs (bilateral haemorrhages, exudates and papilloedema) and the proteinuria.

The treatment of malignant phase hypertension is a medical emergency requiring prompt admission to hospital and effective treatment. Untreated, half the patients with malignant hypertension are dead within 6 months The commonest causes of death are renal failure, cerebral haemorrhage and cardiac failure. Since the earliest days of effective antihypertensive treatment the prognosis has been much improved: two thirds will survive for 5 years and probably much longer if the blood urea is normal, one quarter if it is raised.

Mild to moderate hypertension

Even a mildly elevated blood pressure is associated with an increase in cardiovascular and cerebrovascular mortality. The life expectancy of a 35 year old male is reduced by 9 years if his blood pressure is 140/95 mmHg. This risk is compounded if the patient has other cardiovascular risk factors e.g. cigarette smoking, hypercholesterolaemia.

It does not automatically follow that lowering the blood pressure will improve the prognosis. However, there is good evidence that it will in both males and females, if the diastolic blood pressure is above 110 mm. Also, male patients show considerable benefit if the diastolic is above 105 and some benefit if it is above 90, although the treatment of mild hypertension remains controversial.

It is generally agreed that effective treatment reduces the risk of stroke, renal failure and cardiac failure. In early studies, the incidence of myocardial infarction was not shown to fall despite regression in the electrocardiographic changes of left ventricular hypertrophy. In recent studies, however, it appears to have done so.

Complicated hypertension

The presence of complications affects the prognosis and may also influence the decision about whether or not to start treatment.

Hypertensive encephalopathy

This is a rare complication of malignant hypertension characterized by clouded consciousness, fits and focal neurological signs. It responds dramatically to immediate lowering of the blood pressure, otherwise it is rapidly fatal. It is believed to be due to spasm of the cerebral arterioles.

Angina pectoris

Angina pectoris often coexists with hypertension. The increased suceptibility to coronary atheroma and the increased left ventricular work load are important aetiological factors. It can be eased considerably by lowering the blood pressure, especially if β-adrenergic blocking drugs are used.

Cardiac failure

It is generally considered that in the absence of coexisting cardiac disease, severe hypertension rarely if ever leads to cardiac failure. However, the combination of hypertension, coronary heart disease and cardiac failure is not uncommon and in these circumstances, lowering the blood pressure will help to relieve the failure.

Stroke

Even after a hypertensive patient has sustained a cerebral thrombosis or a cerebral haemorrhage, long term treatment of the hypertension will help to prevent a second stroke. There is, however, no evidence that treatment of the reactive hypertension in a stroke victim who has cerebral oedema or hypoventilation is helpful.

Systolic hypertension

Insurance statistics and population surveys have shown that elevation of the systolic as well as the diastolic blood pressure reduces life expectancy. The systolic pressure correlates slightly better with prognosis than the diastolic pressure, despite the fact that the diastolic pressure is closer to the true mean intra-arterial pressure. It has been argued that systolic pressure reflects the physical stresses on the arteriole and that it should be treated. So far, there is little evidence to support this claim.

Pathological consequences of raised blood pressure

Heart

The increased load on the left ventricle results in

concentric hypertrophy; the individual muscle fibres increase in size. Eventually, progressive left ventricular dilatation occurs, followed by left ventricular failure. Secondary pulmonary hypertension and right heart failure may also develop in the later stages of the disease.

The high blood pressure increases the incidence of atheroma in the coronary arteries so that both chronic ischaemia and acute myocardial infarction are common.

Rarely, renal failure may produce uraemic pericarditis.

Arteries and arterioles

In the aorta, medial necrosis may lead to aortic dissection. Atheroma may result in ulcerated plaques that cause emboli; aneurysms, especially of the abdominal aorta; and stenoses at the mouths of arteries arising from the aorta.

In the smaller muscular arteries and arterioles, the media hypertrophies and the intima thickens. This, together with atheroma, causes widespread damage, especially to the heart, brain, kidneys and limbs.

In addition to medial hypertrophy and atheroma, severe (malignant) hypertension causes two characteristic arteriolar lesions:

- the intima may show concentric layers of proliferation, the so-called 'onion peel thickening'
- focal fibrinoid necrosis may occur in all layers of the arteriolar wall

Brain

Hypertension leads to both cerebral thrombosis, with resultant infarction, and cerebral haemorrhage.

Cerebral infarction is the result of atheroma and does not differ from infarction in normotensive patients.

Cerebral haemorrhage, on the other hand, results from rupture of miliary microaneurysms of the smallest cerebral arteries. These Charcot–Bouchard aneurysms are almost exclusive to hypertension and disappear with antihypertensive treatment.

Subarachnoid haemorrhage from large aneurysms of the circle of Willis occurs with increased frequency in hypertensive patients.

Malignant hypertension can result in spasm of cerebral arterioles and this is thought to explain the clinical syndrome of hypertensive encephalopathy.

Kidney

The earliest lesions occur in the afferent arterioles.

Medial thickening leads to nephrosclerosis characterized by glomerular hyalinization and tubal atrophy, with consequent scarring of the cortex. In longstanding hypertension this reduces the overall size of the kidney and its surface becomes granular in appearance. At this stage, the patient may develop progressive chronic renal failure.

In the malignant phase, the arteriolar lesions progress to onion peel thickening and fibrinoid necrosis, and there may be haemorrhages in the renal substance. The kidneys are usually less shrunken than in chronic renal failure. Renal infarction or acute ischaemia may stimulate the renin–angiotensin system with a consequent increase in the severity of the hypertension.

Retina

The retinal arteries undergo the changes described above. In the malignant phase, fibrinoid necrosis leads to retinal haemorrhages and the escape of protein, causing cottonwool exudates, together with oedema of the optic nerve head (see p. 109).

Investigation of hypertension

Although the majority of patients with high blood pressure require lifelong drug therapy, a small number can be cured. In addition to a full history and physical examination, a few routine investigations are therefore indicated to exclude remediable causes. Additional tests can be used to find and assess complications of raised blood pressure.

Exclusion of an underlying cause

The diagnosis can often be suspected on clinical evidence alone in the following:

- therapy with the contraceptive pill or corticosteroids
- Cushing's syndrome
- polycystic renal disease
- coarctation of the aorta
- pheochromocytoma

Unilateral renal disease, and particularly renal artery stenosis, is best screened for by intravenous urography (IVP). This investigation used to be carried out routinely in all hypertensive patients, but the yield of treatable abnormalities was so small that it is now restricted to patients who are under the age of 40, have severe hypertension or show other evidence of renal disease.

Primary aldosteronism (Conn's syndrome) produces significant hypokalaemia most of the time so that estimation of plasma electrolytes before treatment is a routine investigation.

The exclusion of collagen diseases will be helped by a routine blood count and erythrocyte sedimentation rate (ESR).

If underlying pathology is suspected from the results of any of these screening tests, fuller investigation is indicated.

Estimating the prognosis

A chest X-ray can give useful information about heart size and pulmonary congestion. The electrocardiogram may indicate the degree of left ventricular hypertrophy.

Renal function can be estimated from the blood urea or more exactly by the plasma creatinine concentration or the creatinine clearance.

Other cardiovascular risk factors may be discovered by checking the blood sugar and plasma lipids.

Table 19 shows routine investigations and further tests that are indicated in younger patients and in those with severe hypertension. The more elaborate investigations need only be carried out in special cases.

TABLE 19

In all patients	In young or severe hypertensives	In selected cases only
Urine examination	Plasma creatinine	Plasma cortisols
Plasma urea and electrolytes	Intravenous urography	Plasma renin and aldosterone
Electrocardiograph	Urinary catecholamines	Renography
Chest X-ray	Plasma lipids	Arteriography
Blood count and ESR		

General management and treatment

Therapeutic emergencies

Hypertensive encephalopathy or acute left ventricular failure require immediate intravenous antihypertensive therapy (e.g. with diazoxide, sodium nitrop-russide or labetalol) to lower the blood pressure rapidly to a predetermined level. Overzealous treatment is not without risk. Frequent blood pressure monitoring is required during such emergency therapy and the patient should be nursed in hospital. The head of the bed should be raised to take advantage of any postural fall in blood pressure. As soon as the blood pressure is brought under control, a conventional oral drug regime is commenced.

Patients without these complications, but with Grade III or IV retinopathy, also require treatment that will lower the blood pressure within a few hours. Intravenous drugs are best avoided because a rapid fall in blood pressure may result in permanent neurological damage.

When to treat

Although we know that treatment of hypertension will improve prognosis and, in particular, lessen the likelihood of stroke, it is not possible to say exactly how high the blood pressure should be before treatment is started. The higher the pressure, the greater the potential benefit, but against this must be weighed the inconvenience, side-effects and risks of therapy. Also, that these will vary from patient to patient.

It is conventional to treat hypertension according to the diastolic blood pressure. Simple guidelines are required when deciding whether or not to start treatment. Trials show some benefit from treating those with a diastolic above 90 mm and considerable benefit when the diastolic is above 105 mm. The cut-off should fall between these figures. However, each patient must be considered individually. For example, the case to treat will be stronger in patients who already have evidence of left ventricular hypertrophy and weaker in patients who seem unlikely to comply with the prescribed therapy. Women develop rather fewer complications of hypertension than men and it might be reasonable to select a slightly higher diastolic for them.

General measures

Those who know that they have high blood pressure are usually worried and anxious about it. They require an explanation and reassurance, even when it is decided that treatment is unnecessary. Well-informed patients are likely to be more co-operative and, in those to be treated, it should be stressed that management is aimed at prevention of future complications.

Those who smoke cigarettes should be strongly advised to stop and given help to do so. Those who are obese and those with diabetes should be given dietary advice.

Specific measures

A few patients have remediable hypertension. Even after the cause has been removed their blood pressure should be checked from time to time to make sure it remains normal, because some may require drug therapy and this may not become apparent for some considerable time after the operation.

Drug therapy

Patients who are selected for drug therapy will require it for life. A lot of co-operation is required if treatment is to be successful; so, make sure they understand the reasons for therapy, the risks involved and the consequences of failure to comply.

The aim of drug therapy should be to lower the blood pressure to as near normal as possible for as much of the time and with as few side-effects as possible. In order to achieve this, the prescriber must be fully conversant with the drugs prescribed and with their potential side-effects. It is better to stick to a few drugs and become familiar with them than to use unfamiliar drugs and risk using them wrongly. Although side-effects can often be reduced by using combinations of drugs, the more complex the regime the less likely is the patient to comply with it. A few simple regimes are shown in Table 20.

TABLE 20 **A simple antihypertensive treatment scheme**

Degree of hypertension	Type of regime	Examples
1. Mild	Single drug	Diuretic or β-blocker
2. Moderate	Two drugs	Diuretic plus β-blocker
3. Resistant	Three drugs	Diuretic plus β-blocker plus vasodilator
4. Very resistant	More potent drugs	Diuretic plus β-plus minoxidil or captopril
5. Encephalo-pathy or pulmonary oedema	Intravenous	Diazoxide or sodium nitroprusside or labetalol

In general, when the patient is started on a drug, it is important to achieve good control without side-effects, which often lead to failure to comply with the treatment. If side-effects appear, or control is not good, the regime must be changed. The dose can be increased, a second drug added or an entirely different drug substituted. The individual drugs are discussed on pp. 250–253.

Follow-up

Careful long term follow-up is required for all patients receiving treatment. The interval between visits should not exceed 3 months when control is good and should be considerably shorter if it is not.

During follow-up it is important to ensure good blood pressure control, to check for complications of hypertension, which may require treatment or a change in treatment, and to look for late side-effects of the drugs. There should be a mechanism for detecting patients who default and stop therapy.

RHEUMATIC HEART DISEASE

Rheumatic carditis occurs during the course of acute rheumatism and may lead to chronic rheumatic heart disease.

Acute rheumatism

Acute rheumatism usually presents as rheumatic fever, an acute multisystem disease that affects collagen tissue. Although arthritis is the usual and obvious presenting feature, its important long term consequences are upon the heart.

Rheumatic fever is preceded by a throat infection caused by group A streptococci. A streptococcal antibody response occurs and, in susceptible individuals, the heart becomes involved because 'rheumatogenic' streptococci produce antibodies that react with the sarcolemmic membrane of the cardiac myofibrils.

Prevalence

The prevalence and severity of rheumatic fever has been falling steadily during the past 50 years in the Western world, where it is now seen fairly infrequently. In tropical and subtropical areas such as

Asia and South America it continues unabated and remains a serious health problem.

There are several possible explanations for this decline in Western countries. As the trend started before the introduction of antibiotics, it is likely to reflect a decrease in the virulence of the streptococcus and an improvement in the standard of living, with a consequent increased ability to resist infection. This is to some extent borne out by the difference in hospital admissions between two areas of Scotland, one a Highland community, the other an industrial community that includes large areas of overcrowding and social deprivation (LD-115).

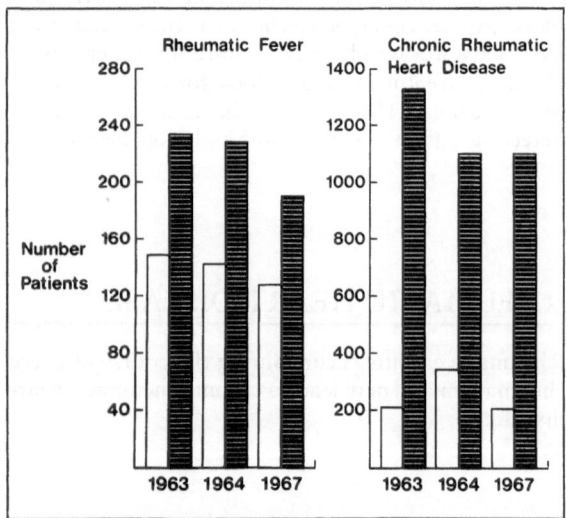

LD-115. *Comparison of discharge rate per 100 000 between northern (Highland) and western (industrial) areas of Scotland. Key:* □ = *northern;* ☰ = *western*

Rheumatic fever tends to occur in families, but this again may be environmental because no genetic susceptibility has been demonstrated and no relationship with HLA antigens has been found.

Rheumatic fever is rare before the age of 5 years and first attacks become increasingly infrequent after the age of 15. Males and females are equally affected by rheumatic fever, but females are more often affected by rheumatic heart disease.

Pathology

In the acute stage there is a generalized subacute inflammation of the whole heart (pancarditis). The early histological changes are non-specific and consist of oedema, lymphocytic infiltration and fibrinoid degeneration and necrosis of collagen. There is also hyperaemia and sometimes capillary haemorrhage. Later, the characteristic histological lesions appear, the Aschoff bodies. First described in 1904, these are found near the smaller branches of the coronary arteries and in the interstitial tissue between bundles of muscle fibres. They consist of a necrotic centre surrounded by Aschoff cells, which are large endotheloid cells with one or several vesicular nuclei and cytoplasm with ragged edges. This area is surrounded by lymphocytes, plasma cells and a variable number of polymorphonuclear leukocytes. A degree of fibroblastic proliferation is always present and, if the condition is severe, it may be followed by significant fibrosis.

These Aschoff lesions are scattered throughout the pericardium, myocardium and heart valves.

During the acute stage, microscopic examination of the valves involved may show fibrinoid degeneration up to the valve margin with overlying fibrinoid vegetations; Aschoff bodies may also be seen. Macroscopic examination shows the valve structures to be swollen and oedematous. Yellowish, warty nodules are often present along the line of cuspal contact and on the chordae tendineae. These changes can lead to fusion of the edges of the cusps with resulting stenosis or to deformity of the cusps with resulting incompetence. The latter is often worsened by fibrotic change in the chordae tendineae, which may shorten and give rise to a funnel deformity. Valves often become both stenosed and incompetent as a result of these changes.

The mitral valve is by far the most commonly affected, followed in frequency by the aortic and the tricuspid valves. The pulmonary valve is seldom involved. In the acute stage, the valves may be involved, not only directly as described above, but also indirectly as a result of cardiac dilation and damage to the valve ring.

Clinical features

The clinical features of rheumatic fever are easily recognized in a florid case, but diagnosis can be difficult and, for that reason, a system based on statistical probabilities has been devised consisting of major criteria (high probability) and minor criteria (lesser probability). A positive diagnosis can be made in the presence of two major or one major and two minor criteria if, in addition, there is evidence of a recent streptococcal infection. This system was first described by Duckett Jones.

Major criteria are:

- carditis
- polyarthritis
- chorea
- erythema marginatum
- subcutaneous nodules

Minor criteria are:

- previous rheumatic fever
- arthralgia
- fever
- raised ESR
- raised white blood count
- prolonged PR interval
- presence of C-reactive protein

Severe cardiac involvement may be present with mild systemic symptoms and it has been said that rheumatic fever 'licks the joints and bites the heart'. Thus, carditis is the most important of the major criteria and evidence of this must be looked for carefully. It includes:

- pericarditis
- myocarditis
- endocarditis

Pericarditis

This is always associated with some degree of underlying myocarditis. In mild cases it is seldom possible to diagnose clinically. The symptoms and signs include:

- pain
  This is characteristically retrosternal and may be referred to the upper abdomen, neck and shoulders. It is often affected by respiration.
- friction
  This is usually best heard at the left lower sternal border and tends to vary with posture and respiration. The to-and-fro sound is clearly related to cardiac action but its timing does not suggest an intracardiac murmur.
- pericardial effusion
  This is best recognized by echocardiography and should be suspected when an X-ray shows increased heart size in a patient with pericardial friction.
- electrocardiogram
  This may show widespread ST elevation in the early stages.

Pericarditis usually indicates severe heart involvement and is good evidence of pancarditis.

Myocarditis

This can be difficult to diagnose and is often inferred from unexplained tachycardia. Evidence of cardiac failure, such as dyspnoea, pulmonary congestion or an elevated central venous pressure, is more reliable.

The electrocardiogram may show prolongation of the PR and QT intervals and the X-ray shows progressive cardiac enlargement.

Endocarditis

Involvement of cardiac valves is suggested by the development of murmurs. But remember that under such circumstances murmurs may also be caused by disturbed myocardial function or simply vigorous heart action in a febrile child.

Mitral valve – systolic murmur

An apical systolic murmur may develop. This is usually pansystolic, conducted towards the axilla, and indicates mitral regurgitation. It may be due to stretching of the valve ring associated with the myocarditis or to damage to the valve cusps, chordae or the valve ring by the rheumatic process.

When the murmur is due to myocarditis, other signs of myocarditis are likely to be present and the murmur will disappear as the condition settles. When due to damage to the valve, the murmur is more likely to persist after the acute phase has passed.

Mitral valve – diastolic murmur

Sometimes a quiet, low pitched, mid-diastolic murmur becomes audible in the mitral area. This was first described in 1924 by Carey Coombs and is caused by turbulence of blood flowing through an oedematous mitral valve. Detection of a Carey Coombs murmur is good evidence of active carditis and it should be listened for carefully, using the bell of the stethoscope. It is not an indication that the patient will subsequently develop mitral stenosis. The murmur usually disappears as the patient's condition improves.

True mitral stenosis is the end result of a slow fibrotic process and does not occur during the relatively short course of acute rheumatic heart disease. Signs of mitral stenosis during an acute attack are evidence of previous affection.

Aortic valve – systolic murmur

This murmur, when heard, is classically ejection in type and is usually due to vigorous cardiac action in a febrile young patient. Aortic stenosis, like mitral stenosis, takes a long time to develop and is not found during the acute phase of a first rheumatic illness.

Aortic valve – diastolic murmur

A short, high pitched early diastolic murmur may become audible at the lower left sternal border. This indicates involvement of the aortic valve and aortic incompetence. It is best heard with the diaphragm of the stethoscope and often persists after the acute illness subsides.

Pulmonary and tricuspid valves

An ejection murmur developing at the pulmonary area is usually innocent and associated with the patient's febrile state. The pulmonary valve is out of fibrous continuity with the rest of the heart and is rarely involved in the rheumatic process.

Tricuspid murmurs are seldom heard unless severe carditis causes cardiac dilatation and right heart failure when the pansystolic murmur of tricuspid regurgitation becomes audible.

Management

The treatment of acute rheumatic heart disease is usually that of the parent condition, but, if the heart is seriously affected, specific treatment may be indicated.

General

As there is no specific therapy, the acute attack is treated along general symptomatic lines paying particular attention to rest, anti-inflammatory agents and residual streptococcal infection.

Rest

Patients should have complete rest until the signs of inflammatory activity have abated as shown by the temperature and ESR.

Anti-inflammatory agents

Pain and pyrexia are greatly helped by acetylsalicylic acid and there is no doubt that the anti-inflammatory effect of this drug speeds recovery.

Steroids should not be used routinely to achieve an anti-inflammatory effect. It has been shown by dividing children with rheumatic fever into three groups, one given acetylsalicylic acid, one given cortisone and one given ACTH, that there is no significant difference in incidence of subsequent valvular disease.

Penicillin

Persistent streptococcal throat infection should be treated with penicillin or another appropriate antibiotic in resistant cases.

Cardiac problems

The only specific treatment available is for cardiac failure. This usually responds to standard treatment with digitalis and diuretics. Occasionally, in the presence of severe carditis, the heart may enlarge progressively despite treatment and steroids must be used.

Period of rest

The duration of bed rest depends on the clinical findings and must be maintained as long as there is any suspicion of carditis. Once the ESR has been normal for at least a week, mobilization may be commenced. Rehabilitation may have to be prolonged for many months to prevent relapse.

Prevention of acute rheumatism

Acute rheumatism is a recurring illness. In one series at least 50% of patients had at least one recurrence and it is estimated that 65% of children with rheumatic fever and 20% of those with chorea will develop chronic rheumatic heart disease. The use of sulphonamides, and later penicillin, has been shown to diminish the recurrence rate greatly and penicillin is now given routinely following the acute attack.

Prophylactic regimes

Phenoxymethyl penicillin 250 mg is given twice daily by mouth or 900 mg of long-acting benzathine penicillin G is given once a month by intramuscular injection. An oral dose of 0.5–1.0 g sulphadiazine daily can be substituted for those sensitive to penicillin.

One of these regimes should be continued until the patient is at least 21 or 25 years of age, or even longer.

Cardiac sequelae of acute rheumatism

The pericarditis heals with no residual damage.

The myocardium may be weakened by fibrotic change.

The main problem in later years results from endocardial damage. Valves that have been swollen, inflamed and deformed during the acute stage undergo gradual fibrotic change with further deformity and disturbance of function. This process may be aggravated by adhesion of the edges of the commissures and, in the case of the mitral valve, shortening and thickening of the chordae tendineae. In addition the valve rings may be affected by scarring. Later the damaged valves may become calcified.

Valves that have been severely damaged may rapidly become and remain incompetent. The signs of mitral and aortic regurgitation may develop during the acute illness and persist after the patient appears to have made a complete recovery.

Stenosis, on the other hand, is the end result of a slow fibrotic process. It takes a long time to develop and often does not become evident until the acute illness has become no more than a memory. Also, because of the heart's considerable reserve capacity, the signs of valve lesions usually precede symptoms by many years.

Although acute rheumatic endocarditis is becoming something of a rarity in this country, chronic rheumatic endocarditis is still the commonest cause of valvar heart disease and will be considered in detail below.

DISORDERS OF CARDIAC VALVES

Mitral valve disease

Anatomy

The mitral valve has two cusps, an anterior cusp and a posterior cusp. They are attached proximally to the atrioventricular valve ring and distally, by the chordae tendineae, to the papillary muscles, which prevent the cusps prolapsing into the left atrium during ventricular systole.

The anterior cusp is the larger of the two and is a most important structure. Its posterior surface forms the anterior surface of the left ventricular inflow tract and its anterior surface forms the posterior surface of the left ventricular outflow tract (LD-17, LD-19). Its upper part is in fibrous continuity with the aortic valve and the root of the aorta.

Mitral stenosis

Causes

There are two types of mitral stenosis, congenital and acquired.

Congenital

This is a very uncommon malformation that usually takes one of two forms:

- a valve with fused cusps similar to that seen in acquired mitral stenosis
- a 'parachute valve' in which the chordae are inserted into a single papillary muscle

Lutembacher's syndrome is mitral stenosis, either congenital or acquired, accompanied by an atrial septal defect.

Acquired

The mitral valve is the one most frequently affected in chronic rheumatic endocarditis. Although only about 50% of patients give a history of rheumatic fever, mitral stenosis is usually the end result of damage caused during and following acute rheumatism. It takes several years to develop and is three times commoner in women than in men.

Pathology

Mitral stenosis is a slow fibrotic process that reduces the size of the valve orifice. It varies in severity from adhesion along the edges of fairly mobile cusps, to dense fibrosis of shrunken cusps with shortened and matted chordae tendineae. Calcification may eventually occur in the fibrosed cusps causing further deformity and, not surprisingly, such stenosed valves are often incompetent as well as stenosed.

Pathophysiology

The normal mitral valve has an orifice of approximately 5 square cm and the heart appears to be able to function normally until this is greatly reduced, to about 1 square cm or less. The strain of compensating for a reduced mitral valve orifice falls initially on the left atrium. The earliest effect is a raised left atrial mean pressure (normal value, 5–12 mmHg). In mild cases, the pressure may be normal at rest but rises rapidly on effort. Later, a raised pressure is required to maintain forward flow even at rest and in severe cases may exceed 25 mmHg.

A raised pressure in the left atrium is matched firstly

by changes in the lungs and later by changes in the right heart. As the resting pressure in the pulmonary veins and capillaries approaches the plasma osmotic pressure (30 mmHg) a potentially dangerous situation exists. A sudden rise in capillary pressure may then cause fluid to pass into the alveoli and cause pulmonary oedema. This may be precipitated by exercise or excitement and is a hazard during pregnancy.

Pulmonary hypertension

Fortunately, left atrial pressure usually rises slowly and certain secondary effects have time to take place. The pulmonary capillary basement membrane tends to become thickened by oedema and collagen, thus affording the alveoli some protection. The pulmonary artery pressure rises in parallel with the pulmonary capillary pressure to a mean of about 30 mmHg. After this, in at least a quarter of cases, the arterial pressure rises sharply in an independent manner as a result of increased pulmonary arteriolar tone. This gives further protection because it prevents a sudden rise in pulmonary capillary pressure and so diminishes the risk of pulmonary oedema.

In the early stages, pulmonary hypertension is reversible if the obstruction at the mitral valve is relieved. Later, fibrosis in the pulmonary arterioles makes a return to normality less and less likely.

Pulmonary hypertension results in right ventricular hypertrophy. If it is severe and sustained, the pulmonary valve ring occasionally becomes dilated and pulmonary regurgitation may occur. Much more commonly, as the right heart fails the tricuspid valve ring dilates and causes tricuspid regurgitation, with systolic pulsation in distended neck veins and an enlarged liver (LD-116).

The above have been described as the 'backward' effects of mitral stenosis. They affect the lungs first and eventually the right heart. The 'forward' effects are caused by reduced cardiac output, which can be considerable when the obstruction is severe. The left ventricle is not affected by 'pure' mitral stenosis.

Symptoms

Most patients do not develop symptoms until many years after the acute rheumatism. In the UK, except during pregnancy, they are usually at least 30 years old before becoming handicapped. The common symptoms include:

- dyspnoea
- haemoptysis
- cardiac pain
- palpitation
- symptoms secondary to right ventricular failure

Dyspnoea

The earliest symptom of mitral stenosis is shortness of breath. At first, this is only troublesome on exertion, but, as time goes by, it becomes more and more easily induced until eventually it is present even at rest. Many clinicians use the following simple method of grading disability according to the New York Heart Association's classification of Cardiac Grade:

- Grade I
  No breathlessness on normal exertion
- Grade II
  Breathlessness on strenuous activity
- Grade III
  Breathlessness on normal activity
- Grade IV
  Breathlessness on less than normal activity or even at rest

Grading is useful both when assessing the severity of the lesion and in following its progress.

Haemoptysis

Haemoptysis is fairly common in patients with mitral stenosis. It may be due to one of several causes.

The commonest cause is probably chest infection,

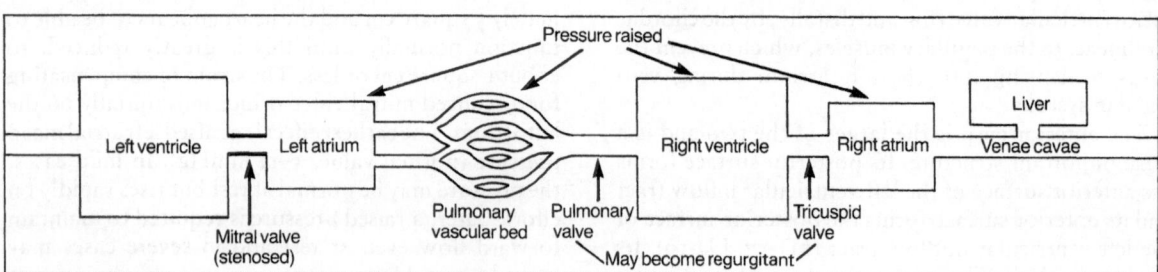

LD-116. *Haemodynamic consequences of mitral stenosis*

to which they are particularly prone. Most of them have winter bronchitis and coughing with congested lungs causes a little bleeding.

Another is rupture of one of the small dilated bronchopulmonary anastomoses that develop as a result of continued high pulmonary venous pressure. Although sometimes alarming, neither of these is of any consequence.

More serious is haemoptysis following pulmonary infarction caused by embolism or thrombosis.

Most serious is the bloodstained frothy sputum that appears in acute pulmonary oedema.

Cardiac pain

Chest pain on effort is fairly common in severe mitral stenosis, usually in older patients, with pulmonary hypertension. In the past, it was thought to be due to low cardiac output with reduced coronary artery flow, but recent studies have shown a high incidence of coronary artery disease in such patients and this must be kept in mind if cardiac surgery is contemplated.

Palpitation

Awareness of rapid heart action or missed beats may occur, especially on effort, and may signal the onset of atrial fibrillation.

Right ventricular failure

When right ventricular failure occurs, symptoms related to venous congestion become troublesome. A large liver causes a feeling of abdominal distension. Engorged gastric and intestinal veins result in nausea and vomiting. The lower limbs become swollen with oedema.

All the symptoms of mitral stenosis may be worsened during pregnancy, chest infections and periods of abnormal cardiac rhythm.

Clinical signs

General examination

The patient's appearance depends on the severity of the lesion. Mild cases appear normal; severe cases may have orthopnoea. Longstanding mitral stenosis with pulmonary hypertension often results in the so-called 'mitral facies' with dusky cyanosed cheeks and cold, rather blue, hands and feet – the peripheral cyanosis being due to low cardiac output and peripheral vasoconstriction.

When the right ventricular pressure is raised, the neck veins are distended and prominent 'a' waves may be seen as the atrium contracts against a poorly compliant right ventricle. This sign is, of course, absent in atrial fibrillation. The raised central venous pressure is usually associated with an enlarged liver and sometimes with ascites. Ankle oedema occurs towards evening in ambulant patients and sacral oedema will be found in those confined to bed.

If the tricuspid valve becomes dilated, the liver will pulsate in systole and prominent 'V' waves will be seen in the internal jugular veins.

Because of pulmonary congestion and frequent infection in the congested lungs, fine crepitations are often heard at the bases of the lungs and signs of bronchitis are scattered throughout the chest.

Cardiac signs

The apex beat is usually normal in position and is classically tapping in nature. The tapping sensation is caused by vigorous closure of the mitral valve, which is held open longer than usual in diastole by the raised left atrial pressure. When the ventricle contracts the cusps have a long way to travel in a short time and make a loud slapping noise on closing because of tension in the chordae. Such an apex beat is evidence of pliant cusps. A severely fibrosed or calcified valve cannot move in this way and the first sound is less obvious. If the stenosis is significant and the chest wall is thin, a thrill may be felt in diastole or presystole.

Elevation of the pulmonary artery pressure causes vigorous closure of the pulmonary valve and this can sometimes be palpated in the second left intercostal space close to the sternum. Right ventricular contraction may also be felt in systole along the left sternal border, the so-called 'right ventricular heave'.

On auscultation, the first sound at the mitral area usually has a loud, slapping quality due to the forcible valve closure already described, and has been called the 'closing snap'. The pulmonary component of the second sound is usually accentuated, making the normal splitting in the pulmonary area easier to detect.

Another high frequency heart sound often follows the second sound. It is best heard at or internal to the apex and is called the 'opening snap'. Again, this is good evidence of a pliable valve. The more severe the stenosis, the earlier the opening snap and so a rough index of severity can be obtained by study of the interval between the second sound and the opening snap.

The classical murmur of mitral stenosis is caused by turbulence when blood flows through the narrow valve during diastole. Flow starts in mid-diastole when the mitral valve opens and rapidly reaches its maximum velocity. The valve is kept open longer than normal by the raised left atrial pressure and the murmur may continue up to the onset of ventricular systole, as indicated by the first heart sound. Flow through the valve depends on the area of the valve orifice and so the length of the murmur is another index of severity. Atrial contraction occurs just prior to ventricular systole and may give the murmur presystolic accentuation – the 'presystolic murmur' of mitral stenosis. With the onset of atrial fibrillation, this murmur disappears because the atrium no longer contracts (LD-117 and 118).

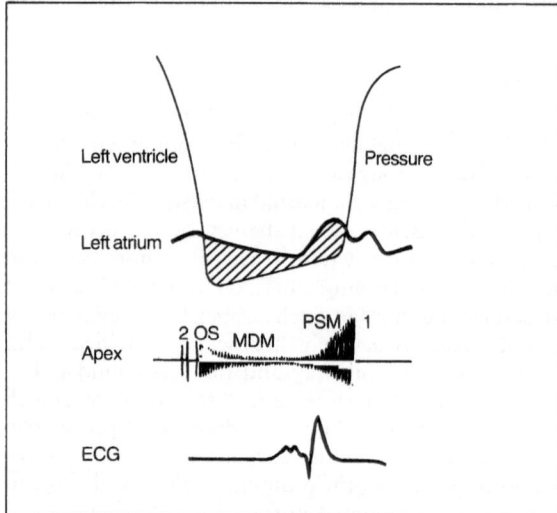

LD-117. Murmur of mitral stenosis – sinus rhythm. Key: 1 and 2, heart sounds; OS, opening snap; MDM, mid-diastolic murmur; PSM, presystolic murmur

In severe pulmonary hypertension, the pulmonary valve ring may dilate and the valve may become incompetent. A high pitched, early diastolic murmur of pulmonary incompetence is then heard along the lower left sternal edge. This murmur was first described by Graham Steell and still bears his name. It is indistinguishable from the murmur of aortic incompetence, a commonly associated lesion, and has to be differentiated from it by looking for other evidence of pulmonary hypertension and the peripheral signs of aortic regurgitation. In such cases right ventricular distension may cause dilatation of the tricuspid valve ring and tricuspid incompetence. This causes a pansystolic murmur in the tricuspid area, which is sometimes confused with the murmur of mitral regurgitation.

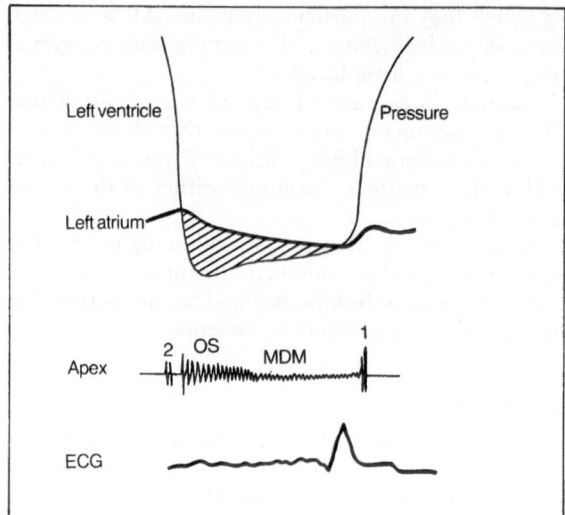

LD-118. Murmur of mitral stenosis – atrial fibrillation

Variations in auscultatory signs

From the above account, it will be obvious that the signs of mitral stenosis vary with the size of the valve orifice, the degree of fibrosis in the cusps and chordae, the extent of calcification and the presence or absence of atrial fibrillation.

The lesion is easily diagnosed in younger patients with sinus rhythm and mobile cusps, when an opening snap is followed by a mid-diastolic murmur that ends with a presystolic crescendo and a loud, slapping first heart sound. It is less easily diagnosed in older patients with atrial fibrillation and shrunken calcified cusps, when a faint rumbling mid-diastolic murmur may be the only abnormal auscultatory sign.

Correct interpretation of the signs can predict the state of the valve mechanism and is important when surgery is being contemplated.

Investigations

Electrocardiogram

In sinus rhythm, evidence of left atrial hypertrophy is usually present. It causes slight prologation of the P wave with a characteristic notched appearance, often referred to as 'P mitrale' (LD-119). This is misleading because any lesion producing left atrial hypertrophy can cause both the right and left atrial P waves to become visible. Signs of right ventricular hypertrophy, right axis deviation with dominant R waves in the right chest leads, are usually conspicuous by their absence, but may be present in those with longstanding pulmonary hypertension.

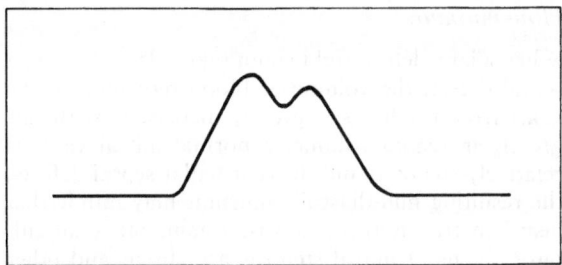

LD-119. '*P mitrale*'

Atrial fibrillation is nearly always present in the later stages.

Chest X-ray

The main features that may be seen in the PA film are:

- an enlarged left atrial appendage
  This fills what is normally a depression on the left cardiac border between the pulmonary trunk and the left ventricle. It may straighten the left cardiac border or give the characteristic appearance of four protrusions: from above downwards, the aorta, the pulmonary trunk, the left atrial appendage and the left ventricle (X-19, arrows).

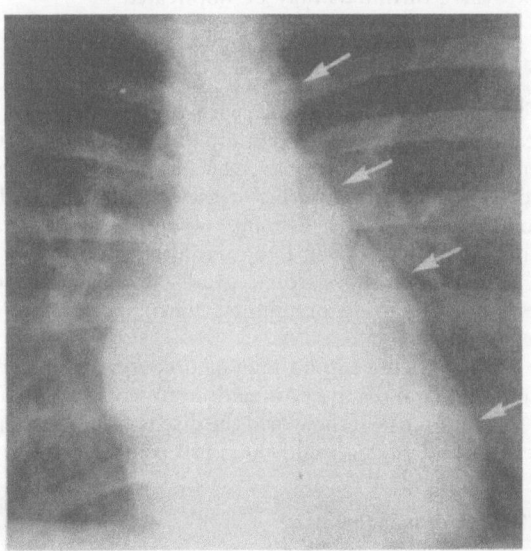

X-19.

- Kerley B lines
  These are seen as little horizontal streaks near the costophrenic angles.
- prominent upper lobe veins

- small pleural effusions
- enlargement of the main pulmonary arteries close to the hilum in pulmonary hypertension
- the fine nodular pattern of pulmonary haemosiderosis that can develop in longstanding cases

The main features in the right anterior oblique (RAO) film are:

- the enlarged left atrium bulges backwards and displaces the barium-filled oesophagus (X-9b)
- calcification may be seen in penetrated films

Echocardiography

The mitral valve cusps, especially the anterior cusp, are easily detected and the rate of closure can be measured. This is slowed in proportion to the severity of the stenosis, especially in sinus rhythm (LD-120). It also detects heavy calcification, which shows as multiple echoes.

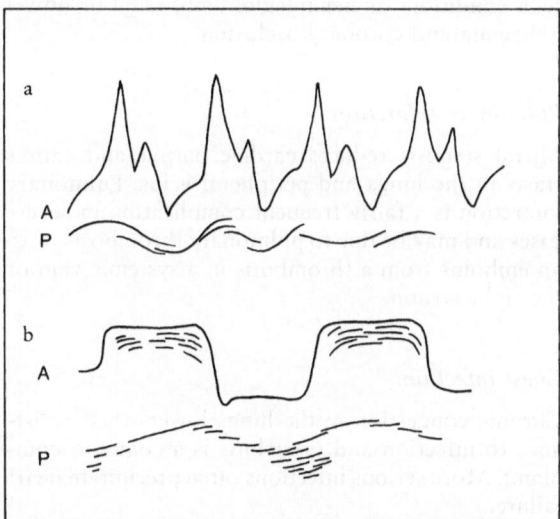

LD-120. *a, Echocardiogram of normal mitral valve. b, Echocardiogram of stenosed mitral valve. Key: as in LD-63 (p. 56). See also text, p. 56*

Cardiac catheterization

If the tip of an end hole cardiac catheter is advanced through the right atrium, right ventricle and main pulmonary artery until it becomes wedged in a small branch of the pulmonary artery, it measures the left atrial pressure via the pulmonary capillary bed. The resting level and the height after a few minutes of leg exercises provide valuable information about the severity of mitral valve obstruction.

The degree of pulmonary and right ventricular hypertension can also be measured and evidence of tricuspid stenosis or regurgitation can be detected from the pressure waves.

Complications of mitral stenosis

Atrial fibrillation

This is common, particularly after the age of 45 years. It may be preceded by a period when atrial ectopic beats are frequent, but its onset can be dramatic and associated with a sudden deterioration in the cardiac grade.

Systemic embolus

This is a constant risk, especially in patients with atrial fibrillation. Stasis within the left atrium encourages clot formation, particularly in the left atrial appendage. The results can be serious, producing such conditions as hemiplegia, limb, renal or bowel ischaemia and coronary occlusion.

Pulmonary infarction

Mitral stenosis reduces cardiac output and causes stasis in the lungs and peripheral veins. Pulmonary infarction is a fairly frequent complication in severe cases and may be due to pulmonary thrombosis or to an embolus from a thrombosis in a systemic vein or the right atrium.

Chest infection

Chronic congestion in the lungs lowers their resistance to infection and bronchitis is a common complaint. More serious infections often precipitate heart failure.

Subacute bacterial endocarditis

This may occur on any valve lesion, but is relatively infrequent in 'pure' mitral stenosis.

Differential diagnosis

Third heart sound

A third heart sound is often mistaken for a mid-diastolic murmur. It occurs at the same time as the onset of the murmur but is short and unaccompanied by other auscultatory signs of mitral stenosis.

Flow murmurs

When a large left to right shunt takes place through a septal defect, the volume of blood returning to the heart from the lungs is greatly increased. With this greatly increased volume, a normal mitral valve is relatively stenosed and, in ventricular septal defects, the resulting mid-diastolic murmur may mimic that heard in true mitral stenosis. Again, other auscultatory signs of mitral stenosis are absent and other features of the malformation readily distinguish between congenital and acquired lesions.

Austin Flint murmur

In severe aortic regurgitation, the anterior cusp of the mitral valve vibrates in diastole and may produce a low pitched sound similar to the murmur heard in mitral stenosis. This can cause difficulty in diagnosis. Echocardiography is helpful in distinguishing between them.

Left atrial myxoma

This relatively uncommon tumour can simulate the murmur of mitral stenosis by obstructing the mitral valve orifice. It usually does so intermittently and is again easily detected by echocardiography. Rarely, a ball valve thrombus may be implicated.

Natural history

The natural history varies with the severity of the lesion. Symptoms develop gradually and the downhill progress is slow. In many, the lesion is discovered accidentally during routine medical examinations. In some, it may only become obvious when atrial fibrillation develops in late middle life.

In women, the cardiac grade may deteriorate temporarily during pregnancy, when special care is required.

Most patients can be managed conservatively for many years and surgery is seldom urgently required.

In some parts of the world the disease is much more serious and runs a rapid downhill course.

Medical management

Atrial fibrillation

Digitalis should be given to control the ventricular rate and increase the cardiac output. If it is paroxysmal before becoming the established rhythm, an antidysrhythmic drug can be used to prevent troublesome attacks.

Heart failure

Heart failure may develop during periods of uncontrolled atrial fibrillation or episodes of acute respiratory infection, which are common in patients with mitral stenosis. These are treated along standard medical lines and the treatment modified when the precipitating factors are brought under control.

Prevention of emboli

All patients with established or intermittent atrial fibrillation should receive anticoagulant therapy to prevent or diminish the incidence of pulmonary and systemic emboli.

Prevention of bacterial endocarditis

Although subacute bacterial endocarditis is not common in 'pure' mitral stenosis, prophylactic antibiotic therapy should be given at times of special risk such as tooth extraction, urological investigation etc.

Prevention of recurrence of rheumatic fever

This has been dealt with, above, p. 158 in the section on acute rheumatism. Remember, that if patients are taking penicillin to prevent recurrences of rheumatic fever, resistant organisms can develop and other antibiotics may be required to prevent bacterial endocarditis.

Surgical management

Surgery is necessary for those who:

- despite adequate medical treatment, remain significantly handicapped
- despite lack of significant symptoms, show evidence of serious complications such as severe pulmonary hypertension

Wherever possible, relief of obstruction should be achieved by mitral valvotomy. Many surgeons now prefer open valvotomy on cardiopulmonary bypass to the traditional closed procedure, which is carried out with a finger in the left atrium and a dilator inserted through the left ventricular apex. An open heart operation should always be advised if the valve is heavily calcified or significantly incompetent, because in these circumstances the valve may have to be replaced if cosmetic surgery is unsuccessful.

Mitral regurgitation (incompetence)

The mitral valve is a complicated structure. To understand its function, it is best thought of in yachting terms as capstans, cables and sails. When the papillary muscles (capstans) contract, the chordae (cables) tighten and the cusps roll against each other like opposing sails to close the atrioventricular orifice. Regurgitation may occur if any of the components fails to function properly or is significantly altered in shape or size. There are, therefore, many causes of mitral incompetence.

Causes

Rheumatic

Until recently, rheumatic heart disease was the commonest cause of mitral regurgitation in this country. It still is in many parts of the world where rheumatic fever is endemic. The cusps are fibrosed, possibly calcified, and the chordae tendineae are often involved in the fibrous process. The result is a rigid valve that moves little during the cardiac cycle and is often stenosed as well as incompetent.

Bacterial endocarditis

Bacterial infection can cause or worsen mitral regurgitation by destroying valve tissue or chordae tendineae.

Papillary muscle dysfunction

This is now recognized as an increasingly frequent cause of mitral incompetence. It may occur with varying severity in all conditions that affect the left ventricle, the commonest being:

- coronary heart disease
- systemic hypertension
- cardiomyopathies

Rupture of a papillary muscle, though much less common, results in acute and often catastrophic left heart failure.

Ruptured chordae tendineae

Rupture of the chordae causes severe mitral regurgitation. It is often dramatic in onset and may be due to bacterial endocarditis, ischaemia, trauma or degenerative disease.

Trauma

The mitral valve may be damaged either by closed chest trauma, such as steering-wheel compression in motor car accidents, or during surgical procedures on the valve itself. Regurgitation may result or be increased when fused cusps are split in operations to relieve mitral stenosis. It may also occur when a prosthetic valve is incorrectly sited or secured.

Congenital

Congenital mitral incompetence may occur in isolation or as one component of complex malformations. Mitral valve prolapse (the floppy valve syndrome) has recently been recognized as a fairly common congenital malformation. Fortunately, it is usually of little consequence.

Functional mitral regurgitation

This has in the past often been ascribed to stretching of the mitral valve ring in conditions that cause dilatation of the left ventricular cavity. It is fairly common in severe cases of acute rheumatism, viral myocarditis, congestive cardiomyopathies, coronary heart disease and hypertension.

Though dilatation may play a part, alteration in the various components of the mitral valve mechanism, as is known to occur in some cases of severe aortic valve disease and obstructive cardiomyopathy, now seems a much more likely explanation for some types of functional mitral incompetence.

Pathophysiology

During left ventricular systole, blood is forced backwards through the incompetent mitral valve into the left atrium. The amount of regurgitation depends upon the degree of incompetence and, to a lesser extent, the compliance of the left atrial chamber. If it is substantial, the left atrium becomes distended and the pressure rises. The increased pressure is transmitted backwards through the pulmonary veins to the pulmonary vascular bed and causes pulmonary hypertension. Unlike that found in severe mitral stenosis, it is usually a fairly passive type of pulmonary hypertension. The pressure is not so high and it does not evoke a great increase in the pulmonary vascular resistance, unless significant mitral stenosis is also present.

Eventually, the left ventricle becomes enlarged and dilated because of the increased work required to maintain an adequate forward output while at the same time compensating for the backward leak. Sooner or later, it will begin to fail in severe cases and,

when this happens, the left atrial and pulmonary artery pressures rise steadily.

When mitral regurgitation occurs suddenly, as in ruptured chordae, the compensating mechanisms for maintaining cardiac output have no time to develop and acute left heart failure often results.

Symptoms

Many patients with modest mitral regurgitation have no symptoms.

In most of those who develop symptoms, the onset is slow. Often, for many years, fatigue is the main complaint, followed by a little breathlessness on exertion. In severe cases, breathlessness becomes increasingly incapacitating and the natural history of the disease may be punctuated by episodes of right heart failure, usually precipitated by intercurrent respiratory infection.

Clinical signs

The pulse is usually normal. In severe cases it may be irregular because of atrial fibrillation.

When pulmonary congestion is present, crepitations are heard on auscultation at the lung bases. Later, signs of right ventricular failure may be present.

Cardiac signs

The physical signs depend upon the degree of regurgitation. In mild cases, an apical systolic murmur may be the only obvious abnormality. In severe cases, the signs are as described below.

Left ventricular hypertrophy is detected by an apex beat that is heaving in character and displaced to the left. In gross cases a systolic thrill may also be felt at the apex.

Regurgitation starts at the onset of ventricular systole and continues till the end of the ejection phase when the second heart sound signals closure of the aortic valve (LD-121). On auscultation, the first sound is usually quiet and often obscured by the classical pansystolic murmur of mitral regurgitation, which is conducted towards the axilla. In chronic cases, the intensity of the murmur gives some indication of the severity of the lesion. In acute cases the regurgitation is often greater than the signs suggest.

Because of the large volume of blood in the left atrium and the high left atrial pressure, blood flows rapidly into the left ventricle when the mitral valve opens in diastole. This is often noisy and produces a third heart sound, usually best heard just medial to the

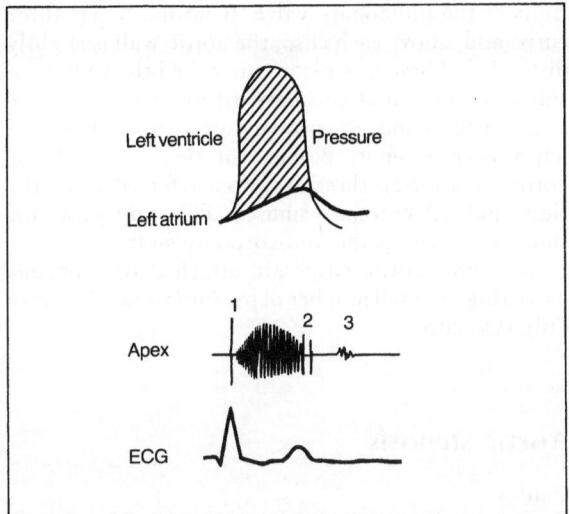

LD-121. *Murmur of mitral regurgitation showing third heart sound*

apex as a short, low pitched sound in mid-diastole.

When regurgitation is due to mitral valve prolapse, the murmur is often confined to late systole and is frequently preceded by a midsystolic click.

The murmur caused by papillary muscle dysfunction is also often heard best in late systole.

Investigations

Electrocardiogram

Left atrial hypertrophy, shown by notching of the P waves, is often present. In severe cases, especially those due to rheumatism, atrial fibrillation commonly becomes the established rhythm in the later stages. Tall R waves in leads reflecting the left ventricle (I, aVL and V_4–V_6) indicate left ventricular hypertrophy. Later, if mitral stenosis is also present, evidence of right ventricular hypertrophy may also develop.

Chest X-ray

The main features are:
- left atrial enlargement
  This is best seen in the right anterior oblique view and may be considerable. It is then called a giant left atrium.
- left ventricular enlargement
  This is seen as an increase in the cardiac shadow downwards and to the left in the PA view and as a posterior bulge in the lateral or left anterior oblique views (X-11).

- Kerley B lines
  These, as previously described above, p. 163, can often be seen at the lungs' bases.
- pulmonary congestion, pleural effusion and, occasionally, pulmonary oedema

A penetrated view may show mitral calcification.

Echocardiography

This is less helpful than in mitral stenosis but often shows marked increase in the diastolic closure rate.

Cardiac catheterization

Apart from measuring pulmonary artery pressure and perhaps demonstrating a large left atrial 'V' wave in the wedge position, right heart catheterization is of little value. Left ventricular cineangiography can be used to make a rough assessment of the degree of regurgitation (mild, moderate or severe) and is fairly reliable in the absence of ventricular ectopic beats, which can cause regurgitation even through a normal mitral valve.

Complications of mitral regurgitation

The main complications are atrial fibrillation, bacterial endocarditis and cardiac failure. Atrial fibrillation is common in rheumatic cases and systemic emboli, though less common than in mitral stenosis, may complicate the clinical course of the disease. Bacterial endocarditis is commoner than in mitral stenosis.

Differential diagnosis

The murmur of mitral regurgitation has to be distinguished from other systolic murmurs which, when loud, may be heard as far out as the apex.

Aortic stenosis

This is recognized by its characteristic mid-systolic crescendo and its radiation to the neck rather than to the axilla. It is often accompanied by a thrill in the aortic area and reversed splitting of the second heart sounds on inspiration may be present.

Tricuspid regurgitation

This is best heard at the left lower sternal border, is accompanied by prominent 'V' waves in the neck and often by hepatic pulsation. It may be increased by inspiration.

Ventricular septal defect

This murmur is best heard along the mid to lower left sternal border. It may be accompanied by a thrill but does not radiate to the axilla.

Natural history

Patients with modest lesions may lead a normal life and have a normal lifespan. Those with more serious lesions often remain relatively symptom-free for many years until the left ventricle gradually begins to fail.

When mitral regurgitation complicates other forms of heart disease it may worsen the prognosis, but this generally remains that of the primary cardiac condition.

The sudden onset of symptoms caused by damaged papillary muscles, torn chordae or ruptured cusps carries a much graver prognosis, although, if the regurgitation is not too severe, the heart may come to terms with it, if assisted by vigorous medical therapy during the acute phase.

Medical management

This consists of supportive treatment for the failing left ventricle with digitalis and diuretics. The threat of recurrent rheumatism should be considered in younger patients and prophylaxis against bacterial endocarditis during dental and other invasive procedures should be advised.

Surgical management

Patients with mitral regurgitation should only be considered for surgical treatment when, despite intensive medical treatment, they are becoming increasingly disabled and no longer able to lead a reasonable life.

Replacement of the damaged valve with a prosthesis is usually necessary and, even when successful, carries its own prognostic problems.

On the other hand, surgery should not be delayed until the patient's clinical condition is so poor that the operation is difficult and dangerous. When timed carefully, open heart surgery can add several years of useful life.

Aortic valve disease

Anatomy

The aortic valve lies behind, below and slightly to the right of the pulmonary valve. It normally has three cusps and, above each cusp, the aortic wall is slightly distended. These distensions are called the sinuses of Valsalva. The right coronary artery arises from the anterior sinus and left coronary artery arises from the left posterior sinus. Because of the origin of the coronary arteries, these are often referred to as the right and left coronary sinuses. The right posterior sinus is known as the non-coronary sinus.

The three aortic cusps are attached to a fibrous valve ring. A small number of people (about 1%) have only two cusps.

Aortic stenosis

Causes

Aortic valve stenosis may be congenital, rheumatic or sclerotic.

Congenital

Most cases of congenital aortic stenosis are due to bicuspid aortic valves. These usually cause no trouble until the cusps become thickened and calcified in late middle life. Occasionally, patients are born with an abnormally small valve orifice that may cause trouble in infancy, childhood or adolescence.

Rheumatic

Aortic stenosis results from adhesion of adjacent cusps, which later thicken and become calcified. The deformed valve may also be incompetent. Rheumatic disease of the aortic valve is often accompanied by involvement of other valves, especially the mitral, which is in close fibrous continuity (LD-17).

Sclerotic

Aortic sclerosis is common in patients over the age of 50 years and may be accompanied by calcification. The aortic valve is the only valve involved and no evidence of rheumatism is found histologically.

Pathophysiology

The normal aortic valve orifice measures about 3 square cm. It has to be reduced to about 0.6 square cm before significant circulatory obstruction occurs. When this happens, the left ventricle has to work harder and takes longer to expel its contents. The peak left ventricular systolic pressure rises to overcome the obstruction. In severe obstruction it may have to be very high to maintain a satisfactory cardiac output.

As a result, left ventricular hypertrophy occurs and, because the overload is systolic, the hypertrophy is concentric in character. This means that the thickness of the left ventricular wall is greatly increased and the size of its cavity is relatively diminished. The thickened ventricle eventually becomes less and less compliant and the left atrium has to work harder to fill the ventricle during diastole.

Symptoms

As with other valve lesions, symptoms depend on severity. In aortic stenosis, a powerful left ventricle lies immediately behind the obstruction and symptoms may not develop until its capacity for further hypertrophy diminishes. Characteristically, patients with severe aortic stenosis may go on for many years unaware of their lesion but, once they develop symptoms, their downhill course is relatively rapid (cf. mitral stenosis).

Dyspnoea

Dyspnoea is usually the first symptom. It is often accompanied by fatigue and may be present for a few years before more serious and ominous symptoms occur. In those who do not die suddenly, it may progress to orthopnoea and paroxysmal nocturnal dyspnoea.

Syncope

Loss of consciousness on exertion is a characteristic late symptom of severe aortic stenosis. This may be due either to a transient dysrhythmia or possibly to excessive peripheral venous pooling.

Pain

Angina is also common in severe aortic stenosis. Like syncope, it is a late symptom and a warning that the coronary arteries are no longer able to supply the increasing mass of myocardium with an adequate blood supply.

Right ventricular failure

Those who survive may eventually develop right heart failure.

Clinical signs

General examination

This is usually unremarkable.

Pulse

In severe cases the pulse is of small volume. It rises slowly and has a plateau wave form (LD-122). The pulse pressure is also small.

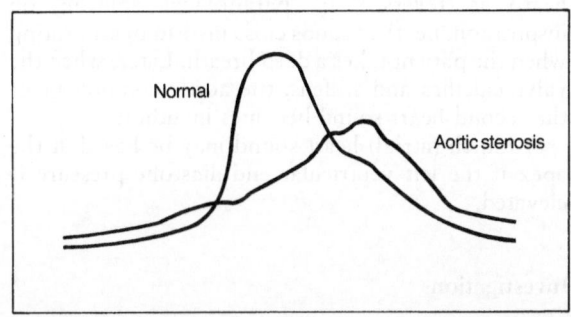

LD-122. *Comparison of normal with slow and small pulse of aortic stenosis*

Cardiac signs

Because concentric hypertrophy does not cause much cardiac enlargement, the apex beat may not be displaced. It is, however, forceful and sustained with a slow heaving quality.

A systolic thrill is often palpable over the right upper precordium and can be felt in the suprasternal notch and the carotid arteries.

On auscultation, the characteristic finding is a loud, harsh, low pitched systolic murmur that reaches its crescendo in mid systole (LD-123). In younger patients, it may be preceded by an early systolic

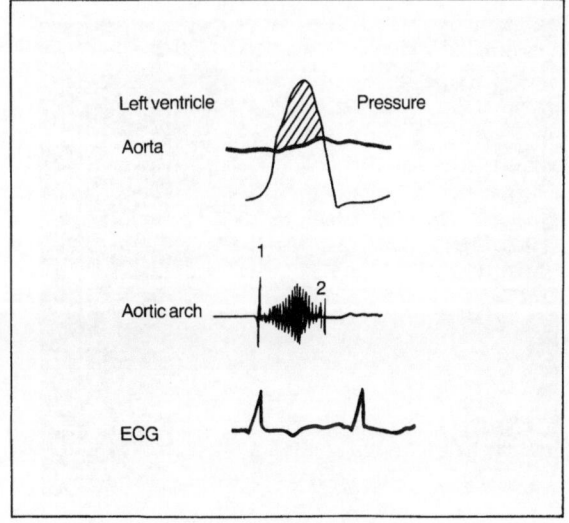

LD-123. *Typical ejection murmur of aortic stenosis*

clicking sound. This ejection click disappears as the valve calcifies and becomes less mobile. In severe cases, the pulmonary component of the second heart sound precedes the aortic component because of the prolonged left ventricular ejection time. This may be heard as 'reversed' or 'paradoxical' splitting on inspiration, i.e. the sounds close instead of separating when the patient takes a deep breath. Later, when the valve calcifies and stiffens, the aortic component of the second heart sound becomes inaudible.

A fourth (atrial) heart sound may be heard at the apex if the left ventricular end-diastolic pressure is elevated.

Investigations

Electrocardiogram

The ECG shows left ventricular hypertrophy.

Chest X-ray

The important features are:

- heart size is usually normal until severe left ventricular failure supervenes
- post-stenotic dilation of the ascending aorta (arrows), a common and useful sign (X-20)
- calcification of the aortic valve is common in patients over the age of 40 and can sometimes be seen, either on a penetrated film or more easily on fluoroscopy.

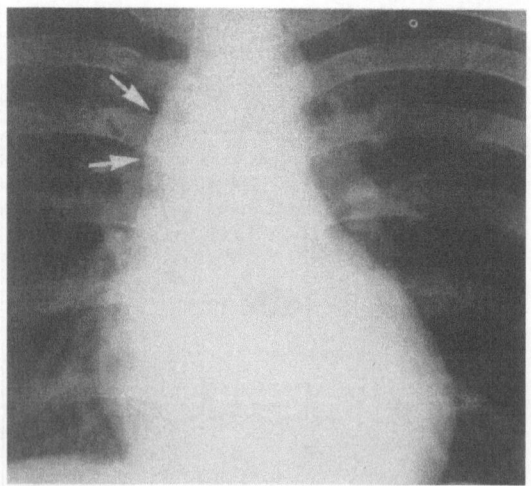

X-20.

Echocardiography

The echo may show:

- signs of thickening and distortion of the cusps
- confirmatory evidence of a bicuspid or stenosed valve
- left ventricular hypertrophy

Cardiac catheterization

When a cardiac catheter is withdrawn from the left ventricle into the first part of the aorta, a systolic pressure gradient is found at the aortic valve. In severe stenosis this will be greater than 50 mmHg at rest. The stenosed valve can be demonstrated by injection of radio-opaque contrast medium into the ventricular cavity.

Complications of aortic valve stenosis

Sudden death

This is always a risk in severe aortic stenosis, even in those without symptoms.

Bacterial endocarditis

This may occur in all types of aortic stenosis regardless of severity. Damage to the valve results in aortic regurgitation.

Differential diagnosis

Subvalvar aortic stenosis

Aortic stenosis may be caused by subvalvar muscle hypertrophy or by a fibrous ring obstructing outflow from the left ventricle. In such patients there is no ejection click and no valve calcification. In hypertrophic obstructive cardiomyopathy, the pulse is often jerky and the heart tends to be larger.

Supravalvar aortic stenosis

This congenital malformation is often accompanied by a typical facies and mental retardation, there is no ejection click and no post-stenotic dilatation on X-ray.

Echocardiography, cardiac catheterization and angiography will help to distinguish these conditions from valvar stenosis.

Aortic sclerosis

This often occurs commonly in the elderly. It is

associated with an elevated systolic blood pressure and calcification of an unfolded aortic arch.

Natural history

Even in severe cases, patients may remain symptom-free for many years. Despite this, it is a progressive disorder caused by gradually increasing fibrosis of a valve that usually becomes calcified in the later stages.

When significant symptoms appear, the course is usually rapidly downhill, death occurs within a few years and is sudden in about 20% of cases.

Management

In symptomless patients, even in children, sudden bursts of exertion and obvious overexertion should be forbidden, to minimize the risk of sudden death.

Patients with symptoms or evidence of severe left ventricular hypertrophy on the electrocardiogram should be fully investigated with a view to surgical treatment.

In those with significant obstruction, the aortic valve should be replaced. This is a satisfactory operation with a low mortality (5% or less). Several types of mechanical and tissue valves can be used. Patients with mechanical prostheses require long term anticoagulant therapy.

In children who require surgery, valvotomy may be used to temporize until they are large enough for a valve that will serve in adult life.

Aortic regurgitation (incompetence)

Causes

Anything that disturbs the normal anatomy of the aortic root (sinuses, valve ring or cusps) may cause the valve to become incompetent. Inflammatory and degenerative lesions account for most cases. Congenital malformations are uncommon except in association with coarctation of the aorta and ventricular septal defect.

Rheumatic heart disease is still the commonest cause but is rapidly becoming a rare cause of serious aortic incompetence in the UK.

Other causes include bacterial endocarditis, syphilitic aortitis, dissecting aneurysm, Marfan's syndrome, ankylosing spondylitis, Reiter's disease and trauma.

Trauma includes not only external injury such as commonly occurs in motor car accidents, but also that occurring during cardiac surgery.

Regurgitation accompanying aortic stenosis is seldom of much haemodynamic significance.

Pathology

This varies with the cause. In rheumatic heart disease the valve is fibrosed, deformed and often calcified. In bacterial endocarditis, one or more cusps may be virtually destroyed. In syphilis, the ascending aorta is ballooned because of aortitis and this stretches the valve ring.

Pathophysiology

Each time the ventricle empties during systole, a proportion of the ejected blood leaks back through the aortic valve during early diastole. To compensate, the left ventricle increases its stroke volume to maintain cardiac output. In severe cases, this leads to dilatation and hypertrophy.

Regurgitation into the left ventricle in diastole results in a low diastolic blood pressure. For this reason, it is relatively easy for the left ventricle to expel its increased volume. As the dilated ventricle also contracts more powerfully than normal against this decreased resistance, the systolic blood pressure is abnormally high. This combination of circumstances produces an abrupt rise in pressure early in systole and a large pulse pressure.

Symptoms

Patients with mild lesions have no symptoms and even those with severe regurgitation can be symptom-free for many years. As in aortic stenosis, once symptoms appear, the downhill course is rapid because they signal left ventricular failure.

Dyspnoea

Breathlessness on exertion is usually the first symptom and is often accompanied by fatigue. Its onset is usually gradual unless the onset of severe regurgitation is acute, as in bacterial endocarditis or trauma.

Angina

This may occur when severe regurgitation greatly reduces the pressure in the aortic root during diastole, but is less common than it is in aortic stenosis.

In syphilitic aortitis, narrowing of the coronary ostia aggravates the situation.

Syncope

Loss of consciousness is rare in aortic incompetence although patients sometimes complain of giddiness.

Clinical signs

In mild cases the only sign may be a short high pitched early diastolic murmur heard over the site of the aortic valve in the middle of the precordium along the left sternal edge and propagated downwards. This is one of the most difficult sounds for the unpractised ear to detect.

When the regurgitation is more serious, most of the signs result from the rapid rise and fall of a high pulse pressure.

At the wrist, the pulse is typically collapsing and is often referred to as a 'water-hammer' pulse (LD-124). It is best appreciated by gripping the raised forearm. In gross cases, this pulse may be visible in the neck.

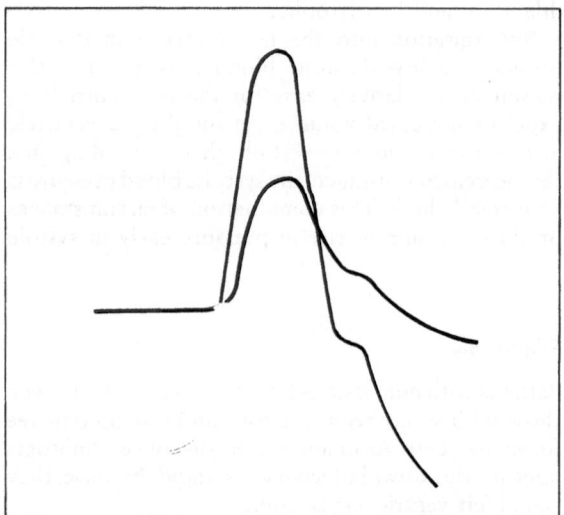

LD-124. Comparison of normal with 'quick rising' or 'collapsing' pulse of aortic regurgitation

In patients with free aortic regurgitation, a to-and-fro murmur and an early systolic pistol-shot sound can sometimes be heard over the femoral arteries.

Capillary pulsation may be observed in the nail beds by pressing gently on the nails or by pressing a glass slide gently on the lips.

Retinal artery pulsation may be seen on ophthalmoscopy.

Cardiac signs

The apex beat is left ventricular in character and is usually displaced downwards and to the left.

On auscultation, the first sound is often quiet because of premature closure of the mitral valve and the aortic component of the second sound is usually absent.

A high pitched diastolic murmur occurs immediately after the second sound. It is best heard down the lower left sternal border with the diaphragm of the stethoscope. The patient should sit up, lean forward and hold the breath in full expiration (LD-125).

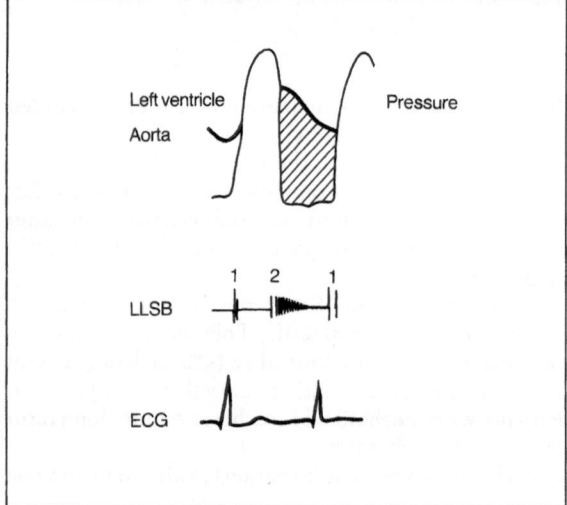

LD-125. Murmur of aortic regurgitation

There may be a short aortic systolic ejection murmur because of the increased volume and velocity of blood flow. This does not necessarily imply that the valve is also stenosed.

A murmur similar to that of mitral stenosis may be heard in pure aortic regurgitation. There are several possible reasons for this, the likeliest being that the regurgitant jet strikes the anterior leaflet of the mitral valve and causes it to oscillate between blood flowing into the ventricle from the left atrium and the regurgitant stream from the aorta. This was first described by Austin Flint, a nineteenth century American physician, and bears his name. It should be diagnosed with caution in rheumatic heart disease because so many patients with aortic regurgitation also have mitral stenosis.

Investigations

Electrocardiogram

This shows left ventricular hypertrophy.

Chest X-ray

Dilatation of the left ventricle is seen when regurgitation is severe. The enlarged heart lies horizontally and there is uniform dilatation of the ascending aorta. Later, signs of left ventricular failure may become apparent.

Echocardiography

During diastole, the anterior leaflet of the mitral valve vibrates in a characteristic manner (LD-126). This helps to distinguish between the Austin Flint murmur occurring with a normal mitral valve and the murmur of organic mitral stenosis.

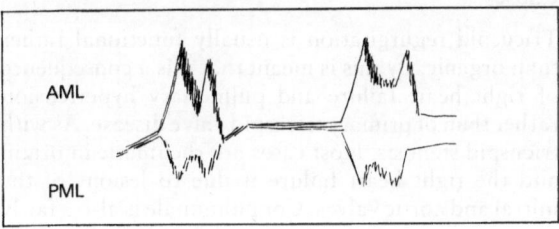

LD-126. *Fine vibrations on anterior leaflet of mitral valve (AML) associated with aortic regurgitation*

Cardiac catheterization

This may be carried out to:
- exclude associated lesions such as aortic or mitral stenosis
- assess left ventricular function
- assess the severity of the regurgitation by cineangiography.

In most cases it is unnecessary.

Complications

Apart from bacterial endocarditis, which is an ever-present risk, complications are seldom seen with pure aortic regurgitation until heart failure develops in severe cases.

Differential diagnosis

The peripheral and auscultatory signs usually make the diagnosis of severe aortic regurgitation easy.

In less severe cases, the other causes of a high pulse pressure must be kept in mind. These include thryotoxicosis, persistence of the ductus arteriosus, other AV fistulae and pregnancy.

In mild cases, the early diastolic murmur must be distinguished from pulmonary incompetence. This is an uncommon lesion except following surgery of the pulmonary valve or in gross pulmonary hypertension, when the other signs of this condition are usually obvious.

Natural history

Minor aortic regurgitation can be regarded as an innocent lesion that will affect neither the quality nor the length of the patient's life. More serious lesions are compatible with many years of symptom-free life. Sudden death seldom occurs and severe symptoms can now be relieved surgically.

Medical management

The medical management is the treatment of left ventricular failure and the prevention and treatment of bacterial endocarditis.

In cases that have an acute onset, intensive medical support with digitalis and diuretics should be used while the left ventricle comes to terms with the unaccustomed volume overload. If it cannot do so, surgery is indicated.

Surgical management

When the symptoms and signs warrant it, the aortic valve should be replaced as in aortic stenosis.

Tricuspid valve disease

Anatomy

The tricuspid valve has three cusps, anterior, posterior and septal. In many ways it resembles the mitral valve but is much less frequently involved in disease processes.

Congenital malformations are rarities, the commonest being atresia and Ebstein's anomaly.

Tricuspid stenosis

Cause

This is almost always rheumatic in origin and is rarely an isolated lesion. The tricuspid valve is said to be involved in about 10% of cases of rheumatic heart disease but, in most, it is of little significance.

Pathology

The pathological process is similar to that seen in mitral stenosis.

Pathophysiology

Tricuspid stenosis obstructs the flow of blood from the right atrium into the right ventricle. The atrial pressure is elevated, at first only during atrial systole but later throughout diastole. This results in a raised venous pressure, hepatomegaly and peripheral oedema as occurs in right ventricular failure.

Symptoms

The symptoms are usually those of accompanying mitral stenosis although restriction of flow through the tricuspid valve diminishes the pulmonary congestion that results from obstruction to flow through the mitral valve.

Clinical signs

Forcible right atrial contraction and elevated right atrial pressure combine to cause a prominent flicking pulsation ('a' wave) in the neck and a congested palpable liver that may pulsate in presystole. With the onset of atrial fibrillation, the pulsation disappears.

Cardiac examination

Palpation of the precordium is usually unremarkable. On auscultation, the first sound over the right lower sternal edge may be loud and a tricuspid opening snap may be audible. The murmur of tricuspid stenosis is mid-diastolic, low pitched and often clearly accentuated by inspiration, which increases the venous return to the right heart.

Investigations

Electrocardiogram

Tall peaked P waves of right atrial hypertrophy are seen especially in leads II, III and aVF.

Chest X-ray

A large right atrium is seen on the right cardiac border in the PA view (X-17a).

Cardiac catheterization

This confirms the high right atrial pressure, the large 'a' wave (in sinus rhythm) and a pressure gradient between the right atrium and the right ventricle during diastole.

Management

Most cases are mild, are difficult to diagnose and require no specific treatment.

In severe cases, surgery is usually carried out at the same time as that for the mitral valve. Unlike mitral stenosis, valvotomy is seldom successful and the valve is usually replaced.

Tricuspid regurgitation

Causes

Tricuspid regurgitation is usually functional rather than organic. By this is meant that it is a consequence of right heart failure and pulmonary hypertension rather than of primary tricuspid valve disease. As with tricuspid stenosis, most cases are rheumatic in origin and the right heart failure is due to lesions of the mitral and aortic valves. Cor pulmonale is also a fairly common cause.

Uncommon causes include trauma, bacterial endocarditis and carcinoid syndrome.

Pathophysiology

When the right ventricle contracts, blood regurgitates back into the right atrium. The right ventricular stroke volume increases to maintain the cardiac output and the right ventricle dilates. The right atrium also becomes larger and the right atrial pressure rises. Eventually, right ventricular failure occurs.

Symptoms

The patient may complain of ankle swelling, epigastric fullness and even epigastric pain after effort. These symptoms are accompanied by marked fatigue.

Clinical signs

With ventricular systole, a prominent 'V' wave is transmitted backwards through the incompetent valve into the atrium. This systolic pulsation is seen in the jugular veins and is often palpable in a large tender liver.

Cardiac examination

A right ventricular heave is often present. The heart

sounds are usually unremarkable, although occasionally a third sound can be heard. The diagnostic finding is a high pitched pansystolic murmur over the lower right sternal edge. With clockwise rotation of the heart, this may be heard well out towards the apex and be confused with the murmur of mitral regurgitation.

Investigations

Electrocardiogram

Right atrial and right ventricular hypertrophy are usually present and often the rhythm is atrial fibrillation.

Chest X-ray

The right atrium is enlarged.

Cardiac catheterization

A large systolic wave is recorded in the atrial pressure pulse. Right ventricular cineangiography confirms the diagnosis and demonstrates the volume of regurgitant flow.

Management

The treatment of functional tricuspid regurgitation is that of the primary condition and is usually, in the first instance, the treatment for congestive cardiac failure. Other causes may rarely require replacement of the tricuspid valve.

Pulmonary valve disease

Anatomy

The pulmonary valve lies anterior and to the left of the aortic valve, but at a higher level. It also has three cusps; anterolateral, anteromedial and posterior. It has little fibrous continuity with the rest of the heart.

Pulmonary stenosis

Causes

Pulmonary stenosis is an uncommon lesion. The pulmonary valve is seldom involved in the rheumatic process, probably because it is out of fibrous continuity with the rest of the heart.

Most cases are congenital in origin. Isolated pulmonary stenosis accounts for about 7% of all congenital cardiac malformations. It is also present in more complex malformations such as Fallot's tetralogy (pulmonary stenosis and ventricular septal defect).

Pathophysiology

To overcome the valvar obstruction, the right ventricle has to contract more forcibly. This causes right ventricular hypertrophy and ultimately right heart failure in severe cases.

Symptoms

Most patients have no symptoms. Those with serious lesions may have increasing fatigue and exertional dyspnoea and, eventually, symptoms of congestive heart failure.

Clinical signs

When obstruction is severe, a prominent 'a' wave is seen in the internal jugular veins. A heaving right ventricle can be palpated along the left sternal border. A systolic thrill can be felt over the upper left precordium where the dominant finding, a coarse systolic ejection murmur, can be heard conducted towards the left shoulder.

Investigations

Electrocardiogram

Mild cases have a normal record. If severe, right ventricular hypertrophy is present and is roughly proportional to the degree of obstruction.

X-ray of chest

The main feature is post-stenotic dilatation of the pulmonary trunk, often seen as a bulge in the PA view (X-17b). In severe cases the pulmonary vascular bed seems almost devoid of blood vessels due to oligaemia.

Cardiac catheterization

Right heart catheterization will demonstrate a raised right ventricular pressure and a systolic gradient across the pulmonary valve. In severe cases, the pulmonary artery pressure is very low and has little wave form.

Natural history

This depends on severity. Mild cases have a normal life expectancy, serious ones eventually develop right ventricular failure.

Management

Pulmonary valvotomy is indicated when the resting right ventricular pressure is greater than 70 mmHg.

Pulmonary regurgitation

Causes

Pulmonary regurgitation is most commonly found secondary to pulmonary hypertension. It can also occur after bacterial infection, as a result of the surgical treatment of pulmonary stenosis by valvotomy and, very rarely, as a congenital malformation.

Clinical signs

An early diastolic murmur is heard in the third left intercostal space close to the sternum. This is the Graham Steell murmur. It is identical to that of aortic regurgitation and may have to be distinguished from it by the presence of other clinical signs such as the loud pulmonary component of the second heart sound in pulmonary hypertension.

Management

Management is that of the primary lesion, the pulmonary regurgitation itself being of little consequence.

PULMONARY HEART DISEASE (COR PULMONALE)

Pulmonary heart disease or 'cor pulmonale', as it is commonly called, are terms used to describe conditions where the heart disease is secondary to diseases of the lungs that cause obstruction to pulmonary blood flow. There are two types of cor pulmonale: acute and chronic.

Acute cor pulmonale

Acute cor pulmonale occurs when there is sudden obstruction of more than 50% of the pulmonary arterial bed by a massive embolus, usually originating from an ileofemoral venous thrombosis. A large clot may occlude the main pulmonary artery or it may fragment and block several smaller arteries causing pulmonary infarction.

Clinical features

The onset is sudden and may be rapidly fatal. Those patients who do not die suddenly develop dyspnoea, cyanosis and circulatory collapse due to low cardiac output. This is accompanied by poor cerebral and coronary perfusion leading to confusion, faintness and central chest pain. There is clinical evidence of right heart failure with a gallop rhythm and congestion of the jugular veins and the liver. The severity of the illness is proportional to the degree of arterial obstruction and the underlying cardiopulmonary state. In less severe cases pulmonary infarction may occur without causing acute right heart failure. In these circumstances the illness presents with:

- pleuritic chest pain
- dyspnoea
- fever
- haemoptysis
- X-ray opacities in the peripheral lung fields and small pleural effusions

Diagnosis

Massive pulmonary embolism occurs most commonly when circumstances favour deep venous thrombosis (DVT) in the lower limb or pelvic veins, e.g.:

- in the postoperative or postpartum period
- following myocardial infarction
- during prolonged bed rest, particularly if this is associated with the factors described on pp. 117–119.

The diagnosis should be considered in any such patient who develops sudden dyspnoea and collapse in the presence of conditions that make DVT and embolism likely. The ECG and chest X-ray may or may not be helpful.

Investigations

Electrocardiogram

The ECG may be normal or show some of the following signs of acute right heart strain (LD-127):

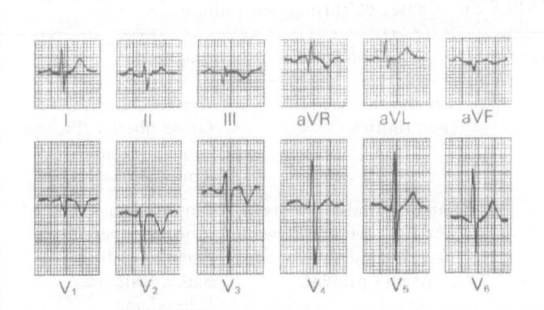

LD-127. An ECG from a patient with acute cor pulmonale following a pulmonary embolism showing SI, QIII, TIII with clockwise rotation and inversion of T waves in chest leads V_1–V_3

- S waves in lead I
- Q waves and inverted T waves in lead III
- high voltage P waves
- the rSR pattern of right bundle branch block
- T wave inversions in the right chest leads

X-rays

X-rays likewise may or may not contribute to the diagnosis, especially in the early stages. The vascular markings in the lung fields may at first show little change. Subsequent pictures may reveal large areas of diminished vascularity and areas with compensatory increased vascular markings. The hilar vascular shadows may be increased in size and the affected arteries may appear to be cut off at the point of obstruction. Occasionally, opacities suggesting pulmonary infarction or collapsed lung are seen (X-21) along with varying degrees of pleural effusion.

Pulmonary arteriography

This is the most certain method of diagnosis but, as it is a major procedure and not without risk, it is only carried out if surgical removal of the embolus is being seriously considered (see Management, below).

Lung scan

Perfusion lung scanning is not normally used as a routine method because it is somewhat non-specific. Newer methods incorporating perfusion and ventilation lung scans are more useful in the differential diagnosis of lesser degrees of pulmonary embolism or infarction.

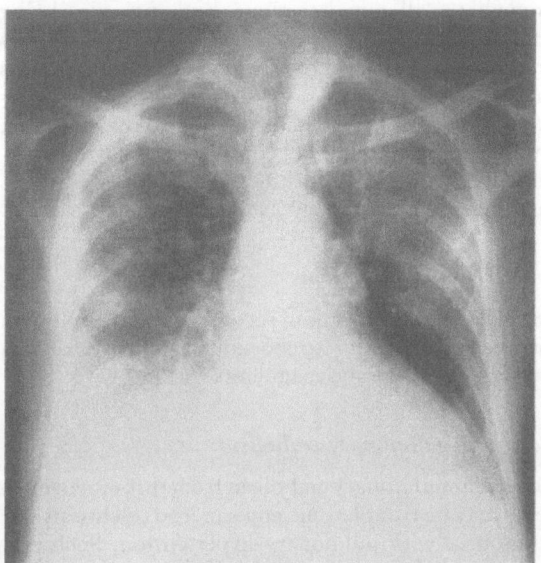

X-21. Acute cor pulmonale due to a postoperative pulmonary embolus showing consolidation in the right lower zone and cardiomegaly in a patient whose heart size had previously been normal

Progress

About 10% of patients die within a few minutes and little can be done to help them. Another 20% die within a few hours or days, but most of those who survive a few hours make a good recovery. This depends, of course, on their underlying clinical state and the prevention of further embolism. Those with existing cardiopulmonary disease may not survive the additional burden of a massive pulmonary embolus.

Management

Oxygen and 10 000 units of intravenous heparin should be given at once. Circulatory collapse may require supportive therapy with dobutamine and digoxin.

Seriously ill patients

In those who do not improve quickly, especially if there is underlying pulmonary or cardiac disease, removal of the clot by thrombolytic or surgical therapy should be urgently considered. In either case, a pulmonary arteriogram is necessary to locate the obstructed vessels.

Thrombolytic therapy with streptokinase or urokinase is the first-choice medical treatment unless there is some contraindication to the use of such agents –

immediate allergic reactions and pyrexia being common. They must be used within the first 48 hours and even then are not always successful. If this therapy fails, or if there is further clinical deterioration before it has had a chance to be effective, embolectomy should be considered, provided experienced surgical staff with cardiopulmonary bypass facilities are immediately available.

Less seriously ill patients

Patients who show signs of recovery should remain on intravenous heparin (10 000 units 6-hourly) for 3–4 days and on oral anticoagulants for 4–6 weeks.

Recurrent pulmonary embolism

Recurrent pulmonary embolism from thrombi in deep veins may be troublesome and can lead to chronic cor pulmonale with pulmonary hypertension. Such episodes may be controlled by long term anticoagulant therapy, but sometimes require surgical treatment such as complete or partial closure of the inferior vena cava. The latter, known as 'plication', leaves three or four small channels open and is marginally more successful than complete closure.

Chronic cor pulmonale

This condition is relatively common. Most frequently, it is secondary to chronic bronchitis and emphysema and may account for one fifth to one quarter of hospital admissions with right heart failure. The various conditions that cause it are shown in Table 21.

Chronic bronchitis and emphysema (CB and E) is a predominantly male disease and 75% of the sufferers are over 50 years of age. Cor pulmonale in a patient under 40 is more likely to be due to one of the other conditions.

Pathogenesis

A number of factors increase the amount of work done by the heart in cor pulmonale. These vary to some extent with the underlying disorder but, basically, they make it more difficult for the right ventricle to pump blood through the lungs. This can be due to physical obliteration or compression of small blood vessels, or to vasoconstriction secondary to reduced pulmonary function. Sooner or later, the right ventricle begins to hypertrophy and eventually, if the

TABLE 21   Causes of chronic cor pulmonale

Group	Basic pathology	Example
1	Structural chest deformities	Kyphoscoliosis Gross obesity (Pickwickian syndrome) Thoracoplasty
2	Parenchymal disorders of the lung (effects depend largely on degree of emphysema present)	Emphysema Fibrotic tuberculosis Pneumoconiosis Sarcoidosis Sclerodema Carcinomatosis
3	Disorders of pulmonary blood vessels	Recurrent pulmonary embolism Thrombosis of pulmonary artery Tumour embolism Pulmonary arteritis Bilharzia Primary pulmonary hypertension

pulmonary disease is of sufficient severity, begins to fail. The principle factors that might influence the development of chronic pulmonale are:

● hypoxia
   This will produce vasoconstriction of the smaller pulmonary arterioles, polycythaemia and an increased blood volume.

● reduction of the pulmonary vascular bed
   This must be in the order of 50% or more to have a significant effect on cardiac function.

● hypercapnia
   This is known to cause vasodilatation elsewhere in the circulation.

It seems likely that pulmonary vasoconstriction caused by hypoxia is the most important factor. The increases in blood and packed cell volume (PCV) are of only minor importance in raising pulmonary vascular resistance although they do contribute to increased cardiac work.

Hypoxia, and the conditions giving rise to it, are therefore of the greatest importance. These conditions (see Table 21) may be:

● structural chest deformities or severe obesity leading to underventilation (Group 1)

● parenchymatous lung disorders usually causing hypoxia in proportion to the degree of emphysema and other features that accompany them. Thus, in chronic bronchitis and emphysema, bronchiolar obstruction, bronchial infection, excessive secretions, decreased lung elasticity and fixation of the rib cage, all combine to reduce pulmonary gas exchange (Group 2)

● less common disorders causing various forms of progressive vascular obstruction or obliteration (Group 3)

Clinical features

In cor pulmonale associated with chronic bronchitis and emphysema, the development of cardiac failure is insidious, being obscured by many of the features of the underlying condition such as cough and dyspnoea.

Cough

The cough becomes more persistent, is worse in the mornings and is often accompanied by yellow or green sputum. Acute exacerbations lead to bouts of heart failure.

Peripheral vasodilation

Unlike other causes of cardiac failure that produce a poor peripheral circulation (e.g. mitral stenosis), hypercapnia causes peripheral vasodilatation with warm hands and dilated veins.

Venous congestion

Congestion of the jugular veins may be misleading because emphysema increases the intrathoracic pressure and they may be congested long before cardiac failure supervenes. In cardiac failure, however, the neck veins will fill rapidly from below after the veins have been compressed. Occasionally, too, a normal liver edge may be palpable because the diaphragm has been pushed downwards by emphysema, again giving a false impression of central venous congestion.

Tachycardia

This may be caused in part by infection and by the use of certain bronchodilator drugs.

Clinical signs

The signs of failure are:

● breathlessness

● cyanosis

● tachycardia and occasional supraventricular dysrhythmias

● a warm periphery and bloodshot eyes

● the presence of sacral or ankle oedema

● varying degrees of clouding of consciousness, from confused states to near coma, as a result of hypercapnia and hypoxia

Progressive weight loss in a bronchitic subject often accompanies the gradual development of heart failure.

Clinical examination

Emphysema makes estimation of heart size difficult because the apex beat cannot be felt. A right ventricular outflow tract heave may be palpable along the left sternal edge.

Noisy breath sounds and added sounds make auscultation difficult also, but the following may be noted:

● a loud pulmonary component of the second heart sound

● a triple rhythm

● a systolic murmur denoting tricuspid valve incompetence

Electrocardiogram

The ECG is variable and may or may not be helpful in diagnosis:

● it may be normal

● it may not differ from that seen in emphysema without cardiac failure, i.e. right axis deviation, clockwise rotation and low voltage

More characteristically, the ECG signs of cor pulmonale may include some or all of the following (LD-128):

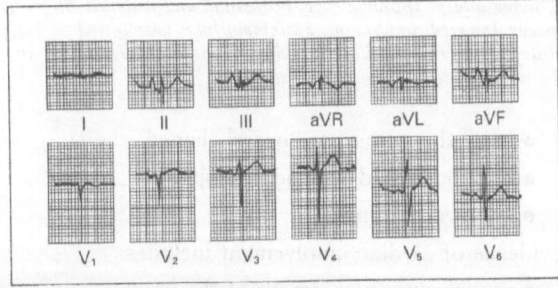

LD-128. An ECG from a patient with chronic cor pulmonale showing low voltage in lead I (often seen in emphysema), peaked P waves in leads II, III and aVF, and marked clockwise rotation in left chest leads

● right axis deviation

● clockwise rotation in the chest leads

- peaked P waves in leads II, III, aVF and over the right ventricle (the so-called P pulmonale)
- tall R waves in aVR
- increased R waves in V_1, but this is a very variable sign and is often absent
- incomplete right bundle branch block (rSR)

X-ray

The radiological features of emphysema often predominate (X-22):

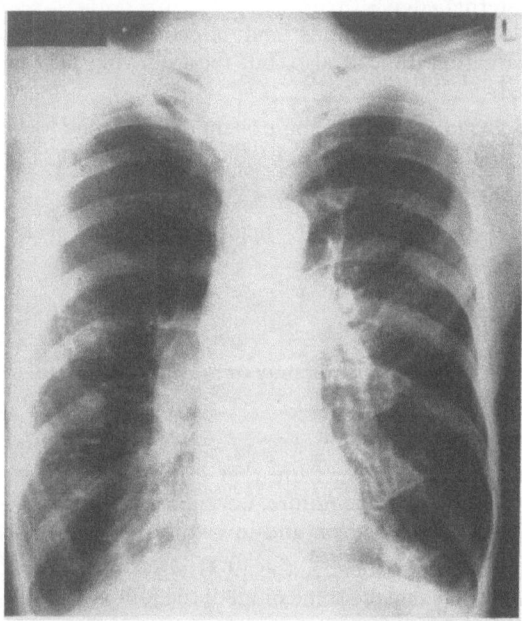

X-22. An X-ray from a patient with an emphysematous chest showing a large thoracic cage, horizontal and widened rib spaces, lowered diaphragm, prominent hilar vessels and absence of peripheral lung markings because of large bullae in the upper zones and left lower zone

- large thoracic cage ('barrel-shaped' chest)
- horizontal and widened rib spaces
- lowered diaphragm

Evidence of cardiac involvement includes:

- progressive enlargement of the heart
- increased pulmonary artery shadows

Blood gases

The P_aCO_2 is raised and the P_aO_2 is low in the majority of cases. The picture is that of a compensated respiratory acidosis.

Blood count

Haematocrit readings show a progressive increase, often to between 50 and 60. Care must be taken to ensure that anaemia with a low mean corpuscular haemoglobin concentration (MCHC) does not occasionally coexist, especially if recurrent venesection is used in management.

Management

The long term prognosis in chronic cor pulmonale remains poor, but is improving slightly as control of infection and understanding of respiratory physiology increases. Many die in an acute exacerbation; others survive for 4 or 5 years with remissions and recurrences, especially in winter time. Treatment may be considered under the following headings:

- hypoxia
- cardiac failure
- special precautions
- venesection
- long term care

Hypoxia

Measures employed include the:

- use of oxygen
- use of bronchodilators
- control of infection
- stimulation of respiration

Cyanotic patients have depressed medullary respiratory centres that are unresponsive to hypercapnia. Their main stimulus to respiration is from the effects of hypoxia on centres in the carotid body. Oxygen will further depress respiration if given too rapidly. It should never be given in concentrations of more than 28%. Special face masks have been designed for this purpose. The P_aCO_2 should be monitored carefully and not permitted to rise.

Many of these patients have severe bronchospasm that further inhibits gas exchange. Various drugs are used as bronchodilators, including aminophylline and its derivatives, the sympathetic amines such as salbutamol and, very occasionally, steroid therapy.

Aminophylline is effective in emergencies by the intravenous route, 250–500 mg being given slowly over 5–10 min. In some patients, aminophylline suppositories, one or two at bedtime, are effective overnight. Oral derivatives of this drug tend to be gastric irritants and this limits their efficacy.

Isoprenaline is not now recommended because of its cardiac stimulant effects, but salbutamol (ventolin) and terbutaline (bricanyl) are selective B_1 stimulators with much less effect on the heart and heart rate. Salbutamol or terbutaline can be given in tablet form or as an aerosol.

Steroids, if used, should be given as prednisolone, starting with 15 mg 8-hourly. The dose should be reduced rapidly as bronchospasm disappears. The indications, however, are much less clear than in bronchial asthma.

It is safe to assume that, in the majority of those presenting with cardiac failure, an exacerbation of bronchitis due to infection is the principal cause of the deterioration. Sputum samples should be sent for culture and antibiotic sensitivity. A broad spectrum antibiotic such as amoxycillin or cotrimoxazole should be given until the results are available.

In severely ill patients, the respiratory drive may be very low. Shallow ineffectual respirations, accompanied by a rising P_aCO_2, demand that all possible steps are taken to stimulate respiration. This includes active physiotherapy as a first and most important step. In some cases, especially where too much oxygen or sedation has been given, respiratory stimulants should be considered. These are nikethamide, vanillic acid diethylamide (Vandid) or doxapram (Dopram). They have a narrow safety margin of efficacy before side-effects occur and all require to be given by carefully monitored continuous intravenous infusion. Doxapram is perhaps the most efficient.

Cardiac failure

This is treated in the normal way using diuretics, digoxin and bed rest. Digoxin must be used with care because there is a more than the usual risk of overdosage and abnormal rhythms.

Special precautions

Beware of giving:

- too much oxygen
- sedatives
  Morphine, codeine and barbiturates should be avoided. The benzodiazepines are also respiratory depressants and should be used with care. Very restless patients should first have their P_aCO_2 checked. Paraldehyde may be occasionally required to quieten the most noisy and restless.

Venesection

In patients with a PCV of more than 55, removal of 1 or 2 units of blood may prove helpful.

Long term care

Discourage cigarette smoking.

Take prophylactic steps against re-infection.

Avoid strenuous exercise and frequent changes of environmental temperature.

Maintain digoxin and diuretic therapy if necessary.

Check the PCV and venesect if it rises above 55.

Watch heart size on X-ray as an indicator of impending heart failure.

CONGENITAL CARDIAC MALFORMATIONS

Incidence

The relative importance of congenital malformations as a cause of infant mortality has increased considerably as other exogenous causes of death have been brought under control.

Approximately 1% of babies are born with congenital cardiac malformations. About one quarter of them have life-threatening malformations that require fairly urgent surgical treatment. About one quarter have malformations that will require medical or surgical treatment later in life. The remainder (one half) have malformations that are not serious, require no treatment and will have little or no effect on either their way of life or their life expectancy.

As the birth rate in the UK is currently around 12 per 1000, this means that between 6000 and 7000 babies with congenital cardiac malformations are born each year; or about ten per month in a city with a million inhabitants.

The incidence of congenital malformations in stillbirths is much higher; possibly three or four times higher if the conceptus is of more than 30 weeks gestation.

Causes

Most congenital cardiac malformations result from damage to the developing embryo between the 6th and 8th week of intra-uterine life. In the vast majority of cases no aetiological agent is discovered. The parents appear to be normal and the mother's health during early pregnancy is said to have been uneventful.

Proved causes, such as viral infections (rubella), drugs, radiation and genetic or chromosomal abnormalities, probably account for less than 10% of the total.

Types of malformations

Malformations may occur in any part of the developing heart during the early weeks of gestation. Some are not compatible even with fetal life and result in abortion. Some do not become manifest until late childhood or adult life. Most of those that have haemodynamic significance are discovered soon after birth. They either cause obstruction to the flow of blood through the normal channels or allow blood to flow through abnormal channels.

Examples of obstruction are:

● pulmonary stenosis
This obstructs the flow of blood from the right ventricle to the lungs.

● coarctation of the aorta
This obstructs the flow of blood from the left ventricle to the trunk and lower limbs.

Examples of abnormal communications are:

● septal defect
This allows communication between the pulmonary and systemic circulations.

● transposition of the great arteries
This allows venous blood to recirculate without passing through the lungs because the aorta arises from the right ventricle and the pulmonary trunk arises from the left ventricle.

In many of the more serious cases both factors operate and, because there is obstruction to the flow of blood through normal channels, it has to pass through abnormal channels as, for example, in:

● Fallot's tetralogy
Here, because of severe pulmonary stenosis, much of the venous return passes from the right ventricle through a defect in the ventricular septum into the left ventricle and escapes via the aorta into the systemic circulation without passing through the lungs.

● tricuspid atresia
Here, because there is no communication

between the right atrium and the right ventricle, the systemic venous return passes from the right atrium through a defect in the atrial septum into the left atrium; usually, some of it then passes back from the left ventricle through a defect in the ventricular septum into the right ventricle and eventually reaches the lungs.

Simple 'hole-in-the-heart' type of malformations,

● atrial septal defect (ASD)

● ventricular septal defect (VSD)

● persisting ductus arteriosus (PDA)

are by far the most common lesions.

Ventricular septal defects alone account for at least one third of all single cardiac malformations and also form an integral part of many complex conditions such as the tetralogy of Fallot, which is basically a large VSD with severe obstruction to right ventricular outflow.

The following seven malformations between them account for 75–80% of the total (the figures in brackets are averages derived from various sources):

● ventricular septal defect (35%)

● atrial septal defect (11%)

● persisting ductus arteriosus (8%)

● pulmonary stenosis (7%)

● coarctation of the aorta (7%)

● transposition of the great arteries (5%)

● the tetralogy of Fallot (5%)

A great deal is said and written about other malformations that are exceedingly uncommon. Many of the most serious are caused by a combination of malformations as, for example, when a coarctation of the aorta is accompanied by a persisting ductus arteriosus and a large defect in the ventricular septum or when pulmonary blood flow depends on an ASD and persistence of the ductus in pulmonary atresia with an intact ventricular septum.

Ventricular septal defect (VSD)

This is far and away the commonest congenital cardiac malformation. Most defects are single and in the membranous part of the septum, some are in its muscular part, and occasionally there is more than one defect. The defects vary in size from large holes, that offer little resistance to the flow of blood between the ventricles, to those that are mere pinholes. As a rule they tend to get smaller or relatively smaller as the patient gets larger and many close spontaneously, usually in infancy or early childhood. Although spontaneous closure is more likely in small defects, closure of defects large enough to have caused heart failure is by no means uncommon.

The haemodynamic effects of the defect and the patient's prognosis depend upon its size. When the hole is large, a large left to right shunt floods the lungs with blood. When it is small, the shunt is of little or no consequence.

In severe cases, the pressure in the pulmonary arteries rises in response to the increased flow through the lungs. After a few years, permanent changes take place in the arterioles and the pulmonary hypertension becomes irreversible if the defect is not closed. A stage is reached when the right and left ventricular pressures are equal and little or no shunting takes place across the defect. Sooner or later, because of progressive resistance to pulmonary blood flow, the pressure in the right ventricle exceeds that in the left and the shunt reverses (right to left). Such patients become cyanosed and have finger clubbing, clinical and electrocardiographic evidence of gross right ventricular hypertrophy and signs of pulmonary hypertension – a condition known as the Eisenmenger syndrome.

In those whose defects are not large enough to cause pulmonary hypertension, the clinical picture depends upon the size of the hole and the volume of the left to right shunt through it. At one end of the spectrum are those with large hearts, distended pulmonary arteries and plethoric lung fields, whose large left to right shunts are evidenced by a systolic murmur and thrill over the lower sternum and a diastolic flow murmur at the apex. They are usually infants who are failing to thrive or who have heart failure precipitated by an intercurrent infection. At the other end of the spectrum are those with normal-sized hearts and normal lung fields, whose only abnormality is a systolic murmur heard along the left lower sternal edge. They are usually healthy children whose murmurs have been discovered during the course of a routine medical examination.

The size of the defect is usually reflected fairly accurately by the physical signs, X-ray and ECG, with the caveat that a small VSD often causes a fairly loud systolic murmur.

Nowadays, the diagnosis is made in most cases soon after birth. Babies with large defects require careful management and in a few the defect has to be closed surgically because of persistent cardiac failure or progressive pulmonary hypertension. The rest are kept under observation either until the defect has closed spontaneously or until it has become clear how large a hole the patient is going to have to live with. In most cases, it becomes relatively smaller and will make little or no difference to the way of life or to life expectancy, provided precautions are taken to guard against the possibility of bacterial endocarditis at times of special risk such as tooth extraction. In a few, it remains large and requires surgical treatment.

Atrial septal defect (ASD)

Atrial septal defects are of two types: holes in the upper part of the septum, usually referred to as secundum type defects, and holes in the lower part of the septum, usually referred to as primum type defects. The latter, being endocardial cushion defects, are often accompanied by a cleft in the anterior cusp of the mitral valve and, occasionally, by a ventricular septal defect as well. Secundum defects are much commoner than primum defects and, although spontaneous closure does occur, it is much less frequent than in VSDs.

The pressure in the left atrium is normally higher than the pressure in the right atrium and blood flows from left to right through the defect. As with defects in the ventricular septum, the haemodynamic effect depends upon the size of the hole. However, because blood flows between the atria throughout the cardiac cycle, resistance to flow is far less than it is between the ventricles during systole, and the left to right shunt can be considerable. With large defects, the amount of blood flowing through the pulmonary arteries may be several times that flowing through the aorta. They are, however, not subjected to the ejectile force of the left ventricle as they are through large VSDs, and can accommodate the increased volume without much increase in pressure.

Pulmonary hypertension is therefore a late feature in the natural history of ASD and usually develops only after the lung vessels have been exposed to high flow for many years.

The physical signs are much less striking than in VSD. Increased flow through the right ventricular outflow tract and pulmonary valve causes a scratchy systolic murmur along the upper left sternal edge. The right ventricle takes longer to empty than the left ventricle, with the result that the pulmonary and aortic components of the second heart sound (the valve closure sounds) are more widely separated than normal. Despite what is so often said, however, the splitting is seldom fixed and usually varies with deep respiration. Increased flow through the defect and the tricuspid valve may cause an early diastolic murmur to be heard along the lower right sternal edge.

The ECG shows a partial right bundle branch block pattern (rSR) in the right chest leads accompanied usually by right axis deviation in secundum defects and by left axis deviation in primum defects.

The X-ray shows dilation of the pulmonary trunk, but the size of the pulmonary arteries and the heart depends upon the size of the defect and the volume of the left to right shunt through it. In severe and longstanding pulmonary hypertension, the dilated hilar vessels do not extend out into the lung fields and give the appearance of a pruned tree.

Atrial septal defects are seldom diagnosed in infancy or early childhood and are overlooked even in older patients because the systolic murmur is often unimpressive and the diastolic murmur, if present, is difficult to hear. The signs are frequently dismissed as innocent noises and this is the reason why no cardiologist will give an opinion about a heart murmur in such cases without first seeing an ECG and X-ray.

The size of the defect and the volume of the shunt through it can be assessed fairly accurately from the physical signs, ECG and X-ray. Small defects should be regarded as innocent lesions. Large defects should be closed, unless pulmonary hypertension makes surgical treatment too hazardous. Those in between should be observed; decisions about the need for surgery and its timing depend on increasing heart size and the onset of symptoms. Many patients with modest lesions live to a ripe old age with little or no disability until the onset of atrial fibrillation in late adult life.

Persistence of the ductus arteriosus (PDA)

The fetal ductus is a large vessel of approximately the same size as the descending aorta. As a rule, it closes spontaneously soon after birth; sometimes it persists. If it persists in its original size, a large left to right shunt develops when the pulmonary vascular resistance falls and allows the left ventricle to pump blood through the ductus into the pulmonary arteries. This is a serious lesion that may cause heart failure and death in the neonatal period, particularly during the course of an intercurrent infection.

In most cases, the ductus at least partially closes. The left to right shunt through it is not large and causes relatively little haemodynamic upset.

The characteristic and easily recognized sign of a persisting ductus is a continuous murmur that builds up to a crescendo in late systole and continues through the second heart sound into diastole. It is heard best in the left upper precordium under the middle and outer thirds of the clavicle. This murmur usually makes the persisting ductus easy to diagnose, although it may sometimes be confused with a venous hum in a normal child. Venous hums, however, are commoner on the right side than on the left and are readily abolished or increased by rotation of the head and neck.

In babies, the murmur is mainly systolic and diagnosis is more difficult. With a large ductus, the femoral pulses often have a bounding or collapsing quality that suggests the diagnosis.

As a rule, the left to right shunt through a ductus is smaller than that through a septal defect. In many cases the patient is an apparently healthy child and the ductus murmur is the only detectable abnormality. In those with relatively large shunts, the X-ray may show a little dilation of the main pulmonary arteries and the ECG is often more obviously left ventricular than is usual in young children.

When a large ductus is detected in a baby, it should be treated surgically without delay by division and suture. In older children with smaller ducts, there is less urgency. Traditional teaching is that they should be ligated before the child goes to school, but once the diagnosis is made and the decision to operate is taken, there seems little point in waiting.

Pulmonary stenosis

When pulmonary stenosis occurs as a single malformation it is nearly always valvar. The cusps are fused together with a small hole in the middle. The severity of the lesion depends on the size of the hole. The right ventricle becomes hypertrophied behind the obstruction because it has to work harder to expel its contents. The pulmonary trunk usually becomes dilated in front of the obstruction because of the effect of the jet of blood passing through it. The pressure in the ventricle is increased and the pressure in the pulmonary arteries is decreased. The sudden difference across the stenosed valve is referred to as the pressure gradient and the severity of the stenosis is judged by the size of this gradient.

The characteristic sign of pulmonary stenosis is a systolic murmur heard over the left upper precordium, propagated upwards and towards the left shoulder. The length and loudness of the murmur depends upon the severity of the stenosis. In mild cases, it does not occupy the whole of systole, an ejection click can be heard soon after the first sound and the pulmonary second sound is audible. In severe cases, it continues throughout systole, it is accompanied by a thrill and the pulmonary second sound is not audible.

The X-ray nearly always shows enlargement of the main pulmonary artery and, with increasing severity, the peripheral lung vessels become progressively less obvious. The ECG, which is often normal in mild cases, also reflects the severity of the lesion by the degree of right ventricular hypertrophy present in the right chest leads.

Pulmonary stenosis rarely causes symptoms in childhood or adolescence. Mild cases can be diagnosed clinically. They are compatible with a normal way of life and a normal life expectancy, and do not require surgical treatment. Severe cases cause increasing disability and heart failure in early adult life. The severity of the obstruction is determined by cardiac catheterization and, where necessary, it is relieved surgically by dividing the cusps along the lines of fusion.

Coarctation of the aorta

This is a serious malformation that narrows or obliterates the aortic lumen. It may occur anywhere in the aorta, but the common site is just beyond the origin of the left subclavian artery near the opening of the ductus arteriosus.

Coarctation of the aorta is the most frequent cause of heart failure in babies without cyanosis. In these circumstances, the ductus usually persists and the lesion is often accompanied by a defect in the ventricular septum. The diagnosis should be suspected when the femoral pulses are absent or delayed.

In later life, signs of a collateral circulation develop in the intercostal arteries and around the scapulae, and the blood pressure in the upper half of the body is elevated.

Surgical correction is life-saving in babies with heart failure, but should otherwise be delayed until around the age of 5 years.

The tetralogy of Fallot

The clinical features of this condition are due to a combination of severe obstruction to right ventricular outflow and a large ventricular septal defect. The right ventricle has less difficulty in discharging some of its contents through the VSD than through the obstruction, which is usually an infundibular stenosis. The result is a large right to left shunt with considerable desaturation of the arterial blood.

Fallot's tetralogy is one of the two common causes of blue babies, but, except in severe cases, the cyanosis is not always apparent immediately after birth. This is because the ductus helps to oxygenate some of the arterial blood until it closes and the infundibular obstruction may become progressively more significant during the first few months of life.

The diagnosis is suggested by clinical cyanosis, a loud systolic murmur, an ECG that shows tall R

waves in V_1 with a sudden change to R and S waves of approximately equal amplitude in V_2 and an X-ray suggesting poor blood supply to the lungs. Detailed studies are carried out by catheterization and angiocardiography before proceeding to palliative or corrective surgical treatment.

Transposition of the great arteries

In this condition the aorta arises from the right ventricle and the pulmonary trunk arises from the left ventricle. The pulmonary and systemic circulations are in closed loops instead of being in series. After birth, the only communication between them is through the ductus arteriosus, unless a septal defect is also present.

Transposition is incompatible with extra-uterine life and most babies survive for only a few days; those with septal defects for a little longer. This is the most common cause of heart failure and death in cyanosed newborn babies and their lives depend upon urgent diagnosis and treatment. It is a situation where hours rather than days are important, because deterioration, when it occurs, is rapid and catastrophic. The diagnosis should be assumed until proved otherwise in all blue babies with heart disease, especially in those without murmurs.

Nowadays, an atrial septal defect is created after emergency cardiac catheterization has confirmed the diagnosis. A communication is made between the pulmonary and systemic circulations by rupturing the septum with a balloon-tipped catheter. This palliative procedure saves life and allows time for carefully planned surgical treatment to be undertaken when the baby is older.

Multiple congenital malformations

Babies with multiple congenital malformations affecting different organs of the body are an increasing cause for concern. They often present grave therapeutic problems, especially when they are associated with serious neurological or mental deficit.

About 30% of those born with congenital cardiac malformations also have malformations of other organs. Of those who do not survive, 45% fall into this category and half of them have multiple non-cardiac malformations.

Nowadays, when it is nearly always possible to maintain life, serious thought should always be given to its likely quality before striving officiously to prolong it.

Mortality

About one in six of those born with serious congenital cardiac malformations do not survive the first month of life and half of them live for only a few days. Of all deaths, 25% take place before the first birthday and thereafter only another 5–10% die during the remainder of childhood and adolescence.

This high mortality during the first few weeks or months of life has, until recently, formed a hard-core problem that is only now beginning to be brought under control by the successful adaptation of open heart surgery to infants and very small children.

Hospital figures, often showing twice this mortality, give a false impression of overall severity because patients are referred from far and wide to specialized units, with the result that they seldom reflect what is happening in the local community.

Of those who do not survive:

- a third die because of their congenital cardiac malformations
- a third die because of congenital malformations in other organs
- a third die from other causes, such as intercurrent infections, that might not have been fatal had they not had serious congenital cardiac malformations

This high early mortality emphasizes the importance of early detection in severe lesions. An accurate diagnosis must be made and treatment initiated as soon as possible after birth. In many cases there are only a few days to spare.

Detection

Profound circulatory changes take place after birth when the lungs take over from the placenta. Throughout this transitional period, the signs produced by many serious congenital cardiac malformations may be considerably modified and the presence of a malformation may delay or alter the haemodynamic adjustments that should normally take place during the neonatal period.

At birth and for the first few days of life, the pressures in both ventricles and both great arterial trunks are approximately equal. While the normal low pressure pulmonary circulation is developing after the lungs expand, many of the intracardiac and extracardiac shunting mechanisms that were used in the fetal circulation (foramen ovale, ductus) may still

function intermittently to produce a little cyanosis when a baby cries or otherwise exerts itself.

Until the pulmonary vascular resistance has fallen well below the systemic vascular resistance, and until the ductus arteriosus and the foramen ovale have closed, some malformations may be difficult to detect at the bedside.

As the cardiovascular and respiratory systems adapt to extra-uterine life, cardiac malformations are more easily recognized. After the first week, the detection rate rises rapidly and, after the first few months, they are seldom overlooked. Most of the real emergencies are over by this time, however, and the natural survivors are discovered during intercurrent infections, because of failure to thrive or at routine medical examinations. Fewer and fewer escape discovery nowadays to present for the first time in childhood or adult life.

The newborn period

Because many malformations that cause or contribute to death in the first few weeks of life are not immediately recognized as such, all babies should be examined soon after birth by a paediatrician and referred to a cardiologist if a cardiac malformation is suspected.

Under these circumstances, cardiac malformations are usually suspected because of heart murmurs, cyanosis or heart failure.

Heart murmurs

These do not necessarily signify cardiac malformations and serious cardiac malformations may exist in the absence of murmurs. Some murmurs heard soon after birth (ductus) will disappear later and some that will persist may not yet have become audible (septal defects). Nevertheless, the presence of a murmur should alert those responsible and no murmur should be disregarded without a careful assessment of the cardiovascular system.

Cyanosis

It is a common misconception that most of those born with serious cardiac malformations are blue babies. In fact, only about 10–15% of serious cases have persistent central cyanosis. Nearly all of them have severe or grave conditions and, until recently, few except Fallots survived the early weeks or months of life. Now that it is possible to help most of them surgically, no time should be lost in establishing a correct diagnosis. All should be treated as medical emergencies, regardless of their clinical condition, because deterioration is often sudden, rapid and catastrophic.

For this reason, central cyanosis must always be taken seriously and an attempt made to discover its cause. Its severity tends to be underestimated in the neonatal period because it often produces a slaty-grey colour rather than the heliotrope-blue seen in older patients.

Remember also that:

- most babies noted to be blue at birth have respiratory rather than cardiac problems
- in central cyanosis due to a congenital cardiac malformation, there is nothing wrong with the oxygenating capacity of the lungs; the problem is that, for one reason or another, the systemic venous return is failing to reach them in adequate amounts
- many babies whose cardiac malformations do not cause persistent cyanosis have intermittent cyanosis when they reverse shunts on exertion
- many normal newborn babies have peripheral cyanosis that may at times give their extremities and particularly the nail beds a dark-blue appearance

Heart failure

Heart failure in infants seldom presents as adult heart failure in miniature. It may pass from the incipient to the frank phase very rapidly and may not be recognized as such until it has become serious.

The first signs are usually an increase of the cardiac and respiratory rates in a baby that is often distressed and irritable. Fine crepitations can usually be heard in the lungs, but liver enlargement is the most obvious site of congestion. Peripheral oedema is seldom seen in babies.

Infancy

Babies with severe cardiac malformations that have not been discovered at or soon after birth usually present with feeding difficulties or failure to thrive.

Symptoms of heart disease (breathlessness and exhaustion) are mostly related to exertion. Babies exert themselves when crying and emptying their bowels, especially if they are constipated, but their main exertion is feeding.

Feeding difficulties occur because the infant becomes tired and falls asleep during feeds. It fails to thrive because so much energy is used up by the heart in its attempt to maintain an adequate cardiac output that there is little left for anything else. A vicious circle

is soon established. The mother, worried by the failure to gain weight, spends more and more time trying to force food into a baby who becomes more and more exhausted by the effort of trying to take it. Such babies should instead, be given small feeds at frequent intervals.

Childhood

Most babies are now born in hospital and most infants attend clinics of one sort or another. As a result, few children with congenital cardiac malformations escape detection. Those who do are usually discovered when a heart murmur is heard while they are being examined for some unconnected reason. Under these circumstances their signs have to be differentiated from the innocent sounds and murmurs that can be heard in so many healthy children if they are examined carefully enough by a skilled auscultator.

The malformations most likely to escape detection are atrial septal defects. These produce few signs in infancy and sometimes fairly unimpressive signs in childhood. Because of this, no heart murmur should be pronounced innocent without seeing an ECG and a chest X-ray.

Adult life

Few malformations are detected for the first time in adults except for those that do not become obvious until adult life.

The most important lesions in this category are bicuspid aortic valves and prolapsing mitral valves. These are probably much commoner than generally appreciated. The bicuspid valves tend to calcify and cause stenosis in late middle life; prolapsing valves cause regurgitation, occasional dysrhythmias and a liability to bacterial endocarditis.

Investigations

So much can be achieved by palliative or corrective surgery that no effort should be spared to make a precise diagnosis as a necessary preliminary to planning future management and treatment.

When symptoms and signs suggesting heart disease are discovered immediately or soon after birth, the presence of a congenital cardiac malformation is almost certain.

Later in life, acquired lesions and innocent murmurs take on an increasing significance in the differential diagnosis.

Few children with congenital cardiac malformations, except for those with central cyanosis, who are usually greatly disabled, have genuine cardiac symptoms. Even those with serious malformations are often described as the wildest member of the family by parents who find it difficult to believe or to accept that there is anything wrong with their child's heart.

Cardiac neurosis, however, is not uncommon in children who know they have heart disease. They sometimes use symptoms to their own advantage. While it is almost impossible not to spoil severely handicapped babies, parents should be warned about this possibility and, where possible, children should be encouraged to lead normal lives.

In most cases, an accurate diagnosis can be made at the bedside by careful clinical examination supplemented by simple ancillary tests such as electrocardiograms, echocardiograms and X-rays.

Cardiac catheterization and angiocardiography are reserved for:

- infants with cyanosis or heart failure
- those whose malformations are thought to be serious enough to justify surgical treatment
- cases in whom diagnosis is difficult

Non-invasive procedures, such as echocardiography and numerical tomography, seem likely to play an increasingly important part in the detailed study of patients with severe malformations.

Management in infants and children

Infants and children with congenital cardiac malformations can be divided into three groups:

- those with insignificant malformations
- those with modest malformations
- those with severe malformations

Insignificant malformations

These require no treatment of any kind. After diagnosis, the facts should be explained to the patients and their parents. They should then be reassured and discharged from medical care. Such patients should be regarded in every way as normal healthy persons. It is extremely important that ideas about heart disease do not become fixed in their psyche. The seeds of cardiac neurosis are already sown and much imaginary heart disease is perpetuated by regular attendance at paediatric and cardiac follow-up clinics.

Modest malformations

These may or may not require treatment. After diagnosis, such patients should be kept under regular surveillance until one or other of the following decisions can be made:

- the malformation is of no significance e.g. the spontaneous reduction in the size of or the closure of a ventricular septal defect.
- the malformation is significant but static and does not require surgical treatment. Such patients may require prophylactic antibiotic therapy at times of special risk (tooth extraction) to guard against the possibility of bacterial endocarditis but, for all other purposes, should be treated as if they had an insignificant malformation, e.g., a modest degree of pulmonary stenosis or a small atrial septal defect
- the malformation is sufficiently severe to require surgical treatment. Most patients in this category have no symptoms and it should be explained that the operation is being done to prevent deterioration in later life when, if the operation was delayed, it might be either too late for surgery or the end result of surgery would be less than satisfactory

Severe malformations

Here surgical treatment is clearly necessary. Infants in this category should have intensive medical therapy followed by full diagnostic studies. In some cases, emergency surgery may prevent considerable loss of life. It gives those with abnormal cardiovascular systems a chance to come to terms with the type of circulation necessary to sustain extra-uterine life.

In some cases, definitive surgery will restore the cardiovascular system to a normal or near normal state. In some cases, palliative surgery will improve or tide patients over until definitive surgery is possible.

In a diminishing number of cases (e.g. hypoplastic left heart, fibroelastosis) surgery still has little or nothing to offer.

After the first few months of life, there is less urgency about treating those even with serious malformations. The timing and the nature of surgery can be planned in the light of local circumstances. In an imperfect world, the choice may be at least partially dictated by what is possible rather than by what would be best.

Aftercare

When patients are placed in one or other of the above

groups, some will be dismissed as insignificant, some will be discharged as cured and some will remain under continuing supervision. Certain guidelines may be helpful:

- all infants should be fully immunized
- children should, whenever possible, go to ordinary school and only in exceptional circumstances, to schools for the disabled
- all should have prophylactic antibiotics at times of special risk of bacterial endocarditis
- patients themselves know best what they are able to do. Apart from obvious overexertion and sudden or sustained exertion, no unnecessary restrictions should be placed on their activities and they should be encouraged to do as much as possible

Management in adults

In adults, the alternative decisions outlined above can usually be made more or less immediately, because the natural history of the malformation has already become obvious.

Course and prognosis

Congenital cardiac malformations vary greatly from those that are barely compatible with life to those that will not affect it.

The course depends on the nature and severity of the malformation and on the effect of surgical treatment upon the natural history of the condition. If present and not relieved, pulmonary hypertension causes irreversible vascular changes in the lungs that greatly influence the long term prognosis.

Those malformations causing central cyanosis at birth are, generally speaking, the most serious. Multiple malformations are more serious than single malformations, which range in severity from serious to inconsequential.

Genetic counselling

Parents ask questions about their affected offspring and both parents and patients ask questions about their possible future offspring. Counselling is of somewhat limited value at present because only about

8% of malformations appear to be genetically determined. However, high risk and low risk situations can be determined.

High risk situations

Fortunately, these are not common. Almost all of them have malformations associated with either chromosomal (e.g., Down's, Turner's) or Mendelian inherited syndromes (e.g., Marfan's, Friedreich's ataxia).

The familial recurrence of chromosomal syndromes is small and counselling is based on the karyotype of the patient or parents or both.

Mendelian disorders account for a very small, though important, subset of congenital cardiac malformations.

Low risk situations

These are the ones usually encountered. The risk is higher for common malformations than for uncommon malformations.

For example, if a patient has a ventricular septal defect, his children are more likely to have a ventricular septal defect than are his brothers' or sisters' children. If he already has one child with a ventricular septal defect, the chances of producing another child with a ventricular septal defect are also greater than normal.

The risk is higher when two first-degree relatives are involved. It is Mendelian or greater when three first-degree relatives are involved and, under these circumstances, the risk can be calculated.

For most practical purposes, however, after the first child with a malformation has arrived on the scene, it is best to say: yes, the risk of having another child with a congenital malformation is a little greater than normal, but not great enough to discourage a further pregnancy. If it happens again, very careful thought should be given to future pregnancies.

Prevention

Prevention is limited to those situations where a preventable aetiological agent can be identified. So far, this is limited to genetic counselling in the few rare cases where a chromosomal or Mendelian inheritance is known and to rubella vaccination, which may prevent a small (2–4%), but readily identifiable, number of lesions. Although in most cases, the cause is unknown, the indications are that further control of infections might bring about a small but significant reduction in their number. A clear association has been demonstrated, for example, between the early weeks of pregnancy of affected mothers and the peak period of common winter ailments.

PERICARDITIS

Pericarditis may be acute or chronic and is often one feature of a generalized process rather than a localized disease. It can cause important clinical effects. In particular:

- the pain of acute pericarditis may simulate the pain of myocardial ischaemia
- the heart may be compressed by an effusion into the space between the visceral and parietal layers of the pericardium
- less commonly, the heart may be constricted by the pericardium if it becomes rigid and fibrotic because of chronic inflammatory disease

Acute pericarditis

Causes

The cause is often not apparent and the condition is then termed 'acute idiopathic or non-specific pericarditis'.

The main causes of pericarditis are:

- infections, viral and bacterial
- myocardial infarction
- rheumatic fever
- neoplastic infiltration
- uraemia
- connective tissue disorders
- rheumatoid arthritis
- disseminated lupus erythematosis
- trauma
- surgery
- radiation

Clinical features

Those due to infection may have a febrile illness. In many others, the primary cause is obvious (e.g., uraemia, surgery).

Pain

Although the main symptom of acute pericarditis is pain, it is not invariably present. The pain is retrosternal and may radiate to the back, neck, shoulders, arms and upper abdomen. It can be distinguished from the pain of myocardial ischaemia because it is often worse on inspiration and exacerbated by rotating the chest. If the cause of pericarditis is myocardial infarction, the pain may have features of both.

Friction

The classical and pathognomonic sign of pericarditis is a friction rub. This, like pericardial pain, is not invariably present. It has a 'scratchy' quality and has been likened to the sound of footsteps in the snow. Pericardial friction is heard over the pracordium along the sternal edges when the heart moves, i.e. in systole when the ventricles contract, in early diastole when the ventricles distend rapidly and in late diastole when the atria contract. It is often difficult to hear and, if it cannot be heard with the patient lying supine, it should be sought with the patient sitting up and leaning forward with the breath expelled.

Effusion

The other signs of acute pericarditis depend on the presence or absence of a pericardial effusion. The circulatory effects of an effusion are dependent, not only on the size of the effusion, but also on the speed with which it accumulates; a rapidly forming effusion having much more marked effects than one that accumulates slowly.

Cardiac tamponade

More rarely, the presenting symptoms of pericarditis are due to cardiac tamponade, the term used to describe compression of the heart by an effusion in the pericardial space. This may develop quickly. The jugular venous pressure becomes markedly elevated and the blood pressure falls. At first there is a reflex tachycardia; later, the heart rate slows progressively with syncope and death from a profound reduction in cardiac output unless some pericardial fluid is removed.

Paradoxical pulses

Two paradoxical pulses should be sought if an effusion is suspected.

An 'arterial pulsus paradoxus' is characterized by a reduction in systolic blood pressure of more than

10 mmHg on normal inspiration. The term is really a misnomer in that a reduction in systolic blood pressure, albeit less than 10 mmHg, normally occurs on inspiration. The sign is not pathognomonic of a pericardial effusion because it is also found in patients with obstructive airways disease. When it occurs with pericardial effusion, it is probably caused by increased venous return during inspiration limiting the available space within the compressed heart for ventricular dilatation. Hence, stroke volume and systolic blood pressure fall.

The 'venous pulsus paradoxus' (Kussmaul's sign) is characterized by a rise in pressure in the neck veins during inspiration instead of the normal fall. The sign is again not specific for pericarditis because it occurs in some patients with venous congestion due to myocardial disease. In pericardial effusion, it is due to limited distension of the right atrium when increased venous return occurs during inspiration.

Investigations

Electrocardiography

The typical electrocardiographic features of acute pericarditis are widespread ST elevations (LD-59) followed after a few days by T wave inversions. Pathological Q waves do not develop. The ECG, however, may or may not be helpful in diagnosis because in many cases it does not show typical features.

Chest X-ray

A large pericardial effusion increases the size of the cardiac shadow on the chest X-ray and gives the heart a globular configuration. Generalized cardiac enlargement from any cause may simulate this appearance (X-6, p. 50) and special techniques such as echocardiography are invaluable in providing a definitive diagnosis of pericardial effusion.

Echocardiography

The pericardial sac is a potential space that fills with fluid when the pericardium is inflamed. Such pericardial effusions are easily detected by echocardiography because the fluid appears as echo-free spaces between the anterior chest wall and the right ventricle and behind the left ventricle (LD-76). Although the echocardiogram can distinguish between large and small pericardial effusions, it cannot indicate if and when emergency pericardiocentesis is required.

Enzymes

Pericarditis may be associated with raised cardiac enzymes, presumably because there is associated inflammation of the underlying heart muscle.

Management

Management of the condition involves:

- relief of symptoms
  e.g. analgesics for chest pain. Those with anti-inflammatory action such as indomethacin are particularly valuable

- treatment of an underlying cause
  e.g. patients with uraemic pericarditis require frequent dialysis

- pericardiocentesis
  This is required when tamponade poses a threat to life

In acute non-specific pericarditis, steroids can often improve the clinical features but they are usually unnecessary and may exacerbate an underlying infection.

Pericardiocentesis may be accomplished by thoracotomy or by percutaneous needle aspiration. The latter technique is dangerous because the needle may lacerate the coronary arteries. It should only be undertaken to prevent death due to tamponade.

Chronic constrictive pericarditis

Chronic pericarditis only causes symptoms when a rigid fibrotic and sometimes calcified pericardium, with or without an associated effusion, constricts the heart. Although it was once thought to be usually caused by tuberculosis, this is now known not to be true.

Chronic constrictive pericarditis may be due to:

- a wide variety of infections, many of which are viral
- collagen disorders
- trauma
- radiation
- uraemia

Although chronic pericarditis commonly follows rheumatic fever, constriction seldom, if ever, occurs and the terms 'chronic pericarditis' and 'constrictive pericarditis' must not be used synonymously.

The clinical features of constrictive pericarditis

resemble those of right heart failure. Often, the first complaint is of abdominal swelling. Dyspnoea on exertion and ankle swelling may also occur. The jugular venous pressure is elevated and the liver is enlarged. Marked ascites is usually present and contrasts with relatively slight peripheral oedema. In addition, there may be features of cardiac compression with paradoxical pulses.

Investigations

Electrocardiography

The ECG may show low voltage complexes and widespread non-specific ST–T wave abnormalities, but it is never diagnostic.

Chest X-ray

The heart size is usually within normal limits. About 50% of cases have calcification of the pericardium, best seen as a shell-like ring in a lateral film. This, however, is not pathognomonic of constrictive pericarditis because calcification can be present without constriction.

Echocardiography

The echocardiogram is of limited value in constrictive pericarditis because the abnormalities that may be seen are also found in other conditions, particularly in patients who have undergone cardiac surgery. The thickened pericardium may be visible. Also, in early diastole, rapid dilatation of the ventricles followed by abrupt cessation of filling may be detected.

Management

Medical treatment is ineffective, except in the short term, and those who are incapacitated should have pericardiectomy. It is unwise to delay, because calcification is progressive and, once extensive, makes surgical relief less effective as it extends into the myocardium.

MYOCARDITIS

Causes

The myocardium is frequently involved in generalized inflammatory conditions. Sometimes, the involve-ment is obvious, as in diphtheria, Chagas disease or toxoplasmosis. Usually, it passes unnoticed, as in influenza, mumps or infectious mononucleosis. Rarely, it is suppurative as in septicaemia.

Myocarditis frequently accompanies common viral infections. It has been reported in association with such diverse conditions as:

- echo and adenovirus infections
- Coxsackie A and B infections
- infectious hepatitis
- poliomyelitis
- varicella
- psittacosis
- mycoplasma pneumoniae
- Q fever

Coxsackie B appears to be the organism most commonly involved in clinically apparent myocarditis. Subclinical involvement of the myocardium is common in many cases of viraemia. Its presence can often be inferred only from ECG changes that usually resolve within a week after the onset of symptoms. These are non-specific ST–T wave abnormalities and dysrhythmias which, along with the transient rise in cardiac enzymes that occurs in many cases, may sometimes cause diagnostic confusion with coronary heart disease. Viral myocarditis must also be distinguished from other diseases such as thyrotoxicosis and sarcoidosis that sometimes involve the heart and cause similar ECG abnormalities.

Clinical features

Myocarditis may occur at any age. When it accompanies the common infectious diseases of childhood, it is seldom serious and usually passes without notice. Clinically overt cases are most common in adult life.

The diagnosis should be considered in any patient with a viraemia, accompanied by disproportionate tachycardia or heart failure, who develops the electrocardiographic abnormalities described above. Although the clinical diagnosis of viraemia is usually relatively easy, the identification of the infecting organism is often very difficult.

Management

Patients with viral myocarditis should be confined to

bed during the acute stage of the illness, because animal studies suggest that the replication of viruses within the heart is enhanced by exercise. As a rule, no specific therapy is required. If heart failure develops, it should be amanged along conventional lines. Once the infection has abated and the tachycardia settled, the patient should be encouraged to get back to normal. In cases with cardiomegaly, the heart often takes a long time to return to its normal size and this should not delay convalescence.

The vast majority of patients recover satisfactorily and show no residual evidence of heart disease.

Rarely, patients with viral myocarditis succumb to severe heart failure a few hours or days after the onset of symptoms. Occasionally a patient dies suddenly, presumably from a cardiac dysrhythmia.

It has recently been suggested that some patients with myocarditis progress to become cases of congestive cardiomyopathy, but the evidence for this remains tentative.

INFECTIVE ENDOCARDITIS

Infective endocarditis is usually caused by bacteria and runs a subacute course. Before the introduction of antibiotics, it was invariably fatal. Even today, treatment is not always successful. The organisms may not be sensitive to the antibiotics and death may occur from such complications as emboli or heart failure even after the lesions have been sterilized.

Although an increasing number of unusual organisms are found in subacute bacterial endocarditis (SBE), the commonest is still *Streptococcus viridans*, which is, fortunately, the easiest to treat. A high index of suspicion is necessary if the correct diagnosis is to be made and appropriate therapy instigated as soon as possible.

Acute endocarditis, as was once to be seen in pneumococcal pneumonia and staphylococcal septicaemia, is now rare, but fungal infections of artificial heart valves pose new therapeutic prolems.

Pathology

This is characterized by friable vegetations that form on the endocardial surface of heart valves or chambers. They usually develop in patients with theumatic heart disease or congenital cardiac malformations. Patients with healthy hearts rarely develop endocar-

ditis, presumably because organisms cannot settle on the smooth surfaces of the heart chambers and valves.

Previous rheumatic heart disease is the most common underlying condition. Vegetations form on the 'downstream' side of an affected valve and, when valves are incompetent, on the surface of the heart where the regurgitant jet impinges on the endocardium. In the case of mitral and tricuspid incompetence, the chordae tendinae may be involved. The infective lesions can destroy the affected cusps and rupture the chordae tendineae. In artificial valves, lesions may form on the prosthesis or on the tissues into which it has been embedded.

In ventricular septal defects, vegetations may form around the defect or where the jet of shunted blood strikes the wall of the right ventricle. Other congenital malformations (persistent ductus arteriosus, coarctation of the aorta) may also become infected.

It has recently become apparent that areas of myxomatous degeneration of the mitral valve are also suceptible to infective endocarditis.

Clinical features

Although many clinical features have been attributed to SBE, some are seldom present and the condition must often be suspected in the absence of florid clinical signs. Unexplained fever for more than a week or ten days in a patient with a significant heart murmur should suggest the possibility.

Patients with endocarditis usually present with vague malaise and other 'flu'-like symptoms; occasionally with increasing breathlessness due to valvular incompetence. Classically, they have a fever, but this may be only intermittently present. Anaemia, a raised WBC and ESR may or may not be present and are at best non-specific.

Petechiae occur in about 40% of cases and often occur in crops. They are found all over the body, in the mucous membrane of the mouth, in the conjunctiva and in the ocular fundi.

Small black streaks called splinter haemorrhages may form under the nails, but are not pathognomonic of infective endocarditis and are frequently caused by trauma. Small tender nodules (Osler's nodes) may be present in the pulps of the fingers and toes. Finger clubbing is a late development in a minority of cases.

About 40% of patients with infective endocarditis develop splenomegaly. The spleen is also the commonest site of embolic infarction and this may cause upper left abdominal pain referred to the left shoulder.

Fragments of the vegetations may become detached and form peripheral emboli. This occurs in about 25% of cases and the effect depends upon the site of impaction. An embolus may cause infarction distal to the site of obstruction or, because it is infected, may result in the formation of an abscess or a mycotic aneurysm.

Emboli in the kidneys result in renal infarction and haematuria. Patients with infective endocarditis may also develop acute glomerulonephritis. This is not directly attributable to emboli. It can occur with endocarditis solely involving the right side of the heart and is probably an immune complex disease.

Because most patients with infective endocarditis have rheumatic or congenital heart disease, the presence of a cardiac murmur is not necessarily indicative of endocarditis, although changing murmurs are suggestive. The rapid development of valvar incompetence or worsening incompetence should suggest endocarditis. Vegetations can cause stenosis, but this is much less common.

Not unexpectedly, in right-sided endocarditis, embolization to the lungs causes predominantly pulmonary symptoms and signs. Cough, pleuritic pain, and signs of pleural friction, pleural effusion and consolidation may develop.

Investigations and management

As the diagnosis of SBE must often depend upon a high degree of suspicion and the disease can still cause death after the infection is under control, no time should be wasted in starting effective antibiotic treatment once the infecting organism has been identified. This is not always easy and the advice of an experienced bacteriologist should always be sought. Blood cultures, if properly carried out, are usually positive. They should be taken at evenly spaced intervals for 2 or 3 days. If the patient is already having an antibiotic, this should be discontinued for 48 hours and appropriate cultures used. Special media are required for brucella and fungal infections. Serological tests should be performed to exclude psittacosis, Coxiella burnetii (Q fever) and viruses.

In some cases positive blood cultures are never obtained and treatment with broad spectrum drugs must be started and controlled according to the clinical response.

The commonest organism causing endocarditis is *S. viridans*. Next in frequency is *Streptococcus faecalis*. These organisms are rarely implicated after heart surgery, when staphylococcal (albus and aureus) and fungal infections are common.

The object of medical treatment is to eradicate the offending organism by giving high doses of appropriate bactericidal (not bacteriostatic) drugs for at least 6 weeks. A combination of antibiotics is usually used. The level of antibiotic in the serum should be measured to ensure that it is at least four times the minimum inhibitory concentration of the offending organism. A close liaison between the clinician and bacteriologist is necessary as new antibiotics are constantly being introduced and sensitivities of organisms change.

For infection with *S. viridans* or *S. faecalis*, a suitable initial regimen is 5 g of penicillin G plus 240 mg of gentamicin per day. The dose of gentamicin must be reduced if renal excretion is poor. Initial therapy is usually by intravenous drip, later changing to the intramuscular or oral route when infection is controlled. Some physicians now use oral therapy from the start.

In those whose infection is not responding, who have severe refractory heart failure or who are continuing to form emboli, surgery must be considered. Although, in principle, prosthetic heart valves should not, ideally, be put into infected areas, surgery under intensive antibiotic cover may provide the only chance of survival in such cases.

Prevention

Bacteraemia is not an uncommon event and why it should be followed by infective endocarditis in some individuals, but not in others, is not clear. However, because patients with rheumatic and congenital heart disease are susceptible to endocarditis, it is reasonable to provide antibiotic cover during procedures that are likely to cause bacteraemia. These include:

- tooth extraction
- genitourinary manipulations such as catheterization and cystoscopy
- abdominal surgery
- abnormal obstetrics

In drug addicts, bacteraemia often follows intravenous injections.

For dental procedures, a single oral dose of 3 g amoxycillin should be given 1 hour before the procedure. Alternatively, erythromycin, vancomycin or cephaloridine can be given (see p. 259).

Before genitourinary, abdominal and obstetric procedures, gentamicin (100 mg) plus ampicillin 1 g should be given intramuscularly 30 minutes before the procedure and the same doses repeated 8 and 16 hours later.

DISORDERS OF RATE, RHYTHM AND CONDUCTION

ECG interpretation of abnormal rhythms

A systematic and deductive approach to the interpretation of abnormal rhythms is much more rewarding than an optimistic attempt at pattern recognition. One should therefore identify:

- all the P waves; their rate, regularity and morphology
- all the QRS complexes; their rate, regularity and morphology
- the relationship between the P waves and the QRS complexes

The atrial rhythm is often most readily apparent during a pause in the RR interval, so pauses should be examined with special care. Alternate P waves can be obscured by the QRS complex. The construction of a ladder diagram often helps in the analysis of an abnormal rhythm as shown in LD-129.

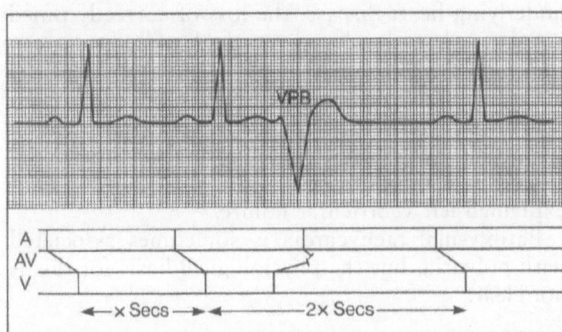

LD-129. *Ladder diagram. The relationship between atrial activation, conduction through the AV node and ventricular activation is shown diagramatically. A ventricular premature beat (VPB) fails to conduct retrogradely to the atrium and the coincident antegrade P wave fails to traverse the AV node to the ventricles. This P wave is obscured in the ECG trace by the ventricular premature beat. The underlying atrial rhythm is undisturbed, so a compensatory pause follows the premature beat*

Normal rhythm

The normal activation sequence of the heart is from the sinus node to the atria and thence through the junctional tissues (AV node and His bundle) to the ventricles. Any deviation from this pattern is an abnormal rhythm. Abnormal rhythms occur frequently in clinical practice. They vary in importance from those that are entirely benign to those that are immediately life-threatening.

Normal sinus rhythm varies between 60 and 100 beats per minute. Rates greater than 100/min are termed 'tachycardias'. Rates less than 60/min are termed 'bradycardias'.

Tachycardias

Tachycardias may be due either to accelerated pacemaker activity or to the mechanism of re-entry.

Accelerated pacemaker

Acceleration of the sinus node pacemaker results in sinus tachycardia. Other areas of potential pacemaker activity are capable of causing ectopic rhythm (see p. 34). Accelerated pacemaker activity in the atrium, AV junctional tissues or ventricles at a rate faster than the prevailing sinus rate will result in an ectopic tachycardia. These sites of potential pacemaker activity can also be the source of escape rhythms should the usual higher pacemaker sites fail.

Re-entry

It is now established that re-entry is the most common mechanism underlying tachycardias. It was first described in 1914 and the mechanism is illustrated in LD-130,1.

If there is inequality of recovery in adjacent limbs of the re-entry circuit, a premature beat can find that although one limb of the circuit is completely refractory, an adjacent limb has partially recovered and is again capable of conduction (LD-130,2). This partially refractory tissue usually conducts slowly (LD-130,3). Provided conduction is sufficiently slow, the previously refractory limb of the circuit has recovered excitability by the time that the advancing impulse arrives and conducts in a retrograde direction (LD-130,4). Activation then re-enters the original partially refractory pathway (LD-130,5) and, with the circuit thus complete, can circulate indefinitely (LD-130,6). Excitation spreads from the circuit to activate the heart.

Re-entry occurs readily within the heart, the most common sites being the AV node, the Purkinje–muscle junction and the ischaemic region surrounding myocardial infarction. If an accessory

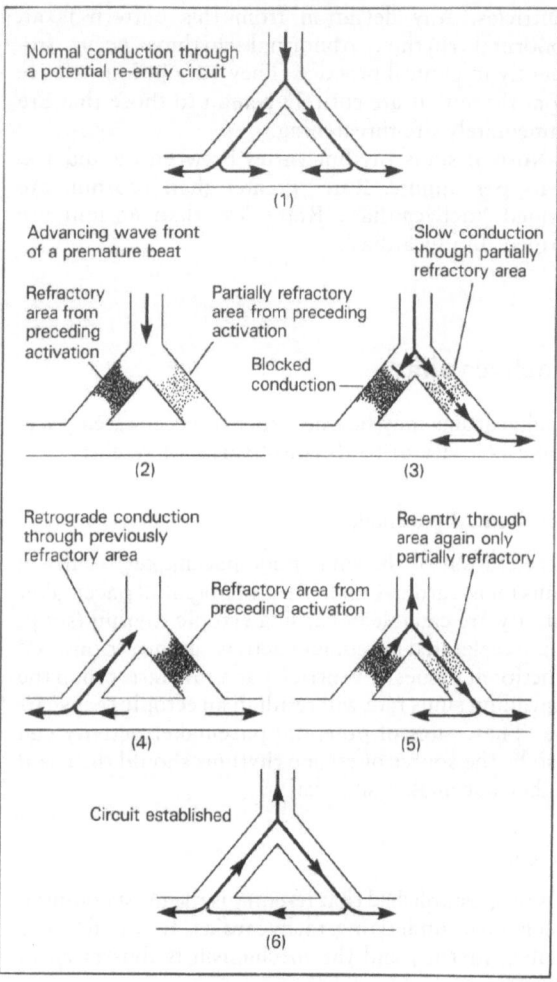

Normal conduction through
a potential re-entry circuit

(1)

Advancing wave front
of a premature beat

Refractory
area from
preceding
activation

Partially refractory
area from preceding
activation

Slow conduction
through partially
refractory area

Blocked
conduction

(2)   (3)

Retrograde conduction
through previously
refractory area

Re-entry through
area again only
partially refractory

Refractory area from
preceding activation

(4)   (5)

Circuit established

(6)

LD-130. A circuit of re-entry. For details, see text

pathway is present, as in the Wolff–Parkinson–White syndrome, a re-entry circuit may be formed comprising the atria, AV node, ventricles and accessory pathway. Although the site may vary, the mechanism is the same.

Re-entry can be terminated either by increased conduction velocity or by prolongation of the refractory period, so that the advancing impulse meets refractory tissue. Termination also occurs if part of the circuit is made refractory by an extraneous beat. These mechanisms can be useful in the treatment of re-entrant rhythms.

Supraventricular tachycardias

Although, strictly speaking, the bundle of His lies in the ventricles, rhythms arising above its bifurcation are termed supraventricular. They usually have a narrow QRS complex. Occasionally, the QRS complex is broadened because of bundle branch block. Characteristics of the supraventricular tachycardias are shown in Table 22.

Symptoms

Some patients are unaware of the dysrhythmia and it can be a coincidental ECG finding.

Because many of the symptoms associated with supraventricular tachycardias are common to the different dysrhythmias, they are considered together. In otherwise normal hearts, supraventricular tachycardia is usually well tolerated but frequently causes palpitations. Patients may find it difficult to describe the rate and rhythm accurately and it can be helpful to have them imitate what they feel by tapping out the rate and rhythm on the tabletop or the sternum. This may suggest the nature of the abnormal rhythm. Description of the onset and termination of an episode may also be helpful.

During the paroxysm of rapid rate, hypotensive symptoms such as dizziness, sweating and, occasionally, syncope may occur. Chest discomfort and dyspnoea are also sometimes present. In patients with underlying heart disease, the loss of correctly timed atrial systole and reduced ventricular filling time can cause marked haemodynamic deterioration. They may precipitate congestive cardiac failure, pulmonary oedema or myocardial ischaemia as major presenting symptoms. For example, an abnormal rhythm should always be considered as a possible cause of unexplained left ventricular failure.

Paroxysmal tachycardia is sometimes associated with polyuria, but the physiological basis for this is not clear.

Vagal stimulation

Vagal stimulation usually results in slowing of the sinus rate, slowing of AV conduction and prolongation of AV node refractoriness. It can be of great diagnostic value in supraventricular tachycardias when the exact diagnosis is uncertain. It should, if possible, be carried out under ECG control so that, if transient changes occur, they will be recorded and available for analysis. Quite commonly, carotid sinus massage (CSM) is ineffective but the diagnostic value of a positive response is such that it should always be performed.

Common methods of stimulating the vagus include gagging, the Valsalva manoeuvre and the one most

TABLE 22 Characteristics of tachycardias

Rhythm	Mechanism	Atrial rate	AV conduction	Response to vagal stimulation
Sinus tachycardia	Accelerated pacemaker	100–200 Rarely > 150 at rest	1:1	Slows
Paroxysmal atrial tachycardia	Accelerated atrial pacemaker or re-entry in atrium or sinus node	140–230	Frequently 2:1 or variable block May be 1:1 at slow rates	Nil or increased AV block
Atrial flutter	Re-entry	250–350 Usually 300	Frequently 2:1 or variable block Rarely 1:1	Nil or increased AV block Rarely causes atrial fib.
Atrial fibrillation	Re-entry	> 350	Variable	Usually nil May slow VR
Junctional tachycardia	Accelerated pacemaker	60–140	Rhythm arises in AV junction AV dissociation may be present	May slow VR
Paroxysmal supraventricular tachycardia	Re-entry in AV node or through accessory pathway	140–240 Usually 150–180 *Ventricular rate*	Rhythm arises in AV junction or utilizes accessory pathway	Nil or may stop
Accelerated idioventricular rhythm	Accelerated pacemaker	60–120 Usually < 100	AV dissociation is usual	Not applicable
Ventricular tachycardia	Accelerated pacemaker and re-entry	120–300	AV dissociation may be present May be 1:1 retrograde (VA) conduction	Not applicable
Ventricular fibrillation	Re-entry	> 300		Not applicable

commonly used, carotid sinus massage. Eyeball pressure is painful and dangerous; it should not be used.

Before proceeding with CSM, the presence of two carotid pulses and the absence of carotid bruits should be confirmed. Each carotid sinus should then be massaged in turn – never simultaneously, as this may reduce cerebral blood flow.

Management

Only the principles of therapy are outlined for each abnormal rhythm in this section. The details will be found in Antidysrhythmic Drugs, pp. 253–256.

Sinus tachycardia

This is a normal response to such things as exercise, stress, pyrexia, thyrotoxicosis and cardiac failure. Young people occasionally achieve rates as high as 200/min with exercise, but the maximum rate falls with age, and at age 60 is about 160/min. Rates at rest in excess of 150/min are unusual.

Sinus tachycardia seldom causes symptoms on its own account and requires no treatment. It may,

however, direct attention to its cause and this may require specific treatment.

ECG diagnosis

Sinus tachycardia is usually readily identified provided the P waves can be clearly visualized. This may require inspection of several leads as the P waves may be obscured by the preceding T waves. In these circumstances, carotid sinus massage may slow the rate sufficiently for the P waves to become obvious. The differential diagnosis includes other regular supraventricular tachycardias and the response may help with diagnosis (see Table 22).

Paroxysmal atrial tachycardia (PAT) (LD-131)

This is due to increased automaticity of atrial pacemaker cells and is usually not truly paroxysmal. The terminology, however, is so well established that the name is retained. It frequently accompanies a variety of underlying clinical conditions, may be due to digitalis toxicity and is occasionally an isolated abnormality.

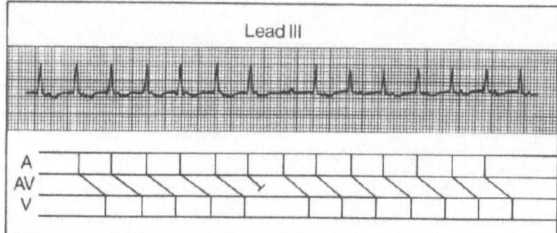

LD-131. Paroxysmal atrial tachycardia. There is a regular supraventricular tachycardia of 240/min with 2:1 AV block. The value of carotid sinus massage (CSM) is illustrated as the atrial tachycardia continues and the nature of the tachycardia can be identified

At relatively slow discharge rates, the AV node may allow 1:1 conduction, usually with a prolonged PR interval. At higher rates, AV conduction usually fails and 2:1 or variable AV block occurs. This is especially common with digitalis toxicity because digitalis slows AV conduction. The ventricular rate, therefore, is variable and may be regular or irregular. Occasionally there are no symptoms, but commonly there is palpitation and symptoms typical of supraventricular tachycardia (see above). If a regular tachycardia occurs in a patient on digitalis therapy, this dysrhythmia should be suspected.

ECG diagnosis

The features to note are:

- The QRS complexes have a normal configuration and the ventricular rate and rhythm vary depending on the underlying atrial rate and AV conduction. Variable AV block may cause an irregular rhythm.
- The configuration of the P waves differs from that in sinus rhythm as they do not originate from the sinus node. They are often small and narrow. The atrial rate varies between 140/min and 230/min.
- CSM increases AV block without terminating the tachycardia and often allows the underlying atrial tachycardia to become apparent.
- PAT is usually distinguished from atrial flutter because the atrial rate is rather slower and by the presence of an isoelectric line between each P wave. Atrial flutter, on the other hand, usually has a continuously varying baseline visible in some ECG leads, although at times, the two dysrhythmias may be indistinguishable.

Management

If PAT is due to digitalis toxicity it should be treated as such (see below). Otherwise, in the absence of symptoms, at relatively slow rates no therapy may be required. At more rapid rates, or when symptoms occur, the ventricular rate should be slowed with digoxin (provided digitalis toxicity has been excluded as its cause), a β-blocker or a combination of both. Where haemodynamic deterioration is present, initial treatment with DC shock should be considered, again provided digitalis toxicity has been excluded.

Junctional tachycardia

Pacemaker activity in the AV junction has a natural rate of 40–60/min. This is normally suppressed by the more rapid sinus rate, though it may manifest itself as an escape rhythm if the sinus rate should slow. In some circumstances, junctional automaticity may be enhanced and exceeds sinus automaticity so that the junctional pacemaker predominates. At rates of 60–100/min, it is termed 'accelerated junctional rhythm' and at rates of 100–130/min it is termed 'junctional tachycardia'.

Common causes of junctional tachycardia are:

- digitalis toxicity
- fever
- myocardial infarction
- carditis
- surgical trauma

These same factors also accelerate sinus rhythm and the rhythm may change to and fro, from sinus tachycardia to junctional tachycardia. Junctional tachycardia *per se* is not usually associated with symptoms, although there may be symptoms of the underlying condition. Occasionally, the loss of correctly timed atrial systole may cause haemodynamic deterioration.

ECG diagnosis

The features to note are:

- the QRS complexes have a normal configuration and the rate is often similar to the underlying sinus rate
- inverted P waves may be present in leads II, III and aVF due to retrograde activation of the atria (LD-132). They may precede, coincide with or follow the QRS complexes, depending on the conduction times in the AV node, but most often the P waves are obscured by the QRS complexes
- the rhythm may be positively identified as junctional if AV dissociation is present

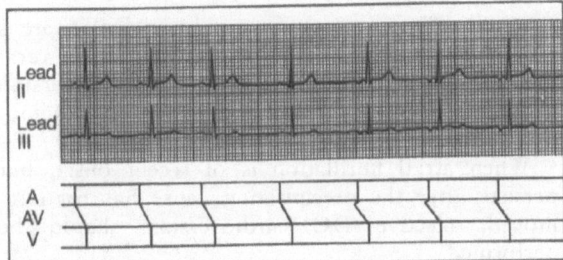

LD-132. Junctional rhythm. The sinus rate slows and after the fourth complex junctional rhythm takes over with a rate of 60/min

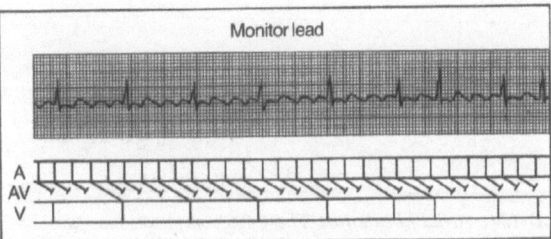

LD-133. Atrial flutter with varying AV block

- CSM may slow the rate and abolish the abnormal rhythm if it falls below the prevailing sinus rate. It usually recurs when CSM is terminated

Management

Usually, in the absence of digitalis toxicity, no treatment is required. If sinus rhythm is desired, atropine or isoprenaline may be given to accelerate the sinus node preferentially or the atrium can be paced.

Atrial flutter (LD-133)

This may be a recurrent or a sustained dysrhythmia. It usually occurs in the presence of heart disease but may occur in an otherwise normal heart. Rheumatic, coronary and thyrotoxic heart disease or cardiomyopathies are commonly responsible. In these circumstances, atrial flutter is frequently precipitated by distension of the left atrium consequent upon incipient left ventricular failure. Its onset may be associated with haemodynamic deterioration due to the loss of atrial systole and a rapid ventricular rate. In others, presenting symptoms may be typical of supraventricular tachycardia (see above). The dysrhythmia is probably due to re-entry within the atrium, giving an atrial rate that is almost always 300/min or thereabouts, but may range from 250–400/min. Occasionally, flutter waves can be seen in the jugular venous pulse.

The ventricular rate depends on AV conduction. In children a 1:1 AV response occasionally occurs, allowing a regular ventricular rate of about 300/min that may be associated with a broad QRS complex due to abnormal conduction. In adults 2:1 conduction is usual and typically gives a regular tachycardia of about 150/min. If higher degrees of AV block are present, a slower rate results and, with variable AV block, the rhythm is irregular.

ECG diagnosis

The features to note are:

- The QRS complexes have a normal configuration and the ventricular rate depends on the degree of AV block, which may vary
- flutter waves are present but are often difficult to identify with 1:1 or 2:1 AV conduction as they tend to be obscured by the T waves and the QRS complexes. Atrial flutter should always be suspected when a regular tachycardia of about 150/min is present and all available leads should be searched for evidence of flutter waves
- CSM may increase AV block and slow the ventricular rate. When effective, the flutter waves can be positively identified.

Management

As atrial flutter is often a recurrent rhythm, the initial treatment of choice is to slow the ventricular rate with digoxin either alone or in a combination with a β-blocker if necessary. If it persists, cardioversion with a low energy DC shock should be performed and is almost always effective. A DC shock is the initial choice if the dysrhythmia is known to be established or if it has caused haemodynamic deterioration.

Atrial fibrillation (LD-134)

This can be paroxysmal, but is commonly sustained. It occurs frequently in:

- rheumatic heart disease
- coronary heart disease
- thyrotoxicosis
- chest infections
- cardiomyopathies
- pericarditis

and also following cardiac surgery.

When present as an isolated feature, it is termed

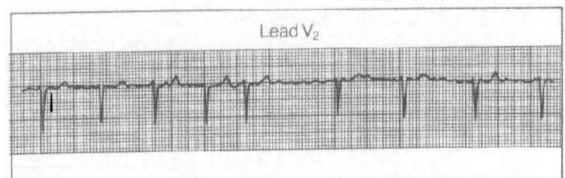

LD-134. *Atrial fibrillation. The QRS complexes have a normal configuration but the rhythm is totally irregular. Irregular baseline activity is present*

'lone atrial fibrillation'. It commonly causes palpitation that is typically totally irregular and may cause other symptoms commonly associated with supraventricular tachycardias (see above). When underlying heart disease is present, such as mitral stenosis, the onset of atrial fibrillation may be associated with marked deterioration in the clinical state because of the rapid ventricular rate and loss of atrial transport function during atrial systole. Systemic embolization occurs readily with the change in rhythm and this may be the presenting feature, especially when mitral valve disease is present.

With atrial fibrillation, the ventricular rate is totally irregular and, because of variation in ventricular filling time, the stroke volume varies. This causes a characteristically abnormal pulse that is totally variable in time and force. A similar peripheral pulse occurs with multiple ectopic beats, though this is less common. When the ventricular rate is rapid many contractions are so weak that they are impalpable in the peripheral pulse. The pulse rate is less than the heart rate, the difference being termed a 'pulse deficit'.

ECG diagnosis

The features to note are:

- the QRS complexes have a normal configuration and the ventricular rate may vary from about 50/min, if digoxin has been given, to 170/min if it is uncontrolled

- the rhythm is totally irregular but, when the ventricular rate is very rapid, variation in the RR intervals is necessarily quite small

- no discrete P wave activity is present. The baseline shows chaotic atrial activity best seen in the longer RR intervals

Management

The ventricular rate should be controlled with digoxin. Occasionally, a β-blocking drug is required in addition, especially in thyrotoxicosis. At times, the ventricular rate is naturally slow and no treatment is

required. When control of a rapid ventricular rate is required urgently, an intravenous β-blocker or verapamil should be given. Immediate DC cardioversion should be considered if there is marked haemodynamic deterioration.

When atrial fibrillation is of recent onset, but persists after the precipitating cause has been removed, elective DC cardioversion should be performed.

Lone atrial fibrillation nearly always recurs following cardioversion.

Antidysrhythmic drugs may help in long term maintenance of sinus rhythm, and some authorities advocate disopyramide or quinidine.

When atrial fibrillation occurs with mitral valve disease or thyrotoxicosis, anticoagulants should be given to reduce the risk of embolism.

Paroxysmal AV node re-entrant tachycardia and circus tachycardia of WPW syndrome (LD-135)

These rhythms differ from paroxysmal atrial tachycardia (PAT) in their mechanism, associated conditions and therapy. As their basis is re-entry, they have been termed 'reciprocating tachycardias'.

The heart is usually normal apart from the predisposition to paroxysmal tachycardia. All ages and both sexes can be affected. These tachycardias seldom have any obvious predisposing cause, are typically abrupt in onset, cause regular palpitation and may or may not end abruptly. The associated symptoms of supraventricular tachycardias are usual (see above).

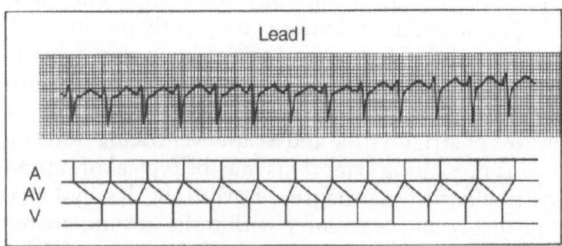

LD-135. *Paroxysmal supraventricular tachycardia. A regular tachycardia with normal QRS configuration is shown. P waves cannot be identified as they are obscured by the QRS complexes. In this example, the tachycardia was shown to utilize an accessory pathway between left ventricle and left atrium for retrograde conduction in a re-entry circuit*

ECG diagnosis

The features to note are:

- regular tachycardia varying from 140 to 240/min, though a rate of 150–180/min is most common. The QRS complexes are usually normal but, at rapid rates, may broaden due to the development of abnormal conduction. A right bundle branch block (RBBB) pattern is more common than left bundle branch block (LBBB) pattern

- P waves cannot usually be identified as they are obscured by the QRS complexes. When identified, they are typically inverted in leads II, III and aVF because of retrograde atrial activation
- CSM may help with diagnosis as it may terminate the tachycardia, thus distinguishing it from PAT, atrial flutter and junctional tachycardia with which it is most readily confused (see Table 22).
- the onset of tachycardia may also be helpful as it is initiated abruptly by an atrial or ventricular ectopic beat
- in the absence of tachycardia, the ECG is usually normal but should be checked for evidence of pre-excitation (see below)

Management

Many attacks are self-terminating and no treatment is required. Patients with frequent paroxysms should be taught how to stimulate the vagus (CSM, Valsalva or gagging). This may be effective, especially if tried early in the attack.

If drug treatment is necessary, the choice depends upon the circumstances. If the patient is not distressed and delay in restoration of sinus rhythm is acceptable, routine digitalization may be all that is required. However, most episodes are distressing if they persist and should be terminated with either an intravenous β-blocker or verapamil under careful supervision. Verapamil should not be given to patients with potential digitalis toxicity because of the risk of asystole or with β-blockers because of their combined negative inotropic effect. If termination is urgently required, DC cardioversion should be used to restore normal rhythm.

These dysrhythmias are typically recurrent and, if attacks are frequent and troublesome, suppressive therapy is indicated. Digoxin alone may be sufficient or a β-blocker may be added. Both interfere with AV node re-entry by prolonging its refractoriness. If ineffective, disopyramide should be tried. This suppresses the ectopic beats that initiate the tachycardia but has little effect on AV node conduction. Oral verapamil, quinidine or amiodarone are alternatives, but a combination of drugs may be required.

If drug therapy is ineffective, a pacemaker can be used to provide an ectopic beat that will interrupt the re-entry pathway by making it refractory.

Rarely, surgical division of the His bundle may be indicated in refractory cases, adequate ventricular rhythm being maintained with a permanent pacemaker.

Wolff–Parkinson–White syndrome (WPW) (pre-excitation)

Originally described in healthy young adults prone to paroxysmal tachycardia, it is now used as a synonym for pre-excitation.

The ECG shows a short PR interval and a prolonged QRS complex due to the presence of an accessory AV connection that bypasses the AV node. This allows premature activation or 'pre-excitation' of the ventricles and accounts for the short PR interval. The broad QRS is due to the presence of a delta wave caused by abnormal ventricular activation via the accessory pathway (LD-136a). Part of the ventricle distant from the accessory pathway may be activated normally via the AV node, and the QRS complex then represents a 'fusion' beat. When the accessory pathway is left sided, the delta wave is positive in V_1 (Type A WPW); when it is right sided, the delta wave is negative in V_1 (Type B WPW) (LD-136b).

Tachycardia can be initiated when an atrial premature beat finds the accessory pathway refractory. The delta wave is then absent and a normal QRS complex follows, due to normal conduction through the AV node. Activation may then be conducted retrogradely to the atrium via the accessory pathway, thus initiating a re-entrant or 'circus' tachycardia that is indistinguishable on the surface ECG from AV nodal re-entrant tachycardia.

It is now appreciated that many patients with paroxysmal supraventricular tachycardia who do not have overt evidence of the WPW syndrome have an accessory pathway that only conducts retrogradely and is responsible for a circus tachycardia. In the absence of tachycardia, the ECG appears normal and the diagnosis can only be made with certainty by intracardiac recording techniques.

ECG diagnosis

The combination of a short PR interval with a broadened QRS complex and a delta wave is pathognomonic (LD-136).

The ECG characteristics of circus tachycardia are identical to AV nodal re-entrant tachycardia, but the abnormal resting ECG indicates the different underlying mechanism.

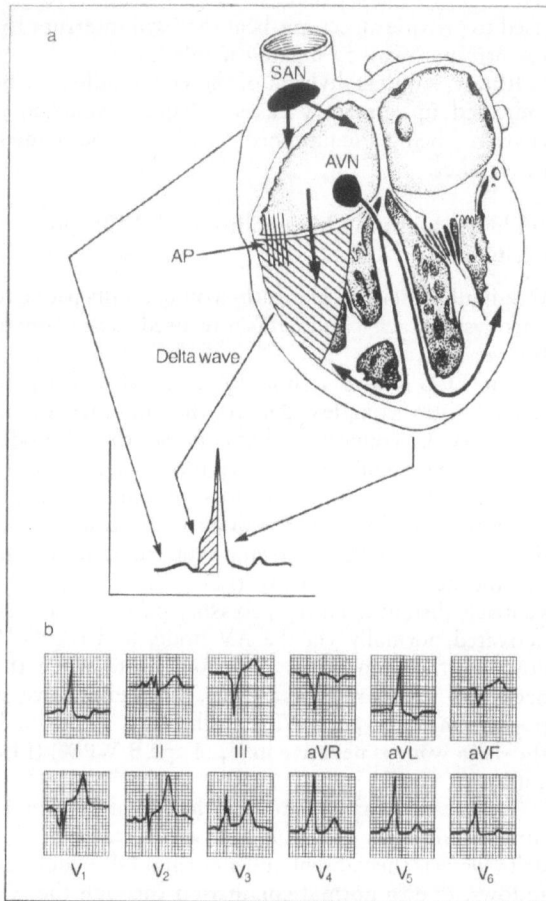

LD-136. *Wolff–Parkinson–White syndrome. a, The short PR interval and broad QRS complex are due to the presence of an accessory pathway (AP) that allows pre-excitation of the ventricles and causes a delta wave on the surface ECG. b, The delta wave is well marked. The QRS pattern superficially resembles left bundle branch block, but the short PR interval is characteristic. The delta wave is negative in V_1 (Type B WPW)*

Management

This is the same as for AV nodal re-entrant tachycardias except that digoxin should be avoided because of the potential danger should ventricular fibrillation occur (see below). Pacing can also be used. Some patients can be cured by surgical division of the accessory pathway.

Atrial flutter and atrial fibrillation with WPW syndrome

The presence of an accessory pathway between the atrium and ventricle may allow transmission of these rapid atrial dysrhythmias to the ventricles and cause very rapid ventricular rates. This occasionally results in ventricular fibrillation and may be one mechanism of sudden death in patients with the WPW syndrome.

ECG diagnosis

The condition should be suspected when rapid dysrhythmias resembling ventricular tachycardia occur in patients with pre-excitation.

Management

A DC shock should be given if the rapid rate is causing haemodynamic deterioration. Alternatively, disopyramide or procainamide should be given intravenously, as these drugs slow conduction in the accessory pathway. Digoxin should be avoided, as it may increase the ventricular rate by shortening the refractory period of the accessory pathway and thus precipitate ventricular fibrillation. When life-threatening dysrhythmias occur, surgical treatment should be considered.

Ventricular tachyrhythmias

Ventricular tachycardia (VT) (LD-137)

This occurs most commonly in acute myocardial infarction, but may also be seen in chronic coronary heart disease and cardiomyopathies and in the absence of identifiable heart disease. It can also be induced by drug toxicity, the most common drugs being digoxin, quinidine and catecholamines.

At rapid rates, VT is less well tolerated than SVT and often causes syncope. At slower rates it may be well tolerated, giving rise to palpitation and symptoms similar to SVT (see above), though polyuria is not a recognized feature. ECG monitoring shows that

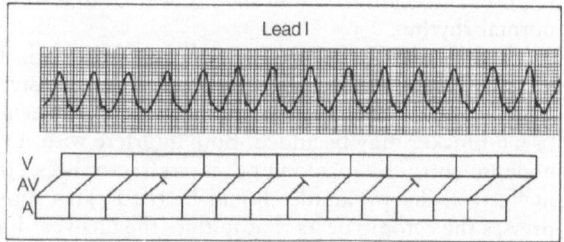

LD-137. *Ventricular tachycardia. The QRS complexes are broad. Intermittent AV dissociation is present and only some QRS complexes are followed by P waves*

short-lived episodes of VT may occur without symptoms. VT may be self-terminating, but may progress to ventricular fibrillation, which is serious and frequently fatal (see LD-139).

VT may occasionally be distinguished clinically from SVT by the presence of cannon waves in the venous pulse and variation in the intensity of the first heart sound. These signs occur because of atrioventricular dissociation. The mechanism is discussed further under Complete Heart Block, p. 208.

ECG diagnosis

The features to note are:

- the QRS configuration is broad, being greater than 0.12 s

- the rate varies between 120 and 300/min

- the rhythm is usually regular, but in some patients slight irregularities occur

- the tachycardia may start with a ventricular ectopic beat, often of the R on T type (see below)

- AV dissociation may occur and is identifiable as independent atrial activity at a slower rate than the tachycardia. When present with the other features, AV dissociation is diagnostic of VT. In some cases the ventricular activation is conducted retrogradely to the atria

- capture beats, with a narrow supraventricular type QRS complex, may be present when an atrial beat manages to capture the ventricle. These are unusual, but are pathognomonic of VT when the other features are present

- fusion beats are partial capure beats due to simultaneous ventricular and supraventricular activation exciting different parts of the ventricle. They are also unusual, but have the same significance as capture beats

It may be difficult to distinguish VT from an SVT with broad QRS complexes due to abnormal conduction (LD-138). A QRS duration of more than 0.14 second favours VT; an RBBB pattern in V_1 favours SVT with abnormal conduction. The presence of AV dissociation, capture beats or fusion beats is diagnostic of VT, but these features are usually absent and a precise diagnosis may require intracardiac recordings.

Management

Ventricular tachycardia should be treated with intravenous lignocaine, mexiletine or disopyramide. If loss of consciousness or haemodynamic deterioration has

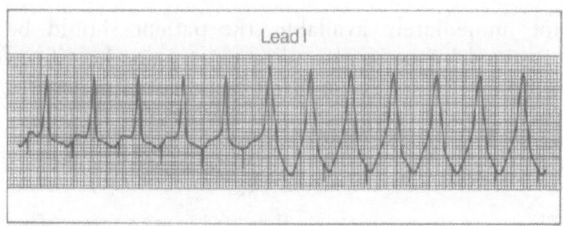

LD-138. *Supraventricular tachycardia with aberrant conduction. With atrial pacing at 190/min a narrow QRS is present but bundle branch block develops giving a rhythm resembling VT*

occurred, immediate DC cardioversion should be used. Occasionally, VT can be terminated by a blow on the chest. Recurrent VT requires therapy with mexiletine, disopyramide, procaineamide, a β-blocker, amiodarone or quinidine, either singly or in combination.

Ventricular fibrillation (VF) (LD-139)

This is a chaotic ventricular rhythm that is occasionally self-terminating but is invariably fatal if it persists. It occurs in the same settings as ventricular tachycardia and is the most frequent cause of death in the early stages following acute myocardial infarction.

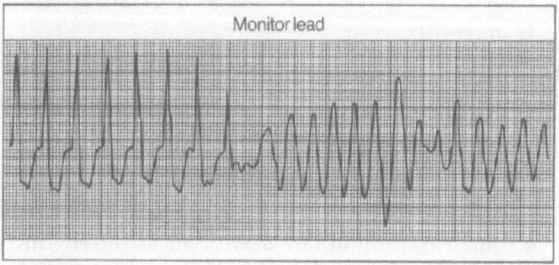

LD-139. *Ventricular tachycardia changing to ventricular fibrillation*

ECG diagnosis

Ventricular fibrillation is easily diagnosed from the presence of rapid chaotic ventricular activity. It may be precipitated by ventricular tachycardia or an R on T ectopic beat, but often occurs spontaneously (see LD-142).

Management

Ventricular fibrillation demands an immediate DC shock to restore normal rhythm. Subsequent prophylactic therapy is given as for VT. If a defibrillator is not immediately available, the patient should be sustained by external cardiac massage and artificial ventilation until DC cardioversion is available (see pp. 266–268).

Accelerated idioventricular rhythm (LD-140)

This is an uncommon rhythm and is seen most often after acute myocardial infarction. Ventricular pacemaker activity is enhanced and a ventricular rhythm with a rate of 60–100/min, or occasionally more, is faster than the prevailing sinus rate. Episodes commonly last for between four and 30 beats. As the rate is not rapid, it is unusual for associated symptoms to occur. It is usually benign and seldom precipitates more dangerous dysrhythmias.

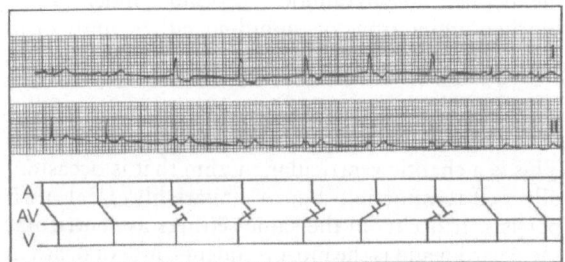

LD-140. *Accelerated idioventricular rhythm. The record shows a transient change from sinus to idioventricular rhythm*

ECG diagnosis

The features to note are:

- the QRS configuration is broad, being greater than 0.12 s in duration
- the rate is usually between 60 and 100/min but is occasionally more rapid
- some variation in rate may occur as the rhythm often initially accelerates and then slows before being superseded by sinus rhythm. The rhythm may come and go as the sinus and ventricular rates vary
- AV dissociation is usually present
- fusion beats and capture beats may occur

Management

As a rule no therapy is required. Atropine may be used to abolish the ventricular rhythm by increasing the sinus rate.

Ectopic beats

Ectopic beats are those that arise from any site other than the sinus node. Although they are not necessarily either extra or premature, the terms 'ectopic beat', 'extrasystole' and 'premature beat' are commonly used synonymously. They may be single or multiple and frequently cause palpitation. Patients complain of 'missed beats', although they are usually unaware of the ectopic beat and are conscious of the compensatory pause that follows (LD-130). They may also notice 'thumps' because the post-extrasystolic beats have a larger than normal stroke volume as a result of this longer filling time.

An early premature beat may be associated with such a small stroke volume that no peripheral pulse is palpable and the ectopic beat is detected clinically as a 'dropped beat'. On auscultation, however, the ectopic beat is audible. Occasionally, cannon waves are present in the neck veins when the atrium contracts against a closed tricuspid valve.

Supraventricular and ventricular ectopic beats are common in normal people but are seen more frequently in those with heart disease. The term 'coupled beats' is used when each sinus beat is followed by an ectopic beat.

ECG diagnosis of supraventricular ectopic beats (LD-141)

The features to note are:

- premature beats with a normal QRS morphology are present
- a preceding atrial ectopic beat may be identifiable as an abnormal P wave though it may be difficult to distinguish from the preceding T wave
- the premature QRS complex is followed by a pause that may be compensatory or less than compensatory depending on whether or not the premature atrial beat has interfered with sinus node function. A compensatory pause is of such duration that the premature beat does not 'reset' the basic sinus rhythm (LD-129).
- occasionally, early atrial ectopic beats are fol-

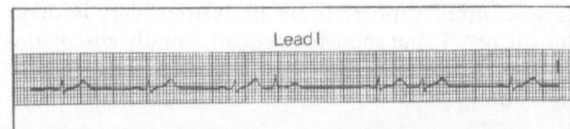

LD-141. *Junctional ectopic beats. The fourth and sixth beats are premature. The fourth beat is followed by a P wave but the sixth has no visibly related P wave. The fourth beat also has a slightly different QRS configuration due to aberrant conduction*

lowed by a broad QRS complex due to aberrant conduction caused by incomplete recovery of one or other of the bundle branches. An RBBB pattern is more common than an LBBB pattern

● very early atrial ectopic beats may fail to traverse the AV node if it has not recovered from the preceding beat. This blocked atrial ectopic beat is therefore not followed by a QRS complex and there is a less than compensatory pause before sinus rhythm resumes

ECG diagnosis of junctional ectopic beats

These have the same characteristics as supraventricular ectopic beats, but may be identified as arising in the AV junction because they are preceded or followed by inverted P waves in leads II, III and aVF. The P waves are inverted because of retrograde atrial activation and their timing is dependent upon VA conduction time as discussed above, in Junctional Tachycardia (p. 198) (LD-131).

Management

Supraventricular and junctional ectopic beats usually require no therapy. If palpitation is troublesome, it can usually be suppressed with a β-blocker, or disopyramide.

Wandering atrial pacemaker

This can be recognized by P waves of varying morphology when activation is initiated at varying atrial sites. No specific therapy is indicated.

ECG diagnosis of ventricular ectopic beats

The features on ECG are:

● premature beats of broad configuration with no preceding P wave and usually with a T wave of opposite sign.

● the premature beat is usually followed by a compensatory pause as the basic sinus rhythm is not disturbed

Coupling (ventricular bigeminy) is said to occur when each sinus beat is followed by an ectopic beat. This is commonly a sign of digitalis toxicity and other features of digitalis toxicity may be present. When an ectopic beat occurs on the T wave of the preceding beat, it is termed an 'R on T' ectopic beat. Such beats can initiate ventricular tachycardia and ventricular fibrillation (LD-142).

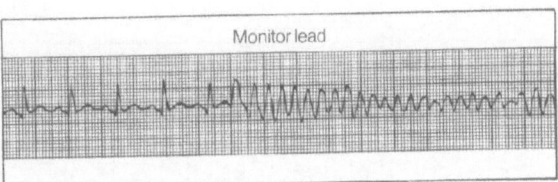

LD-142. *R on T ectopic beat. The sixth beat is a premature ventricular ectopic beat and occurs on the T wave of the preceding complex, initiating ventricular fibrillation*

Management

Isolated ventricular ectopic beats are common and require no therapy. When associated with symptoms, they will often respond to one of the drugs used to treat ventricular tachycardia (see above). R on T ectopic beats should usually be treated, as they may precipitate more serious dysrhythmias.

Conduction abnormalities

AV block

AV block occurs when there is impaired conduction between the atria and the ventricles (LD-143). It can vary in severity from slowing (prolongation of the PR interval) to failure of AV conduction (complete heart block).

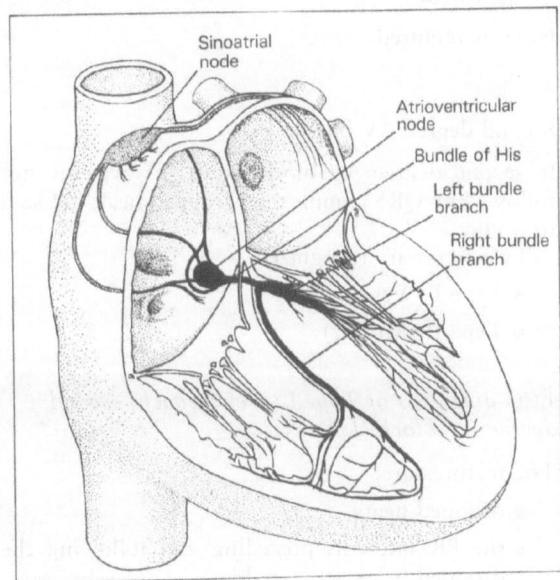

LD-143. *The conduction system*

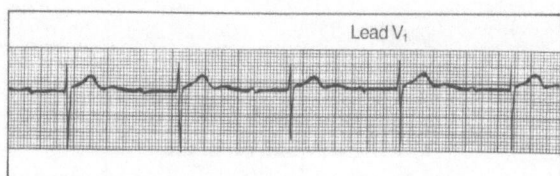

LD-144. *Sinus bradycardia and first degree AV block. The ventricular rate is 47/min and PR is 0.42 s*

First degree AV block (LD-144)

First degree AV block is present when the PR interval is prolonged beyond the upper limit of normal (0.20 second). The delay in conduction normally occurs in the AV node but it can occur rarely in the His–Purkinje system.

The most common causes are:

- digitalis toxicity
- myocardial infarction (especially when this is inferior)
- calcific disease of the aortic valve

In young people, more common causes are acute rheumatic fever and diphtheria. At times, no obvious cause is evident.

ECG diagnosis

The PR interval is prolonged.

Management

None is required.

Second degree AV block

In second degree AV block, some P waves are not followed by QRS complexes. Dropped beats are said to occur.

Two types are recognized:

- Type I (Wenckebach)
- Type II (Mobitz)

ECG diagnosis of Type I (Wenckebach) second degree AV block (LD-145)

The features are:

- dropped beats
- the PR intervals preceding and following the dropped beats are variable

Classically, the PR interval prolongs with success-

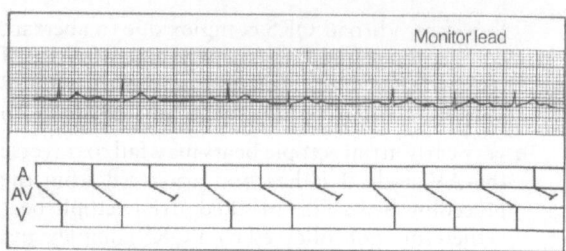

LD-145. *Type I (Wenckebach) second degree AV block. The PR interval lengthens progressively until a dropped beat occurs*

ive beats until a dropped beat occurs, i.e. a P wave is not followed by a QRS complex. Following this, the PR interval shortens again and the cycle repeats itself. The diagnosis is often missed because the relation between P waves and QRS complexes is not appreciated. Construction of a ladder diagram helps to clarify the diagnosis. Wenckebach AV block should be suspected when QRS complexes repeatedly occur in groups followed by a pause. This is called 'group beating'.

The conduction delay almost always occurs in the AV node. It may progress to complete heart block and, when this occurs, a relatively rapid junctional escape rhythm usually takes over. The condition is, therefore, relatively benign.

The most common cause is inferior myocardial infarction. Occasionally, digitalis toxicity is responsible. It can also occur with excess vagal tone.

Management

Usually, no therapy is required. Atropine may restore sinus rhythm. Pacing is indicated only if haemodynamic deterioration occurs. If digitalis toxicity is implicated, this requires specific therapy.

ECG diagnosis of Type II (Mobitz) second degree AV block (LD-146)

The features are:

- dropped beats

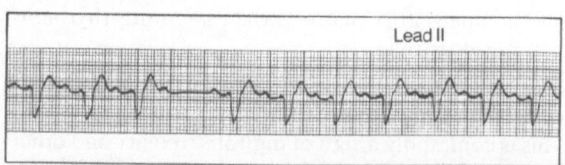

LD-146. *Mobitz Type II second degree AV block. A single dropped beat occurs and there is no significant change in the subsequent PR interval which is prolonged at 0.24 s. Left bundle branch block is also present indicating trifascicular block*

- the PR intervals preceding and following the dropped beats are constant

This is much more serious than Type I. The conduction abnormality is usually in the His–Purkinje system where conduction tends to be all or none. A single dropped beat may therefore presage complete failure of conduction. As the block in conduction is relatively distal, a subsidiary pacemaker may fail to emerge or, if it does emerge, may have a very slow rate. Asystole or AV block with a very slow ventricular rate will result. Type II second degree AV block is uncommon and occurs mainly in patients with acute myocardial infarction.

Management

A pacemaker should be inserted.

2:1 Second degree AV block (LD-147)

In this condition only alternate P waves are followed by QRS complexes and alternate beats are dropped. It must therefore be distinguished from Type II second degree AV block in which only single beats are dropped. The site of block is most commonly in the AV node but it can also occur more distally. 2:1 AV block is seen after acute myocardial infarction and in chronic degenerative disease of the conduction system. It may progress to complete heart block and may be associated with Adams–Stokes attacks if conduction fails completely.

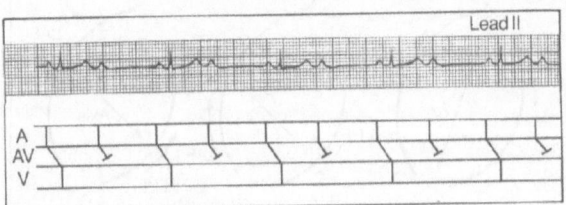

LD-147. *2:1 second degree AV block. The atrial rate is 74/min and the ventricular rate 37/min*

ECG diagnosis

The atrial rate is twice the ventricular rate and there is a fixed relation between the P waves and the QRS complexes.

Management

Pacing is indicated if symptoms occur.

Complete AV block (LD-148)

With complete AV block, the atrial and ventricular rhythms are independent of each other and the ventricular rate depends on the rate of the subsidiary pacemaker. Usually, this is about 40/min, but faster and slower rates occur.

Complete heart block is most commonly due to degenerative disease in the conduction system. It also occurs in coronary heart disease, calcific aortic valve disease and following heart surgery. Congenital heart block is rare, but is the likely aetiology when the condition is seen in young people.

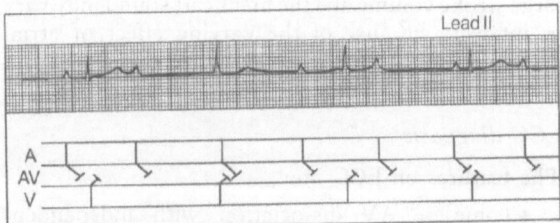

LD-148. *Complete AV block. Note how the obscured P wave can deform the QRS complex and T wave. The atrial rate is 62/min and the ventricular rate 37/min*

Clinical features

The most common symptom of complete heart block is syncope due to Adams–Stokes attacks. These usually occur either when the rate becomes very slow or when asystole occurs and cerebral perfusion becomes inadequate. Most patients remain asymptomatic while the heart rate is maintained above 40/min. A few develop congestive cardiac failure due to bradycardia and, occasionally, in the elderly, dementia results from poor cerebral perfusion.

Adams–Stokes attacks are syncopal attacks caused by cardiac dysrhythmias. Though most commonly due to asystole, other rhythms such as ventricular tachycardia or ventricular fibrillation may be responsible. They give identical clinical features. All ages can be affected but attacks are more common in the elderly, the average age being about 70. Syncopal attacks are typically recurrent. They may occur at any time and at widely varying intervals, without provocation and at rest or on exertion. There may be momentary warning lightheadedness before loss of consciousness, but usually the onset is abrupt and, not uncommonly, the patient is injured when falling. The duration of unconsciousness varies from a few seconds to several minutes. Recovery may be slow or rapid. Sometimes minor attacks of dizziness and unsteadiness occur without loss of consciousness.

The patient is typically 'deathly pale' and pulseless and, if the attack is prolonged, may have a fit. Recovery is associated with flushing of the face due to resumption of blood flow through dilated skin vessels and this, in association with the initial pallor, is virtually diagnostic of the condition.

In complete heart block, there is a slow, regular pulse. A heart rate of around 40/min should suggest the diagnosis. Cannon waves are usually present in the jugular venous pulse. These are seen as intermittent large systolic waves caused when the atrium contracts against a closed tricuspid valve. On auscultation, there is often a systolic murmur due to the large stroke volume and the first heart sound may vary in intensity because of the varying effect of atrial systole on mitral and tricuspid valve closure.

ECG diagnosis

The features on ECG are:

- complete AV dissociation with independent atrial and ventricular rhythms
- the ventricular rate is regular and uninfluenced by atrial activity which, being faster, 'walks through' the QRS complexes
- the QRS complexes are narrow if ventricular activation is initiated above the bifurcation of the bundle of His, and broad if bundle branch block is present or if activation arises distal to the bifurcation

Management

An artificial pacemaker should be inserted when complete heart block is associated with symptoms. In acute myocardial infarction, only temporary pacing is usually required but, in other circumstances, permanent pacing is indicated.

AV dissociation

AV dissociation occurs when the atrial and ventricular rhythms behave independently. AV block, either second degree or complete, is one cause of AV dissociation, but other mechanisms can also give rise to it when AV conduction remains intact. The atrial rate either becomes slower than the rate of a subsidiary pacemaker or the subsidiary pacemaker rate becomes faster than the atrial rate, as in accelerated junctional rhythm or accelerated idioventricular rhythm. The atrial and ventricular rhythms run independently because the ventricular rhythm is not conducted retrogradely to the atrium. However, when the atrial and ventricular rhythms come into phase, appropriate P waves can be conducted to the ventricles and initiate a QRS complex; the atrium is

said to capture the ventricle. Under these circumstances, the QRS rhythm is not quite regular. If the atrial rate is increased by atrial pacing or atropine, normal sinus rhythm will result when it becomes faster than the junctional or idioventricular rate. The abnormality is, therefore, quite different from AV block.

AV dissociation is seen in acute myocardial infarction and also with excessive vagal stimulation. It is benign in the absence of AV block and so it is important to determine whether or not AV block is present.

The hemiblocks

The concept has evolved that the left bundle branch comprises an anterior and posterior fascicle, each of which is susceptible to conduction abnormality. Block in the anterior fascicle is termed 'left anterior hemiblock' and, in the posterior fascicle, 'left posterior hemiblock'. Left anterior hemiblock is identified by left axis deviation. This occurs because, with block in the anterior fascicle, activation of the anterobasal portion of the heart is delayed, resulting in a shift in the mean QRS vector to the left (LD-149). Left posterior hemiblock is identified by right axis deviation. This occurs because block in the posterior fascicle causes delay in activation of the posterobasal portion of the heart and a shift in mean QRS vector to the right.

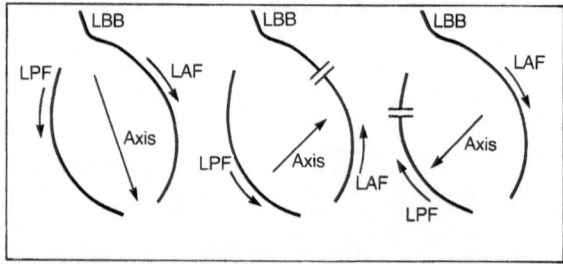

LD-149. *Diagram showing how the normal axis is altered by left anterior and left posterior hemiblock*

Axis deviation as an isolated finding has little clinical significance except in congenital heart disease where left axis deviation is associated with endocardial cushion defects and tricuspid atresia.

Bifascicular blocks (LD-150)

When right bundle branch block occurs in conjunction with left axis deviation (left anterior fascicle block) or right axis deviation (left posterior fascicle block) bifascicular block is said to be present; the

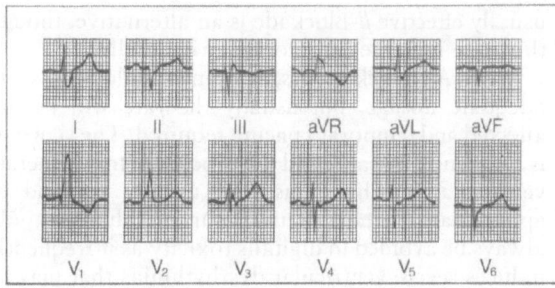

LD-150. *Bifascicular block. Right bundle branch block with left axis deviation. The PR interval is normal*

right bundle is regarded as the third fascicle. Conduction depends on the integrity of the remaining fascicle. In myocardial infarction this is associated with an increased risk of complete AV block or asystole and is usually an indication for prophylactic pacing. Bifascicular block as an isolated finding in the absence of myocardial infarction, however, has a relatively good prognosis and usually requires no treatment unless associated with evidence of more severe conduction abnormalities.

Trifascicular block

When bifascicular block is associated with evidence of abnormal conduction in the remaining fascicle (first degree AV block) trifascicular block is present (LD-146). This may be seen as first degree AV block with RBBB and either right or left axis deviation or first degree AV block and LBBB. These patterns are more serious abnormalities than bifascicular block.

Sick sinus syndrome

The term 'sick sinus syndrome' has been used to embrace several abnormalities of sinus node function. These are:

- inappropriate sinus bradycardia (a sinus rate of less than 60/min)
- sinus arrest
- sinoatrial block
- alternating bradycardia and tachycardia

Failure of sinus node function or prolonged sinus arrest without the emergence of an adequate escape rhythm is a not uncommon cause of Adams–Stokes attacks. In some patients, abnormal sinus node function is associated with paroxysmal supraventricular tachycardia, atrial flutter or atrial fibrillation, and these may be responsible for major symptoms (see above). When the paroxysmal tachycardia stops,

asystole may occur due to overdrive suppression of the sinus node and can result in syncope. Bradycardia and tachycardia may then alternate, giving the name 'bradycardia–tachycardia syndrome'. The varying atrial rhythm appears to predispose to systemic embolization and, occasionally, this may be the presenting feature.

Sinus bradycardia and, occasionally, sinus arrest and sinoatrial block can be physiological and may be extreme, because of excess vagal tone. They are sometimes associated with digitalis toxicity and also occur in acute myocardial infarction. It may be difficult at times to determine whether a finding is physiological or pathological. It should be considered pathological if it is severe, recurrent or associated with Adams–Stokes attacks or when associated with other evidence of cardiac disease.

ECG diagnosis of sinus arrest (LD-151)

There is abrupt failure of sinus node function resulting in a pause with no PQRST activity. The pause is not a multiple of the basic RR interval. It may be terminated by resumption of sinus rhythm or by emergence of an escape rhythm that is usually junctional.

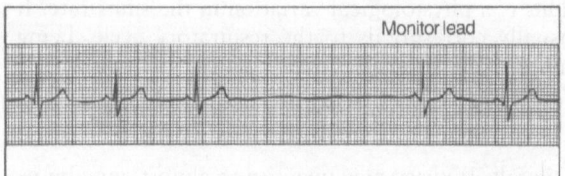

Monitor lead

LD-151. *Sinus arrest. There is complete absence of PQRST activity. The pause is not a multiple of the underlying RR interval*

ECG diagnosis of sinoatrial block (LD-152)

This is due to failure of conduction between the sinus node and atrial tissue and results in a pause that is an exact, or nearly exact, multiple of the basic RR interval.

Management

When symptoms are absent, abnormalities of sinus node function require no treatment. In acute situations, when excess vagal tone is the prime aetiological factor, intravenous atropine is usually effective. If bradycardia is associated with non-specific symptoms of lethargy, slow release isoprenaline (Saventrine) is often effective in increasing the sinus rate but, if Adams–Stokes attacks have occurred, permanent

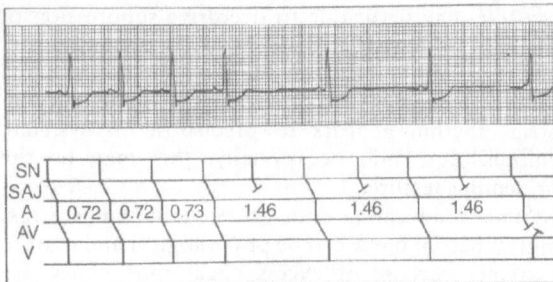

LD-152. 2:1 *sinoatrial block. The atrial rate abruptly halves. The seventh beat is a junctional escape beat; the preceding P wave is a sinus P wave (see ladder diagram)*

pacing is obligatory and medical treatment should not be contemplated. Occasionally, atrial pacing is employed, although ventricular pacing is technically easier and is usually preferred.

In bradycardia–tachycardia syndrome, appropriate therapy is indicated for the tachycardia. This may exacerbate the bradycardia by further slowing the sinus rate. Symptoms can then be controlled by pacing in combination with antidysrhythmic therapy.

Sinus arrhythmia

This is a physiological variation in the sinus rate. It usually corresponds to the respiratory cycle, being more rapid in inspiration.

Dysrhythmias of digitalis toxicity

Digitalis toxicity may give rise to almost any abnormal rhythm but several are especially common. These are paroxysmal atrial tachycardia (PAT) with AV block, frequent ventricular premature beats, ventricular bigeminy, ventricular tachycardia and junctional tachycardia. Less commonly, AV block (first degree, second degree or complete) and abnormal sinus node function occur. If the patient is receiving a digitalis preparation when such a dysrhythmia occurs, digitalis toxicity should always be suspected and excluded.

Management

With non-life-threatening dysrhythmias, it is sufficient to discontinue digitalis, check serum potassium levels and, if necessary, restore this and any other electrolyte or fluid imbalance to normal. The serum digoxin level should also be checked.

When rapid rhythms of sufficient severity to require treatment are present, e.g. PAT with AV block or ventricular tachycardia, intravenous phenytoin is

usually effective β-Blockade is an alternative, though this may increase AV block detrimentally.

When AV block occurs, atropine should be given in adequate dosage, but usually the rate will be unaffected and temporary pacing required. The ventricle is frequently irritable and the procedure may generate ventricular dysrhythmias that usually respond to appropriate therapy. Direct current shock should always be avoided in digitalis toxicity as it frequently induces severe ventricular dysrhythmias that may be totally unresponsive to therapy. When massive overdosage is present, gastric lavage should be considered.

CARDIAC COMPLICATIONS OF SYSTEMIC DISEASE

The heart may be affected by diseases arising in other parts of the body.

These include:

- infections
- endocrine and metabolic disorders
- anaemia
- general systemic diseases
- familial neuromuscular diseases

Infective endocarditis and pericarditis are dealt with elsewhere. Many other conditions occur only rarely. Some (thyrotoxicosis, anaemia) are relatively common and should be excluded routinely by clinical or other tests.

Infections

With greater control of bacterial infections, the number of cases with cardiac complications has been greatly reduced.

Cardiac involvement in infection can be due to:

- direct invasion by organisms
- toxic myocarditis
- effects on peripheral vasculature
- effects on the vasomotor centres

Bacterial infections

These can involve the cardiovascular system in any of the ways mentioned above, but are less frequently seen nowadays in Britain.

Diphtheria

The heart is involved in about one fifth of those affected and this is an extremely serious complication, especially in infants and children. Destruction of the myocardial cells by the exotoxin causes tachycardia and triple rhythm, and later varying degrees of heart block, cardiac enlargement and heart failure. In those who recover, there is little evidence of permanent cardiac damage.

Pneumonia

Pneumonia, particularly in the elderly, may cause toxaemic cardiac failure, and is also occasionally the cause of acute bacterial endocarditis.

Tuberculosis

This mainly affects the heart by causing pericarditis which, on healing, may cause severe fibrosis.

Syphilis

The ascending aorta becomes dilated in some cases of tertiary syphilis. This may result in the formation of aneurysms and aortic regurgitation.

Virus infections

These cause both pericarditis and myocarditis. Involvement of the heart in acute viral infections may have to be differentiated from myocardial infarction. The viruses most often concerned are Coxsackie B and, occasionally, polio, influenza and those causing infectious mononucleosis. The exact diagnosis is difficult and can only be made by stool culture in the first week of the illness or later by routine examination of sera at 10-day intervals for rising titres. Myocarditis is often preceded by pericarditis and other evidence of viral infection such as upper respiratory infection, fever, malaise and muscular pains. Evidence of myocarditis is given by tachycardia, triple rhythm, cardiac enlargement and sometimes failure. ECGs may reveal conduction abnormalities and ST–T wave changes. Complete recovery is usual but some may develop constrictive pericarditis or cardiomyopathies in later life.

Protozoal disorders

Trypanosomiasis (Chagas disease) and toxoplasmosis may also affect the heart.

Endocrine and metabolic disorders

Over- or underactivity of the thyroid gland can produce cardiac disorders that may complicate other forms of heart disease and, like anaemia, require to be excluded in any case of cardiac failure or angina.

Hyperthyroidism

In this condition, heat production and oxygen consumption are increased. Thyroxin also has a direct effect on the heart and all these factors raise cardiac output, mainly by increasing its rate and contractility rather than by increasing its stroke volume. A normal heart may tolerate this, an abnormal one may not. Thus, particularly in older patients and especially in those with coronary, hypertensive or rheumatic heart disease, the symptoms and signs of heart failure may predominate in thyrotoxicosis. Occasionally, there is no underlying heart disease, but in these cases the thyrotoxicosis is severe and longstanding. Atrial fibrillation is common and is probably due to a direct effect of thyroxine on the myocardium. Palpitation and tachycardia are common in thyrotoxicosis and may make differentiation from anxiety and cardiac neurosis difficult.

The pulse is of large volume and collapsing. The systolic pressure is elevated. The heart sounds are loud. A pulmonary systolic murmur can often be heard, reflecting increased flow through the right ventricular outflow tract. The whole picture suggests hyperactivity.

Unexplained sinus tachycardia, atrial fibrillation or flutter, cardiac failure or persistent angina should lead one to suspect hyperthyroidism.

The ECG is not helpful. Diagnosis is confirmed by the usual tests of thyroid activity.

Antithyroid drugs, surgery or radio-iodine therapy are appropriate to individual patients. β-Blocking drugs are now used to moderate cardiac side-effects of hyperthyroidism, but must be given cautiously in the presence of cardiac failure. Atrial fibrillation only responds well to digoxin after hyperthyroidism is controlled. It may then revert spontaneously to sinus rhythm. The prognosis is good but may depend on underlying cardiac disorders.

Hypothyroidism

Although hypothyroidism may affect the heart and cardiovascular system in several ways, with the exception of angina due to underlying ischaemic disease, it causes relatively few cardiac symptoms.

Lowered metabolism results in a low cardiac

output, diminished peripheral blood flow and a slow pulse. Lack of thyroid hormone can cause interstitial oedema and pericardial effusion. Hypercholesterolaemia may exacerbate existing coronary artery disease.

The pulse rate is usually 50–60/min. The heart sounds are soft and the apex difficult to define. The ECG may show low voltage complexes and flat or inverted T waves.

Treatment has to be cautious because of the fear of causing heart failure or provoking severe angina. Thyroxin 0.05 mg per day should be the initial dose and β-blockers can be given to minimize its cardiac effects.

Carcinoid

Rarely, cardiac lesions can be caused by the actions of kinins or 5-hydroxytryptamine secreted by metastatic carcinoid tumours in the liver. Pulmonary or tricuspid valve stenosis and right heart failure may occasionally result. Diagnosis is confirmed by the detection of 5-hydroxyindoleacetic acid in the urine.

Amyloid disease

Amyloid disease of the heart is usually primary and produces a form of cardiomyopathy.

Beriberi

This is due to a dietary deficiency of thiamine. It can be caused by eating a diet of polished rice but may be seen in other forms of malnutrition. It causes a high cardiac output with a low peripheral resistance. Patients complain of fatigue, palpitations, breathlessness and peripheral oedema. The heart rate is rapid, the pulse pressure is high and the heart is enlarged. Peripheral neuritis usually coexists and diagnosis depends on this association with a poor nutritional history. Thiamine and a high protein diet produce immediate improvement.

Alcohol

Alcohol with associated nutritional deficiency may produce a thiamine deficiency type of cardiac failure as outlined above. It may also have a direct toxic effect on heart muscle causing all types of dysrhythmias and in some cases alcoholic cardiomyopathy with low output cardiac failure.

Contraceptive pill

There are two slight risks to the cardiovascular system from the oestrogen content of the pill. One is hypertension, the other thromboembolism. Neither risk is great, but alternative contraceptive methods are preferred in older women and those with hypertension or at risk from thromboembolism.

Anaemia

Anaemia, particularly if severe and longstanding, demands an increased cardiac output. It may produce or aggravate cardiac failure or angina and should be excluded in all cases of heart disease.

General systemic diseases

Practically all of the connective tissue disorders may involve the heart.

Rheumatoid arthritis

This may occasionally affect the valves or cause a pericardial effusion, but is detected rather infrequently except at autopsy.

Disseminated lupus erythematosus

This often involves the heart, although rarely as a presenting sign. Pericarditis, myocarditis and a specific form of endocarditis with large vegetations on the valves are the forms taken.

Systemic sclerosis

This may cause a form of constrictive cardiomyopathy or a picture resembling cor pulmonale due to diffuse pulmonary fibrosis.

Infiltrative disorders

Infiltrative disorders and granulomas such as leukaemia and sarcoidosis can cause conduction defects, dysrhythmias, sudden death and cardiac failure.

Tumour tissue

Tumour tissue from adjacent organs such as the bronchi may invade the heart and cause dysrhythmias or pericardial effusion.

Familial neuromuscular diseases

Friedreich's ataxia, progressive muscular dystrophy and myotonia atrophica may all affect the heart.

CARDIOMYOPATHIES

The main causes of myocardial disease are:

- ischaemic
- hypertensive
- rheumatic
- pulmonary

Sometimes, however, a patient is encountered with heart muscle disease that cannot be explained by any of these main causes. It is then loosely, if conveniently, described as a 'cardiomyopathy'.

Cardiomyopathies are difficult to diagnose. If, after exhaustive investigations, no cause can be found, the cardiomyopathy is termed 'primary' or 'idiopathic'; the diagnosis being made by exclusion.

If the heart is already the seat of acquired or congenital disease, or has been damaged by trauma or drugs, the cardiomyopathy is termed 'secondary'. Table 23 shows a few examples of some of the commoner causes of secondary cardiomyopathy.

TABLE 23   Secondary cardiomyopathies

Cause	Examples
Neurological	Muscular dystrophies (e.g. Duchenne), Friedreich's ataxia
Storage disorders	Glycogen storage disease, haemochromatosis
Primary amyloidosis	
Infections	All types of organisms (especially Coxsackie B virus)
Sarcoidosis	
Collagen disorders	Many varieties
Endocrine disorders	Thyrotoxicosis, myxoedema, acromegaly
Nutritional	Starvation, anaemia, beriberi
Tumours	Primaries are rare
Drugs	Alcohol, emetine

Clinical classification

A useful and widely used classification of cardiomyopathies is based on their clinical presentation.

Patients whose clinical features are those of right or left heart failure are said to have 'congestive' cardiomyopathy, those whose features suggest constrictive pericarditis are said to have 'constrictive' cardiomyopathy and those whose features resemble aortic or pulmonary stenosis are said to have 'obstructive' cardiomyopathy. Constrictive cardiomyopathy is not common in the UK.

Congestive cardiomyopathy

The patient gives a history of increasing breathlessness and, on examination, has a large heart, triple rhythm and high venous pressure. There is evidence of mitral or tricuspid incompetence or both, because of dilated ventricles and papillary muscle dysfunction. Atrial fibrillation is often present and the ECG shows low voltage complexes with non-specific changes in the ST–T wave segments. Cardiac catheterization shows raised right atrial pressure with evidence of tricuspid incompetence.

The majority of cases in this group have idiopathic cardiomyopathy, but some have secondary cardiomyopathy, such as primary amyloidosis, viral myocarditis and, in some South American countries, Chagas disease (South American trypanosomiasis).

Constrictive cardiomyopathy

Constriction of the myocardium can be caused by abnormalities of the pericardium, as in constrictive pericarditis, by a thickened endocardium or by a myocardium whose compliance is reduced by a diffuse disease process. Haemodynamically, and therefore to some extent clinically, the site of constriction does not greatly influence the end result.

Clinically, such patients present with the picture of conventional right ventricular failure together with certain particular features. The jugular venous pressure is raised out of all proportion to the heart size; the y descent is unusually prominent and 'paradoxical pulsation' of the venous pulse may be present, i.e. it rises on inspiration.

Causes of endocardial constriction include endocardial fibroelastosis and, in equatorial Africa, endomyocardial fibrosis.

Obstructive cardiomyopathy

The commonest example of obstructive cardiomyopathy is that known in Britain as hypertrophic obstructive cardiomyopathy (HOCM). This condition, sometimes sporadic but often familial, consists of hypertrophy of the left ventricle and the ventricular septum.

The history is that of breathlessness, but occasionally there is effort syncope and sometimes angina. There may be a family history and there is a risk of sudden death.

The clinical picture is that of obstruction to left ventricular outflow, which is often phasic and variable. It may therefore mimic aortic stenosis and, because patients with HOCM often have associated mitral incompetence, the mistaken diagnosis of rheumatic heart disease is sometimes made. The arterial pulse in aortic stenosis, however, is slow-rising, whereas in HOCM it is jerky. The ejection systolic murmur in HOCM is late in systole, it is maximal at the left sternal edge and usually there is no aortic diastolic murmur.

Certain drugs and manoeuvres increase the obstruction and therefore influence the murmur. For example, positive inotropic drugs such as digitalis and isoprenaline make the obstruction greater and increase the murmur. Negative inotropic drugs such as β-blockers, and peripheral vasodilators such as nitrites, relax the obstruction.

The ECG shows left ventricular hypertrophy or a pathological Q wave in central chest leads. The chest X-ray may be normal or show a cardiac silhouette that has a rather 'plump' left ventricle or gross left ventricular enlargement. Echos show characteristic changes in the ventricular wall, especially in the septum, and in the function of the anterior cusp of the mitral valve. At cardiac catheterization, the pressure gradient is shown to be in the left ventricle rather than between the left ventricle and the aortic valve.

Management

In most cases all that can be done is to give symptomatic treatment with supportive measures such as rest, digitalis (not in HOCM) and diuretics. Usually, by the time symptoms develop, the disease is far advanced and all that can be expected is transient improvement in the progressive downhill course.

Patients with obstructive cardiomyopathy may improve with β-blockade. A few require surgical treatment.

HEART DISEASE IN PREGNANCY

During the past few decades, several factors have brought about considerable changes in the nature and management of heart disease in pregnancy.

The most important of these has been the dramatic reduction in the prevalence of rheumatic heart disease, which in the past accounted for the vast majority of cases. Nowadays, such patients are few and far between and have much less serious lesions.

Along with this decrease in rheumatic heart disease has come a small but steady increase in the number of women with congenital cardiac malformations who have had successful surgical treatment.

Equally remarkable are the advances in therapeutics that have accompanied these changes. Antibiotics, effective diuretics, safer anaesthetics, cardiac surgery and intensive care facilities, together with the liberalization of attitudes towards contraception, abortion and sterilization, now permit a much more rational approach to childbearing for the relatively small number who still have significant heart disease.

Young women known to have heart disease should be encouraged to seek cardiological advice before pregnancy, so that the risks can be assessed and the necessary measures taken to minimize or avoid them. Otherwise, they should be examined as soon as possible after conception before the hyperkinetic circulatory state that accompanies pregnancy becomes fully developed, modifies the signs of heart disease and makes accurate diagnosis difficult.

The effects of pregnancy

Profound circulatory changes occur during pregnancy that greatly increase the amount of work required of the heart.

Beginning early in the second month, cardiac output increases rapidly by about 30% and remains at this level until term. The increased cardiac output is required by the uterus for the large placental circulation, by the kidneys for the increased elimination of soluble waste products and by the skin for the dissipation of heat generated by the increased metabolic rate. It is achieved by increasing the blood volume (mainly its plasma component), the heart rate and the stroke volume.

A normal heart readily responds and adapts to the increased demands of this hyperkinetic circulatory state; an abnormal one may find itself under considerable strain. The consequent symptoms often focus attention upon the cardiovascular system for the first time and reveal a pre-existing cardiac lesion.

Clinical features

Warm flushed hands, with easily felt pulsation in the digital arteries, signal the greatly increased peripheral blood flow.

The resting pulse rate is increased by about 15 beats/min and the pulse pressure is usually raised because decreased peripheral vascular resistance causes a slight fall in the diastolic blood pressure.

The central venous pressure may be slightly raised. Obvious signs of a high venous pressure in the lower half of the body are caused mainly by the gravid uterus obstructing venous return through the iliac veins and the inferior vena cava.

The heart feels active on palpation and may be slightly enlarged even after allowance is made for the raised diaphragm. The increased flow of blood through it is frequently manifest by a third heart sound at the apex and a soft early systolic murmur along the left sternal edge – physiological signs that are frequently mistaken for evidence of heart disease.

Assessment of risk

Few women with heart disease fail to survive pregnancy if they are properly cared for by those with the necessary experience and resources.

In assessing the risks and deciding what measures should be taken to minimize them, many factors are taken into account.

The first, and the most important of these, is the nature and severity of the cardiac lesion itself. For example, mild mitral regurgitation is of little or no consequence, whereas tight mitral stenosis may demand urgent attention. Atrial fibrillation or cardiomegaly indicate fairly advanced disease and limited cardiac reserves. Gross pulmonary hypertension, especially when associated with congenital malformations, carries a maternal mortality rate of around 40–50% with a poor prospect of a live baby, even in those who survive. Severe central cyanosis is also associated with a high fetal mortality.

The age and parity of the patient are important because, by and large, the younger she is, the better will she tolerate her pregnancy. Also, experience in previous pregnancies provides useful information about the likely outcome of future pregnancies.

Social, ethical and religious attitudes often require careful consideration.

Management during pregnancy

After the nature and severity of the lesion have been determined, management depends upon the assessment of the risks involved.

All patients with heart disease should be seen regularly by cardiologists at antenatal clinics where their progress can be monitored by sequential evaluation of the cardiac grade.

Ideally, patients with severe lesions should have surgical treatment before they become pregnant. If they are seen for the first time very early in pregnancy, this may still be possible without interruption of the pregnancy. If not, it is often best to terminate the pregnancy and start again following successful cardiac surgery which, though still possible later in pregnancy, is probably more hazardous than intensive medical therapy.

The cardiac grade

This is a scale based upon functional capacity:

- those in grade I have no symptoms
- those in grade II have symptoms only on fairly strenuous exertion
- those in grade III have symptoms when carrying out everyday activities
- those in grade IV have symptoms on the slightest exertion or even at rest and may have signs of heart failure

A modest deterioration in cardiac grade is to be expected as pregnancy progresses, even in healthy women. In women with heart disease, it usually starts earlier and progresses more rapidly. Thus, barring unforeseen circumstances, patients with mild mitral stenosis, who have had no symptoms and may have been unaware of their cardiac condition, would be expected to develop symptoms fairly late in pregnancy. In those already incapacitated by more serious lesions, deterioration would be expected earlier.

Regular and careful monitoring of the cardiac grade indicates if and when treatment is necessary.

Treatment, when necessary, is aimed primarily at giving the heart less work to do. The patient is advised to avoid rapid weight gain and overexertion. She should rest in the afternoon, go early to bed and rise late in the morning. If she must get up early, she can go back to bed when the family has gone.

If, despite these measures, her cardiac grade deteriorates, breathlessness and pulmonary congestion usually respond to diuretic therapy. In more serious circumstances, temporary admission to hospital may be necessary. Cases with frank heart failure require vigorous medical treatment and should remain in hospital under careful medical supervision for the remainder of the pregnancy.

All patients with significant heart disease should be admitted for rest a week or two before term and a plan made for their delivery.

Management during labour

Patients with mild heart disease can be treated as normal and no special precautions are necessary.

Patients with more serious lesions should be protected as much as possible from the strain imposed upon the cardiovascular system by labour and delivery. The third stage of labour is particularly hazardous because it is a time of profound and rapid circulatory readjustment that requires careful supervision.

With the techniques now available, an increasing number will have elective caesarean section, provided the cardiac lesion is of sufficient severity to warrant such a course of action.

Management during the puerperium

As during labour, patients with modest lesion require no special treatment.

Those with more serious heart disease require a longer period of rest and rehabilitation. Arrangements should be made for help at home and advice given about family planning before they are discharged from hospital.

Postnatal assessment

A careful reassessment should be made 3 months after delivery when the cardiovascular system has returned to normal and the patient has readjusted to life with a young baby. Following this, she should be advised about future pregnancies and general medical supervision.

Family planning

Careful family planning is a top priority for women with heart disease.

Even those who have relatively little disability during pregnancy may become unduly fatigued with two young infants to care for. They require advice about both the size and spacing of the family. The aim should be to have the first one toddling before starting off on the second.

Those with significant lesions are advised to settle for two healthy babies and then be sterilized.

During the period when the family is being planned, oral contraceptives are probably best if the patient is young. The risks are small and the method is reliable. For older women, and for those who do not wish to be sterilized, other long term methods should be considered.

HEART DISEASE IN CHILDREN

Acquired heart disease

In Britain much of the heart disease seen in children differs from that seen in adults and, with the virtual disappearance of rheumatic heart disease, the number of children with acquired heart disease has become greatly reduced.

Infections

The control of infections that may affect the heart, such as those responsible for diphtheria, poliomyelitis and acute glomerulonephritis, has also contributed to a reduction in numbers.

Other types of acquired heart disease still seen include myocarditis and pericarditis. Frequently occurring together, they can cause grave illness in babies and young children. As they are usually due to viruses, often of the Coxsackie group, little can be done except to give supportive therapy. Most cases make a complete recovery, although it may take a long time for the heart size to return to normal.

The heart may be involved in any of the common infectious diseases, but seldom seriously, and the involvement is usually discovered accidentally, often on a routine ECG.

Rarely, cardiomyopathies of both the obstructive and congestive types are found in children who present with heart failure of unknown aetiology.

In the tropics

Reference is made below, pp. 219–221, to the ravages of heart disease in children who live in tropical and subtropical countries. Many are afflicted by serious forms of the diseases seen in the temperate zone, particularly by virulent rheumatic heart disease, many have diseases peculiar to their own parts of the world and many suffer from diseases associated with social deprivation and malnutrition.

Coronary heart disease

This is not yet seen in children although the age at which it first presents is gradually creeping downwards. Young men in their twenties are appearing in coronary care units and routine autopsies on battle casualties have shown that extensive coronary artery atheroma is not uncommon in apparently healthy young people.

Children with familial hypercholesterolaemia thought to be at high risk of developing coronary atheroma are being identified and treated with lipid lowering agents in some centres.

The danger of cigarette smoking as a risk factor, especially in those with a family history of coronary artery disease, cannot be overemphasized.

Systemic hypertension

This is not common in children and, until recently, few paediatricians routinely measured the arterial blood pressure. It occurs as a secondary phenomenon in a wide variety of relatively rare conditions, mostly related to renal and adrenal disease, but primary or essential hypertension, as it is usually called, is not generally regarded as a disease of childhood. Considerable interest is currently being shown in detecting those who might later develop this all-too-frequent condition and tables of normal values at different ages are now readily available.

Congenital malformations

Paediatric practice in Britain and similar countries is increasingly concerned with congenital cardiac malformations and, as many of those who are born with serious malformations do not survive the first year of life, the concern is for younger and younger patients.

The various lesions and their management in different age groups have been discussed on pp. 181–190. Most of those with serious malformations are dealt with surgically in infancy or childhood and most of those who do not require surgical treatment do not require continuing medical care. The result is that fewer and fewer patients with significant congenital malformations are seen in adult cardiac clinics.

Disturbances of rhythm and conduction

Disturbances of rhythm are not uncommon and are seen at all ages from the neonatal period onwards. They are mostly paroxysmal supraventricular tachycardias and are troublesome rather than serious. Some that are associated with ventricular pre-excitation occasionally have more sinister implications.

Many require no treatment. Of those that do, the majority are easy to control and a few are very difficult to control. Fortunately, they nearly always grow out of trouble.

Life-threatening ventricular dysrhythmias are uncommon in childhood, as are serious abnormalities of conduction. Heart block is rare and nearly always congenital. When it is associated with other congenital cardiac malformations, the outlook is uncertain. When it occurs as an isolated finding, the prognosis is relatively good.

Suspected heart disease

Children with suspected heart disease are far more numerous than those who have it. As was pointed out on pp. 110–111, large numbers of healthy children have auscultatory signs that can easily be misinterpreted and cast suspicion on the heart. They are usually detected at well-baby clinics, at school medical examinations or by family doctors during the course of some minor illness, often a respiratory infection.

Systolic murmurs are the usual culprits. Many of them arise outside the heart (venous hums) or over its surface (pleuropericardial noises). A few are caused by insignificant lesions, but in the majority no abnormality can be detected even when extensive investigations are carried out. It is best to regard them as innocent noises and to say nothing about them either to the patient or to the parents. Most of them will disappear as the child grows older and those that do not are unlikely to be of any consequence.

If the presence of a murmur is already known, the strongest possible reassurance should be given to dispel parental anxiety and to ensure that the child does not develop a cardiac neurosis, the seeds of which can be sown at a very early age.

HEART DISEASE IN THE ELDERLY

Cardiovascular disease is common in the ageing population although its effects are often less obvious than in younger patients.

No one escapes injury and disease. Their cumulative effects, often accompanied by an acute episode, lead to death. There is no such thing as 'physiological' death or the body 'wearing out'. Most elderly patients have several diseases and it is often difficult to say which is the main cause of death even when disease is largely confined to the cardiovascular system.

The common cardiac disorders in old age are:

- coronary heart disease
- hypertensive heart disease
- degenerative calcification of the mitral and aortic valves
- fibrosis of the AV conduction pathways
- senile cardiac amyloidosis

The less common cardiac disorders in old age are:

- rheumatic heart disease
- calcific aortic stenosis
- cardiomyopathy
- mucoid degeneration of mitral valve
- subacute bacterial endocarditis
- cor pulmonale
- thyrotoxic heart disease
- myxoedematous heart disease

Special features of heart disease in the elderly

Coronary disease

Over the age of 60, male predominance becomes progressively less evident and death from coronary disease is common in the elderly of both sexes. It is the most important cardiac cause of death. Multiple small infarcts, without frank clinical episodes of myocardial infarction, result in extensive left ventricular scarring and may cause heart failure. Breathlessness, faintness or syncope, weakness or general deterioration of health with rather indefinite complaints of chest pain, may make clinical diagnosis difficult. In such circumstances, coronary heart disease should always be suspected.

Associated strokes, thromboembolic disorders, confusional states, vomiting and other alimentary symptoms, may lead to diagnostic difficulty. Dysrhythmias, heart block, heart failure and cardiac shock are also much commoner in the older age groups.

Sensitive discrimination is needed when consider-ing the admission of elderly patients to coronary care units, having regard on the one hand, to the kindest and most sensible management of the patient and on the other, to the appropriate use of scarce resources.

Diastolic hypertension

It is important to differentiate between classical hypertension (in which systolic, mean and diastolic BP are elevated) and pure systolic hypertension.

Pathophysiology

The prevalence of diastolic hypertension increases steadily up to the sixth decade and then steadies out or declines. It probably continues to be a significant risk factor for coronary disease and stroke. The decision regarding whether or not to treat it and, if so, what the treatment should be, will depend on an assessment of the individual case. This will include:

- degree of hypertension
- age
- general health
- domestic and social circumstances

Management

Weight reduction may be all that is needed in obese patients. If the diastolic blood pressure lies between 90 and 110 mmHg, some physicians prescribe diuretic therapy; others will not prescribe at this level of hypertension. In more severe cases, particularly where there is evidence of hypertensive heart disease or retinopathy, it may be necessary to combine diuretic therapy with one or more other drugs (e.g. β-blocker, hydrallazine, methyldopa, clonidine). Adrenergic blockers (bethanidine, debrisoquine) cause postural hypotension, particularly in the elderly, and should not be used.

Pure systolic hypertension

Here, the systolic BP is greater than 160 mmHg and the diastolic BP is less than 90 mmHg.

Pathophysiology

Whereas the incidence of diastolic hypertension stops increasing or actually declines after the age of 60, the incidence of systolic hypertension continues to increase with advancing age. Pure systolic hypertension is usually associated with extensive arteriosclerosis of major blood vessels and is perhaps merely a haemodynamic response to the rigid walls of the arterial system (cf. the disproportionately high systolic BP in coarctation of the aorta, where the left ventricle delivers blood into a small reservoir aorta above the coarcted segment).

A systolic BP of more than 180 mmHg carries with it an increased incidence of coronary events and strokes. However, it is difficult to say whether systolic hypertension is the cause or merely an accompaniment of extensive coronary and cerebral vascular disease.

Management

The benefit of treating pure systolic hypertension is doubtful and the side-effect of postural hypotension is particularly hazardous. Elderly patients, particularly females, tolerate high pressures for many years.

Cardiac amyloidosis

Amyloid disease confined to the heart or, less commonly, to the heart and the pulmonary vasculature, is surprisingly common in the elderly. Often, it has no effect on function, but occasionally it is sufficiently extensive to constitute a cardiomyopathy and leads to heart failure. It may also involve the specialized conducting tissues and cause heart block.

Valvar disease

Valvar disease is common in the elderly. It may be a delayed manifestation of rheumatic heart disease (mitral or aortic) or of congenital heart disease (bicuspid aortic valve). More commonly, it results from degenerative calcification affecting the aortic or mitral valve or both. Often, the effect on function is not great. Stenosis is the likelier consequence on the aortic valve, incompetence in the case of the mitral. Mitral incompetence in old age is much less commonly due to a prolapsing valve.

Subacute bacterial endocarditis

Over the past few decades, there has been a steady increase in the proportion of elderly patients suffering from this disease and the peak incidence is now in the 50s or 60s. Degenerative valve lesions, often producing insigificant signs and little effect on cardiac function, may be the site of infection. Also, cardiac pacing, valve replacement and coronary bypass surgery are being increasingly performed in the elderly and are sources of infection.

Congenital heart disease

Some malformations whose effect on function is not great are surprisingly well tolerated into the later decades. An atrial septal defect is the one most likely to be encountered in the over 70s.

Complete heart block

Patients with complete heart block are seen with increasing frequency as the population ages. Cardiac pacing has greatly improved their well-being and prognosis. Previously, most of them were confined to bed or to close quarters as a result of a low cardiac output or for fear of syncopal attacks. They required a great deal of expensive care and attention. Nowadays, after the insertion of a permanent pacemaker, they take on a new lease of life, becoming independent and able once again to look after themselves. Although the initial capital cost of pacing is considerable, it is easily justified as the cheaper option because most elderly patients who require pacing live to a ripe old age.

HEART DISEASE IN THE TROPICS

Although most of the heart disease seen in Europe and North America is now fairly well documented, a great deal remains to be learned about the different types of heart disease seen in tropical and subtropical countries. These vast zones encompass many different races and the terrain varies from humid jungle to arid desert. Large numbers of the inhabitants are undernourished and exposed to a multiplicity of parasites, viruses and other organisms seldom encountered in colder climates.

While these ethnic and environmental factors undoubtedly account for some of the differences in the types of heart disease seen, others are probably more apparent than real. In many parts of the world, health services, as we know them, are virtually non-existent. Experience in developing countries has demonstrated over and over again that, when medical care becomes available, diseases thought to be rare or non-existent often become relatively commonplace, while others, thought to be specific, turn out to be local variations of relatively commonplace conditions.

For example, rheumatic fever and rheumatic heart disease, said to be diseases of the temperate zone, are now known to be rife in many other parts of the world where coronary heart disease and high blood pressure, diseases of so-called Western civilization, are also being diagnosed with increasing frequency, as the expectation of life rises. And, despite early reports to the contrary, the prevalence of the various types of congenital cardiac malformation are found to be remarkably constant wherever properly-conducted population studies are carried out by experienced examiners.

Some heart diseases, however, do appear to be peculiar to the tropics and some, also found elsewhere, have a somewhat different form when they are seen in the tropics. Many cases are complex and multi-factorial, as in the strange cardiopathies that occur in grossly undernourished patients living under appalling circumstances, whose resistance to infection is poor and who are severely anaemic because of malaria and infestation with hookworms and other parasites. In some such patients, malnutrition, infection and anaemia are clearly important aetiological factors but, in others, the aetiology is completely unknown.

Malnutrition

Many names have been used to describe the myocardial disorders seen in those who are grossly undernourished. Those like beriberi heart disease, which is due to thiamine deficiency and common where polished rice is the staple diet, are fairly well understood. Others are less well defined. The complex inter-relationships between dietary deficiency, electrolyte imbalance, anaemia and toxicity from associated infection, remain to be resolved. The end results vary from small, thin walled, flabby hearts to those that show considerable enlargement and hypertrophy.

The generic term 'cardiomyopathy' is probably the best one to use in the present uncertain state of our knowledge about most of them.

Infection

Heart diseases associated with bacterial, viral and parasitic infections are commonplace. Not all are peculiar to the tropics, as witnessed by the ravages of tuberculous pericarditis, diphtheritic myocarditis and syphilitic endocarditis. Many viruses affect the heart, some quite seriously and much more seriously than they would in Britain. Parasites of all types abound and a few of them have severe cardiovascular consequences.

American trypanosomiasis (Chagas disease), wide-spread in South America, is a good example of the type of heart disease caused by parasites: in this instance by *Trypanosoma cruzi*. In the acute form, which often occurs in young children, a febrile illness is accompanied by myocarditis and a mortality of up to 10%. In the chronic form, a slow but steady replacement fibrosis leads to progressive cardiomegaly with disturbances of rhythm and conduction, and eventually to heart failure and death. It is a serious condition resulting in severe cardiac disability for which there is no effective treatment.

Anaemia

Severe anaemia is common in the tropics. It is an important cause of cardiac pathology either in its own right or as a complicating factor in other diseases.

The anaemia may be due to a wide variety of causes such as:

- chronic malarial and bacterial infections
- dietary deficiencies of iron and folic acid, that are often contributed to by chronic gastroenteritis
- chronic blood loss because of intestinal infestation
- hereditary disorders of haemoglobin synthesis, e.g. the thalassaemias and sickle cell anaemias

Pulmonary heart disease

The prevalence of heart disease secondary to respiratory disorders is said to vary considerably in different parts of the world. It tends to be thought of mainly as a complication of chronic bronchitis and emphysema, brought about by a combination of cold weather, air pollution and cigarette smoking.

There is ample evidence that this form of heart disease is everywhere underdiagnosed.

Pulmonary heart disease is common in many tropical countries because gross respiratory disease is common. Pulmonary tuberculosis still ravages many communities. Parasites are again important; this time the schistosoma, which causes massive and repeated pulmonary infarcts and granulomata, in areas where the infection is endemic.

Diseases of unknown cause

Reference has already been made to the various

tropical cardiomyopathies. Their aetiology is still far from clear, although the differences between them may be fewer than was first appreciated.

A few examples of the many other types of cardiovascular diseases seldom or never seen in the UK are given below.

Endomyocardial fibrosis

This is a strange disease in which the cavities of the heart are progressively obliterated by dense fibrous tissue. First described in Uganda, it is now found in many parts of equatorial Africa; mostly among Negroes, but no race is immune.

Left ventricular aneurysms

These occur just below the aortic and mitral valves and extend through the fibrous annulus into the substance of the heart. First reported from Nigeria, they have now been reported from many other parts of the world.

Idiopathic arteritis

This is seen much more frequently in the tropics than in the temperate zones. It may affect any part of the aorta and its branches in one or many places, causing both stenoses and aneurysms.

Peripartum heart failure

This follows about 1% of deliveries in Northern Nigeria. Asymptomatic postpartum hypertension occurs in about 60% of normal Hausa women in West Africa. Peripartum heart failure may be due to a combination of the pressure overload caused by the hypertension, with a volume overload caused by the sodium-rich diet customarily eaten during the puerperium when it is traditional for the women to overheat themselves in what is already a very hot climate.

DEEP VENOUS THROMBOSIS

Thrombosis results in the formation of a blood clot (thrombus) in an artery or vein. The solid thrombus is formed from constituents of the liquid blood. These include platelets, fibrin, and red and white blood cells; the first two are the most important. A thrombus characteristically has a white head, where leukocytes and platelets predominate, and a red tail, where the red cells predominate.

Causes

Thrombosis may be due to change in the vessel wall, in the flow of blood through it or in the formed elements of the blood itself. Of these, the platelets appear to play an essential role. It is not known for certain why a thrombus develops, but the present view favours damage to the wall of the vein by phlebitis, external pressures that cause slowing of the blood with possible intimal damage, and haemoconcentration caused by dehydration. One or more of these may lead to an accumulation of platelets at the site of injury to plug the defect. A reaction occurs between the platelets and the subendothelial tissues. Collagen in the tissues combines with the platelets to release various vasoactive substances that cause further platelet aggregation (Table 24).

TABLE 24 Factors affecting platelets

Aggregating agents	Inhibitory agents
Adenosine diphosphate (ADP)	Adenosine
Prostaglandin E_2	Prostaglandin PG_1
PGG_2, PGH_2	PGI_2
Thromboxane A_2	Aspirin
	Phenylbutazone

Phospholipids from the platelets and the tissue thromboplastins initiate the formation of a fibrin mesh. Further platelet aggregation activates the blood-coagulating mechanism and this increases the size of the thrombus. Although a slow blood flow potentiates thrombus formation, some flow is necessary because, in vivo, a thrombus will not form in stationary blood.

Fate of thrombus

Once formed, a thrombus may:
- gradually increase in size and length
  An arterial thrombus extends along the vessel as far as the next major branch of the artery. A venous thrombus tends to extend much further because of the slower blood flow
- undergo thrombolysis
  Fibrinolysin released from the wall of the vessel breaks down the fibrin. This is especially true in veins, whose walls contain much fibrinolysin
- become organized
  Fibrous tissue is laid down in the blood clot.

Recanalization takes place at the same time so that the thrombus may be penetrated by numerous vascular channels

- be covered by endothelium
  It is then incorporated into the vessel wall. With a small localized arterial thrombus, this may be the first stage in the development of an atheromatous plaque

- form an embolus
  This happens when a portion breaks off and passes into the blood stream

Predisposing factors

Certain factors appear to predispose to venous thrombosis:

- obesity
- ageing
- prolonged immobility
- varicose veins
- malignancy

In patients undergoing operation, coagulation is more likely because of an increase in the number of platelets and their adhesiveness. The fibrinogen level in the blood is also increased with a corresponding fall in fibrinolytic activity. The tendency to coagulate is more marked in polycythaemia, dehydration and shock. Certain operations such as prostatectomy and pinning of a fractured neck of femur carry a high risk of deep vein thrombosis.

Upper limb thrombosis is uncommon and rarely of serious consequence. It most frequently happens after intravenous therapy or the insertion of a transvenous line or a cardiac pacing catheter. It may also occur spontaneously in the axillary or subclavian veins and may be a consequence of thoracic outlet compression.

Thrombosis of the superior vena cava is rare. It most often occurs as a result of malignant disease. It may also be secondary to peripheral vein thrombosis, trauma or severe infection.

Clinical features

Lower limb thrombosis, by far the commonest, occurs in approximately 30% of all patients undergoing general surgical procedures. It is useful to classify the deep veins anatomically into the:

- distal or peripheral venous segment
- proximal or iliofemoral (pelvic) venous segment

The peripheral segment, especially the calf, is most commonly implicated. Pain, tenderness and oedema, together with shininess of the skin, may result. However, these features are by no means always present and clinical diagnosis can be difficult. On the other hand, 30–50% of patients suspected clinically of having deep vein thrombosis appear normal when tested with ^{125}I fibrinogen scanning or phlebography.

Iliofemoral venous thrombosis may be occlusive or non-occlusive. If non-occlusive, the diagnosis may be difficult although groin tenderness may be present over the common femoral vein. A pulmonary embolism may be the first sign of thrombosis in this segment.

Occlusive iliofemoral venous thrombosis usually results in a grossly swollen, oedematous and tense limb. Superficial venous prominence develops a few days after the initial event. Occasionally, the venous engorgement is severe enough to compromise the arterial inflow, resulting in the picture of phlegmasia cerulea dolens (blue phlebitis). If untreated, venous gangrene may ensue.

Venous thrombosis is a multifocal process, the calf, popliteal, common femoral and iliac veins being involved, either independently or in combination. Propagation of thrombus is more frequent from calf to iliac veins than vice versa.

Differential diagnoses include:

- lymphoedema
- rupture of the soleus or gastrocnemius muscles
- lymphangitis
- cellulitis

The latter two are usually characterized by fever.

Acute upper limb thrombosis results in pain, swelling and obvious venous engorgement of the superficial veins with delay in venous emptying on elevation of the arm. Claudication on exercise may also be a feature.

Superior vena cava thrombosis manifests itself by oedema of the head, neck and upper extremities.

Investigations

Clinical diagnosis in severe cases is straightforward but, as already described, substantial diagnostic error is found when more objective criteria are applied.

Fortunately, about 80% of those patients with deep

calf vein thrombosis resolve spontaneously and no special investigation is required.

Phlebography

When pulmonary embolism is the presenting feature, or where the diagnosis is in doubt, phlebography remains the definitive investigation. Ascending phlebography via a dorsal foot vein will accurately delineate the deep veins to the level of the groin. To visualize the iliofemoral venous segment adequately, bilateral percutaneous iliofemoral phlebography is usually necessary. This examination is most frequently performed under local anaesthesia. On occasions, perosseous phlebography is necessary and this requires general anaesthesia with all its attendant risks. Phlebography is necessary before carrying out surgical therapy.

^{125}I fibrinogen test

This is extremely sensitive below the level of the groin but less so with the pelvic veins. It is a simple test and shows where active thrombus formation is occurring. The incidence of thrombosis in postoperative cases detected by this test varies from 15% in gynaecological operations to over 75% in fracture of the neck of femur. It has also shown that, in over 50% of cases, thrombosis commences during the operation.

Doppler ultrasound

This is a simple, non-invasive and useful technique for detecting recent occlusive thrombosis of deep veins cephalad to, and including, the popliteal. Detection of thrombi within the calf veins by this technique is imprecise.

Haemotological indices

Full blood count, ESR and coagulation screening should be carried out.

Management

The most important aim is to prevent thrombosis and its sequelae: acute pulmonary embolism, chronic venous outflow obstruction, valve damage and leg ulceration.

Prophylaxis

Great emphasis is placed on prophylaxis. Simple methods to increase the venous blood flow by leg elevation and compression bandaging help. Early ambulation and postoperative exercises are also worthwhile. But none of these measures is really effective. Peroperative stimulation of the calf muscle pump, either by electrical or pneumatic means, has been employed and has been shown to help, but these methods are cumbersome and not practical in the postoperative period, which is also critical.

The best method of prophylaxis is to alter blood coagulability. This may be effected through full systemic heparinization, though this has to be suspended during the operative period. Prothrombin depressants (warfarin and phenindione) can be used during this period so long as the prothrombin time is not more than about twice normal. However, low-dose subcutaneous heparin, 5000 iu twice daily for 5–7 days, commencing just before the operation, has been shown to be effective in lowering the incidence of deep vein thrombosis and subsequent pulmonary embolism.

Dextran 70 also reduces the incidence of deep vein thrombosis and pulmonary embolism, although its exact antithrombotic effect remains largely unknown. A 500 ml infusion is commenced just before and maintained throughout the operative period. Thereafter, 500 ml is given over 6 hours for the next 4 postoperative days. The benefit of such therapy far outweighs the very infrequent complications of circulatory overload, bleeding or anaphylactic reaction.

Antiplatelet drugs, such as aspirin or persantin, used as prophylactic agents, are generally agreed to be non-effective.

In practice, only anticoagulants and dextran have been shown significantly to reduce the incidence of postoperative deep vein thrombosis and subsequent pulmonary embolism.

Established deep vein thrombosis

The treatment of established deep vein thrombosis has two objectives:

- to prevent further thrombus formation
- to promote fibrinolysis of thrombus already formed

Anticoagulation is initiated by heparinizing the patient for approximately 7 days and following this with oral anticoagulants. These are continued for at least 6 weeks.

Fibrinolysis, using plasminogen activators such as streptokinase, is effective in achieving complete lysis of the thrombus in about 25% of patients. It is, however, expensive, requires careful laboratory monitoring and cannot be used in the immediate post-operative period. Anaphylactic reaction and bleeding are the main complications.

Removal of the thrombus, venous thrombectomy, has a role to play. Where a large non-occlusive thrombus is demonstrated in the iliofemoral venous segment and is thought to be potentially life-threatening, it should be removed. This is done under local anaesthesia via the common femoral vein in the groin using a Fogarty catheter. Where occlusive iliofemoral venous thrombosis threatens the viability of the limb or where there is evidence of impending venous gangrene, decompression of that segment via the same route is indicated. However, the incidence of rethrombosis is high following this procedure. Interruption of the inferior vena cava either by plication or division carries a high morbidity and mortality. More recently, the Mobin umbrella caval filter, inserted under local anaesthesia with X-ray screening, has been used with some success, but it is expensive and is also not without hazard.

In simple calf vein thrombosis, which occurs in the majority of cases, supportive measures in the form of adequate compression stockings, leg elevation and early ambulation are all that is required.

Upper limb thrombosis should be treated by elevation of the affected limb and systemic heparinization. Thrombolytic therapy may also be employed, the drug being given by regional perfusion through an indwelling cannula. Decompression by venous thrombectomy is rarely necessary. Surgical correction of any amenable thoracic outlet problem is indicated as necessary. By and large, the venous collaterals of the upper limb will usually, in time, act as an efficient bypass much sooner than will those of the lower limb.

ARTERIAL EMBOLISM

Arterial embolism is the most frequent cause of acute ischaemia. It may be completely reversible if diagnosed and treated promptly.

Causes

Emboli nearly always originate from thrombi in a heart chamber. Rarer forms are tumour emboli, air emboli and those resulting from the injection of particulate matter into the bloodstream. Most of them arise centrally and may lodge in any part of the body, commonly obstructing a vessel at a bifurcation. The majority travel to the lower extremities and often end up in the common femoral artery.

The patients are usually elderly and frail, almost 80% of them having some form of cardiac decompensation. About half will have atrial fibrillation, most frequently in association with coronary heart disease. Other causes of atrial fibrillation such as rheumatic heart disease, thyrotoxicosis and hypertension are less frequently implicated. One third will have had a recent myocardial infarct, one quarter have diabetes and a further quarter have had a previous embolism.

Other sources of emboli are:

- Atherosclerotic lesions in major vessels
- bacterial endocarditis (often produces multiple emboli)
- prosthetic heart valves

Common sites of blockage affecting the legs are the:

- bifurcation of the abdominal aorta
- common femoral artery
- popliteal artery

In the upper limb, emboli commonly impact in the axillary, subclavian or brachial arteries.

Thrombosis occurs at the site of impaction, first distally and then proximally.

Clinical features

The diagnosis is usually straightforward. Thrombosis and embolism are easily distinguished from one another. Difficulty may arise, however, about the cause of ischaemia where there is no obvious source of embolus, especially if there is a background of known peripheral vascular disease. In such cases of acute-on-chronic ischaemia, arteriography is of great help in establishing the diagnosis and determining the correct treatment.

Obstruction of the circulation produces sudden ischaemia of the affected part which, if not relieved, may result in gangrene. The degree of ischaemia depends on the site and duration of the obstruction and the nature of the collateral circulation. Pain, followed by coldness, pallor and numbness and a varying degree of paralysis, is the rule. Not infrequently the embolic event occurs during sleep. Occasionally too, 'silent embolism' occurs, the patient being unaware of the condition.

Clinical examination usually reveals a waxy pallor, empty veins, coldness and absence of pulses distal to the site of obstruction. Motor and sensory loss of varying degree are also evident. Differential diagnosis should not prove much of a problem. The chief conditions to be borne in mind are:

- acute arterial thrombosis
- dissecting aneurysm
- deep vein thrombosis
- venous gangrene
- drug abuse

Investigation

A careful history and physical examination is usually enough to establish the diagnosis in most patients. Because of the frequency of underlying cardiac problems, electrocardiography and chest X-ray should be arranged. Doppler ultrasound assessment of the affected limb may be helpful. Arteriography is only necessary when there is doubt about whether the problem is embolic or thrombotic.

Management

Bearing in mind that many of the patients will be elderly and have heart disease, the prime consideration should be for life rather than for limb. Having made the diagnosis, it is important to institute supportive measures to correct any existing cardiac decompensation as far as possible. Digitalis, diuretics and antidysrrhythmic drugs are used as necessary. Maintenance of adequate blood pressure is also vital. Unless contraindicated, systemic heparinization should be implemented immediately. This helps to prevent further propagation of thrombosis and also, hopefully, lessens the chance of an associated deep vein thrombosis. Since the advent of the Fogarty catheter, limb salvage has improved dramatically, but the overall mortality remains approximately 25%. Arterial embolectomy is usually carried out under local anaesthesia. Only when embolism is associated with a near terminal event, or when massive gangrene is already present, is it contraindicated.

As a general rule, the longer the duration of occlusion the greater the degree of ischaemia, but there are frequent and significant exceptions to this concept. The condition of the patient's limb when initially seen is the real determinant of limb salvage. When there is advanced ischaemia, as evidenced by early rigor, the amputation rate is high although limb salvage not impossible. Lack of motor activity associated with a 'wooden' feel to the muscle bulk is a contraindication to surgery. Complications resulting from restoration of flow in such cases are related to the return of acidotic blood to the heart, hypotension and fatal dysrrhythmias. Maintenance of blood pressure by volume replacement and cardiac support are necessary.

The common femoral, profunda and superficial femoral arteries are approached via a vertical groin incision. An arteriotomy made over the common femoral artery is adequate in nearly all cases to allow removal of emboli. Once the occlusion has been removed, operative arteriography should be performed to ensure that the distal arterial tree is patent, because back-bleeding is not a reliable sign. The procedure takes but a few minutes. Heparin therapy is usually continued postoperatively for 2–3 days and the patient then maintained on oral anticoagulants for 6 months.

Saddle embolism of the abdominal aortic bifurcation is dealt with by the same approach carried out simultaneously in both groins. Again, operative arteriography should be employed to ensure that the distal arterial trees are patent.

Embolism of the upper limb is a less frequent event. Although the collateral supply to the upper limb is better than that to the lower limb, embolectomy should be performed in the majority of cases. Embolic material lodges in approximately equal proportions in the subclavian, axillary and brachial arteries. Using local anaesthesia, an arteriotomy made over the axillary artery allows adequate access both proximally and distally. Operative arteriography is carried out to ensure patency of the distal arterial tree. So long as either the radial or ulnar artery is patent, the viability of the limb is ensured. A close check should be kept on the pulses after restoration of the blood flow as further embolism or thrombosis may occur.

Very occasionally, systemic heparinization (2000–4000 units hourly) may result in limb salvage where surgery is contraindicated. Thrombolytic agents such as streptokinase have little or no role in the management of acute arterial embolism.

Where signs of irreversible ischaemia exist in the limb, e.g. fixed mottling of the skin, muscle involvement or joint contractures, early amputation at the appropriate level is indicated.

Overall, the results of embolectomy for acute arterial embolism are rewarding and justify an aggressive approach towards both medical and surgical management.

DISEASES OF THE AORTA

Dilatation of the aorta

Simple dilatation of the arch of the aorta, usually associated with arteriosclerosis, with or without longstanding hypertension, is common in older patients. It gives rise to no symptoms but is seen on a PA X-ray of the chest and commonly reported as 'unfolding of the aorta'.

Aortic aneurysm

Aortic aneurysms can be 'saccular', a pouch-like sac projecting from the side of the aorta, or 'fusiform', a spindle-shaped dilatation involving the whole circumference of the aorta. In a 'true aneurysm', one or all of the layers of the aorta make up the sac. If the aortic wall is destroyed, without fatal haemorrhage, a pulsating haematoma may make up the wall of the aortic enlargement; this is called a 'false aneurysm'.

The commonest cause of aortic aneurysm in Western countries to-day is atherosclerosis. Tertiary syphilis used to be a common cause and still is in countries where early recognition and adequate treatment of syphilis are less common. Most aortic aneurysms are found in older patients (40–70 years) and more often in men than in women.

The thoracic aorta lies in relation to many important structures, so the signs and symptoms of an aneurysm depend upon its size and location.

Aneurysm of ascending aorta

There may be no symptoms or there may be pain from pressure erosion of the sternum or nearby ribs. Visible pulsation or even an obvious pulsating tumour may be seen on either side of the sternum or in the suprasternal notch.

There may be a systolic bruit with or without a thrill. X-rays of the chest show a mass that may be seen to pulsate on fluoroscopy. Compression of the superior vena cava may distend the jugular veins and cause oedema of the face, neck and shoulders.

Aneurysm of the arch of the aorta

Depending upon the size and site of the aneurysm, almost any structure in or near the superior mediastinum may be compressed, giving physical signs or symptoms.

Pressure on a subclavian artery may cause differences between the pulses and blood pressures in the arms.

Pressure on the left bronchus may cause pulmonary collapse and the bronchus may be depressed with each pulsation, pulling the trachea downwards during systole and causing the physical sign known as 'tracheal tug'. Pressure on the trachea may cause cough, stridor or other respiratory obstruction. Pressure on the left recurrent laryngeal nerve may cause paralysis of the left vocal cord and a 'brassy' cough.

Pressure on the oesophagus may cause dysphagia. Involvement of the left sympathetic chain can produce Horner's syndrome.

Pressure on nerve roots and the spine may cause nerve or bone pain.

Over 90% of patients with thoracic aneurysms that are untreated die within 5 years, frequently from haemorrhage into the bronchi, pleural space, pericardium or trachea.

Aneurysm of the abdominal aorta

Abdominal aneurysms are usually atherosclerotic and fusiform. Often there are no symptoms until rupture occurs, but the patient or doctor may find the aneurysm as a pulsating mass when examining the abdomen. It may cause pain in the upper abdomen, lower back, groin and, sometimes, in the testes. This is usually because of sudden enlargement or a rupture or leak into the retroperitoneal space.

A plain X-ray of the abdomen often shows the aneurysm because of the calcification in the aortic wall. About a third of the patients with untreated abdominal aneurysms die within a year of diagnosis, again, usually from rupture.

Management

Patients with small aneurysms and no symptoms may survive for many years and should merely be kept under observation. Those with large aneurysms, those whose small aneurysms are getting larger and those with symptoms, should be considered for surgical treatment, if an experienced vascular surgeon is available. Although techniques have improved considerably in recent years, it should be remembered that such patients usually have extensive cardiovascular disease and are bad operative risks.

Dissecting aneurysm of the aorta

The name is slightly misleading. The dilatation ('aneurysm') of the aorta is the result of bleeding into the aortic wall that splits the media upwards and downwards from the site of origin. It is really a haematoma that restricts or obliterates the lumen of the aorta and the mouths of its main branches as the dissection forms and progresses.

Aortic dissection is two or three times commoner in men than in women and is commonest in the fourth to seventh decades. Although many patients have atherosclerosis and preceding hypertension, the causal lesions lie in the media of the aorta: there are cystic gaps in the elastic lamina filled with mucoid material and a decrease in muscle fibres with increased intercellular mucoid material ('cystic medial necrosis'). Such lesions commonly occur in patients with Marfan's syndrome.

Usually a transverse tear in the intima just above the aortic valve allows blood under high pressure to enter the vessel wall and split the media, usually distally, but sometimes backward towards the aortic valve. The dissection varies in extent and in time; it may occur for a short distance or involve the whole length of the aorta including its main branches.

Clinical features

The location and extent of the dissection determine the symptoms and signs. It frequently mimics myocardial infarction and when the dissection extends proximally to involve the coronary ostia, myocardial infarction can result. Involvement of the ostia of the carotid arteries, the renal and mesenteric arteries, and the main arteries to the limbs, while forming a useful lead to the correct diagnosis may, on the other hand, confuse the clinical picture with the result that diagnoses of cerebrovascular accidents, peripheral vascular occlusions and acute abdominal emergencies may be made.

Aortic dissection is accompanied by pain that may be episodic as the dissection advances. It may be both excruciating and short-lived, for death is often rapid: 90% of patients have severe retrosternal pain that is usually maximal at onset and which radiates to the back, abdomen, legs or other parts of the body to which radiation of the pain of myocardial infarction is uncommon. Although patients often look shocked, their blood pressure is usually raised. Peripheral pulsations vary from hour to hour because of ostial occlusions and arterial spasm. Aortic systolic and diastolic murmurs develop in 10–15% of cases and the development of an early diastolic murmur is an important diagnostic finding. Neurological abnormalities from ischaemia of the brain and spinal cord are common. There may be confusion or coma, weakness of a limb, with or without pain, paraesthesia and even hemiplegia or paralysis of both legs.

Investigation

A PA X-ray of the chest may show widening of the aorta. The ECG shows non-specific ST–T wave changes, unless the retrograde extension of the dissection has caused myocardial infarction. A leukocytosis is common. Renal artery occlusion results in oliguria with red cells, protein and casts in the urine.

Prognosis

A large aortic dissection can be rapidly fatal and the diagnosis is often made in the postmortem room. Sometimes, the dissection progresses more slowly, during a few hours or even days, and allows time for elective surgical treatment.

Management

The medical management is supportive (the relief of pain, the administration of blood and of oxygen, etc.) while plans are made for surgery, where this seems indicated.

Syphilitic aortitis

Aortic incompetence

Tertiary syphilis causes dilatation of the aortic root, separation of the aortic cusps at their commissures and valvar incompetence. In the UK, 40 years ago, about a third of all cases of aortic valve disease, and about half of those in patients between the ages of 40–60, were due to syphilis. Nowadays, it is so uncommon that it is often overlooked when considering the aetiology of aortic valve disease. Syphilis is still common in some parts of the world and should always be kept in mind when a patient presents with aortic incompetence. Often the incompetence is considerable, but it is never accompanied by stenosis. Angina pectoris occurs if the mouths of the coronary arteries become stenosed. Calcification of a dilated ascending aorta in a chest X-ray should suggest the diagnosis.

Syphilitic aortic aneurysm

Syphilitic aneurysms are usually saccular and involve the arch of the aorta. They tend to occur in younger patients than do atherosclerotic aneurysms. Sometimes syphilitic aortitis causes dilatation of the ascending aorta that may almost assume aneurysmal dimensions.

CEREBROVASCULAR DISEASE

Incidence

Cerebrovascular disease is the third most common cause of death in Western countries. It affects both sexes equally and no convincing racial differences have been described. The annual incidence of new cases is between 1.3 and 1.9 per 1000 of the population. At any one time, six patients per 1000 population will have experienced a stroke.

Pathology

Atheroma

Generalized atheroma (see p. 32) affects the cerebral vessels where the results can be catastrophic. It is more common in the presence of diabetes mellitus, lipid abnormalities, cigarette smoking and hypertension. Plaques in the major arteries of the neck, particularly at the origin of the internal carotid artery, may ulcerate and become a source of microemboli to the cerebral circulation or retina and cause transient ischaemic attacks. Progressive atheroma may result in thrombosis and cause cerebral infarction, particularly if the collateral circulation is impaired by atheroma or a congenital abnormality in the circle of Willis.

Hypertensive vascular disease

Hypertension accelerates the development of atheroma. Severe hypertension may cause fibrinoid necrosis of the arterioles. Vasomotor changes in the arterioles (probably spasm) may cause hypertensive encephalopathy.

The other important change in hypertension is the development of microaneurysms at the point of division of smaller vessels. These are particularly common in the area of the internal capsule and are of importance because their rupture leads to cerebral haemorrhage. They are characteristic of hypertension and their number decreases with successful antihypertensive therapy. Sometimes vessels adjoining these aneurysms become thrombosed, probably the result of thrombus propagated from the aneurysm. These small vessel thrombi lead to small infarcts (lacunae).

Intracerebral haemorrhage

Rupture of a microaneurysm leads to sudden extravasation of arterial blood and disrupts surrounding brain tissue. The size of the haemorrhage and the amount of damage it causes is very variable. A large haemorrhage may rupture into the ventricles and cause bloodstaining of the cerebrospinal fluid. The usual site is the internal capsule, but the cerebellum or brainstem may be involved.

Cerebral haemorrhage is less common in normotensive patients. When it does occur, it is in the elderly, but the site and course are similar.

Clinical features

The patient sometimes has warning signs a few minutes or hours before the haemorrhage, but the onset is abrupt. The size and site of the haemorrhage determine its effects. A large haemorrhage or one in the brainstem will lead to loss of consciousness and early death. Smaller haemorrhages around the internal capsule lead to hemiplegia, hemianaesthesia and hemianopia. Headache may be a feature. The patient may have a raised blood pressure. That this contributed to the haemorrhage may be shown by evidence of left ventricular hypertrophy or fundal changes.

Management

Treatment in the early stages is largely nursing, with attention to the airway, skin and bladder. Surgery is rarely indicated to remove a haematoma. As recovery progresses, an active combined approach with the physiotherapist, speech therapist and occupational therapist gives the best functional result. If the patient is hypertensive, this should be treated to help prevent further episodes.

Cerebral infarction

The commonest sites for cerebral artery thrombosis are at the origin of the common carotid, at the origin of the internal carotid or in the syphon and at the origin of the middle cerebral artery. All lead to infarction of the motor and sensory areas particularly related to the upper limb, face and, on the dominant side, speech.

Clinical features

The symptoms and signs will depend largely on the

size and site of the infarct. The onset is usually abrupt, but may develop over several minutes and occasionally over several hours (stroke in evolution). Progression over several days suggests a space-occupying lesion as the cause of the symptoms. Severe lesions will lead to loss of consciousness with the head and eyes deviated towards the lesion and contralateral flaccid paralysis. If the patient is conscious, the presence of hemianaesthesia, hemianopia or dysphasia may be noted. The common infarct of the middle cerebral artery territory will affect the arm and face (and speech, if on the dominant side) more than the leg and will be associated with sensory and visual field loss if it is extensive.

Management

Treatment for cerebral infarction, like that for cerebral haemorrhage, consists of nursing in the early stages followed by progressive active mobilization and re-education by the rehabilitation team. In the first 48 hours, blood pressure may be elevated because of cerebral oedema or hypoventilation, but hypertension persisting after this will require treatment along the usual lines.

Subarachnoid haemorrhage

Subarachnoid haemorrhage most often comes from a large berry aneurysm on the circle of Willis. Both berry aneurysms and subarachnoid haemorrhage are associated with hypertension and particularly with coarctation of the aorta and polycystic renal disease. A congenital arteriovenous anomaly is a less common cause of subarachnoid haemorrhage.

The rupture leads to sudden bleeding into the subarachnoid space. The force of the bleed may cause extension of the haemorrhage into the brain. The blood in the cerebrospinal fluid leads to irritation of the meninges and arterial spasm that can be intense enough to produce cerebral infarction.

Clinical features

Typically, patients develop severe headache of instantaneous onset. Some describe an 'explosion' inside the skull or what feels like a blow on the head. They may lose consciousness temporarily or remain comatose. Intracerebral extension of the bleed or infarction will produce symptoms and signs depending on the site. Neck stiffness and a positive Kernig's sign are usually, but not invariably, present. Occasionally, a sub-hyaloid haemorrhage may be seen in the optic fundus.

A cranial bruit may be heard if an arteriovenous anomaly is present. The cerebrospinal fluid will be evenly bloodstained and, after 24 hours, will show xanthochromia.

Management

Early management consists of nursing care and bed rest. Analgesics may be needed, but the narcotics are best avoided because of respiratory depression. When the patient is fully conscious, arteriography should be considered with a view to treating the aneurysm surgically to prevent further bleeding, which is a particular risk in the first 4–6 weeks. Hypertension will require standard treatment.

Cerebral embolism

Arterial emboli are discussed on pp. 224–225. They may lodge in the cerebral circulation and cause infarction. The middle cerebral artery territory is the one most frequently involved.

The onset is sudden, often with loss of consciousness. A search should always be made for a site of an embolus in patients with cerebrovascular disease.

Treatment consists of general measures, together with anticoagulant therapy to prevent further thrombus and emboli. Because of the risk of a second embolus, immediate anticoagulation with heparin is usually favoured although it carries a small risk of haemorrhage into the infarct.

Transient cerebral ischaemic attacks

Cerebral ischaemia without infarction may result in transient loss of function. The ischaemia is usually associated with severe atheroma, platelet emboli and stenosis of a major vessel. Severe hypertension may also produce transient ischaemic attacks (TIA). This is probably because of vascular spasm. Transient cardiac dysrhythmias, by producing a fall in blood pressure, are also important causes of TIAs. The vertebral arteries, particularly, may be subjected to mechanical compression in the neck and this is another important cause.

Clinical features

Carotid artery TIAs produce transient contralateral hemiparesis, often with sensory and speech loss. They usually last for 5–30 minutes, but occasionally for 24 hours. If the common carotid is the source, vision may be lost in the ipsilateral eye and platelet emboli can sometimes be observed in the retinal vessels. Carotid TIAs may herald a cerebral infarct.

Vertebrobasilar TIAs produce transient vertigo, often with other brainstem symptoms and signs. They carry a better prognosis than carotid TIAs.

Management

Attacks can be reduced by giving antiplatelet agents, e.g. dipyridamole or aspirin, and by carotid artery surgery, but there is no evidence that this affects the long term prognosis. Vertebrobasilar attacks can often be helped by wearing a collar to restrict neck movements.

DISEASES OF PERIPHERAL ARTERIES AND VEINS

Occlusive arterial disease

This term includes any type of arterial disease that produces occlusion of an artery, notably:

- atherosclerosis (the main cause)
- diabetic arteriopathy
- Buerger's disease

The main techniques used to relieve the obstruction are:

- disobliteration or endarterectomy
- patch angioplasty
- bypass operations

These are best discussed in relation to the various sites of obstruction detailed below.

Carotid stenosis

One must distinguish between complete occlusion and stenosis, which is a narrowing of the vessel.

Stenosis of the internal carotid artery may cause no symptoms and be detected when a bruit is heard in the neck or when it gives rise to transient ischaemic attacks (TIA). The latter are sometimes called the 'little

stroke syndrome' because of a brief loss of consciousness and paralysis. They are due to chronic ischaemia from narrowing of the artery and platelet emboli that pass upwards to the brain. The clinical diagnosis is made by detecting the thrill and bruit at the angle of the mandible and is confirmed by arteriography.

Management

There is still some debate about whether it is better to operate and remove the obstruction or to deal with the problem medically with antiplatelet drugs, such as aspirin or sulphinpyrazone.

If surgical treatment is decided upon, the artery is opened up and the atheromatous plaque excised (endarterectomy). It may be sufficient then to suture the vessel but, as this in itself produces some narrowing, a patch of vein or synthetic material is usually sewn in to widen the lumen of the vessel (patch angioplasty).

Aortic arch disease

The vessels coming off the aortic arch may become narrowed. Most often, this affects the subclavian artery where a patch of atheroma either narrows or completely blocks the vessel. The limb then depends on collateral circulation for survival. As this is usually good in the upper limbs, gangrene is not a problem but two conditions may arise:

- claudication of the arm muscles
- the subclavian steal syndrome

Claudication of arm muscles

This comes on especially when the forearm muscles are actively exercised for a prolonged time. The pain is usually felt only after fairly strenuous exercise and is relieved by rest.

Subclavian steal syndrome

Here, one of the main collateral vessels, the vertebral artery, siphons off blood from the basilar artery system when movement of the arm demands more blood. This blood is supplied at the cost of the supply to the base of the brain and causes attacks of diplopia, blurring of vision, ataxia and collapse.

Occlusion of the subclavian artery can be detected by unequal radial pulses. The diagnosis is supported by a difference in the arm blood pressures and is established by arteriography.

Management

The obstruction can be relieved by patch endarterectomy, but more commonly now by using a length of vein or prosthetic material to connect the common carotid artery to the subclavian artery beyond the block.

Renal artery stenosis

This is usually discovered when arteriography is used in the assessment of a patient with hypertension. The lesion is usually due to atheroma or fibromuscular dysplasia and, in over 30% of cases, is bilateral.

Management

Management is by nephrectomy or by arterial surgery; either endarterectomy with a patch or a bypass between the renal artery and the aorta to improve the renal blood flow.

Abdominal angina

This is a condition often suspected but rarely proved where the patient complains of abdominal pain coming on about 10–30 minutes after a meal. It may be of such severity that it causes severe weight loss. A bruit may be heard over the upper abdomen and arteriography may show narrowing of the arteries supplying the gut: coeliac, superior mesenteric, inferior mesenteric and rectal arteries. As the interconnections between these vessels are numerous, it is suggested that more than one of these major vessels should be affected before the diagnosis is sustained.

Management

Treatment is by endarterectomy or by resection of the narrowed or occluded segment and the insertion of a graft.

Aorto-iliac disease

Severe atheromatous disease of the aorto-iliac segment is not uncommon. If occlusion is complete, there is marked ischaemia of both limbs with atrophy of muscles, claudication in the buttocks as well as in the lower limb muscles and impotence (Leriche syndrome). Less severe narrowing will produce less severe symptoms. The femoral pulses will either be absent in complete occlusion or diminished on one or both sides, depending on the extent of the disease. A thrill felt over the femoral artery with a bruit suggests proximal stenosis. The extent of the disease is demonstrated by aortography.

Management

In a localized lesion, endarterectomy with suture or a patch may be possible but, in extensive disease, a bypass between the aorta and both femoral arteries will be necessary, using a trouser graft of Dacron.

Lower limb stenosis

The commonest area of narrowing or blockage is the lower end of the superficial femoral artery above the adductor opening. The occlusion may extend proximally to involve much, if not all, of the femoral artery up to the common femoral or it may progress distally to block the popliteal artery. Less common, but of major significance, is narrowing of the profunda femoris artery as this is the main supply to the limb when the superficial femoral is blocked.

The patient complains of intermittent claudication of the calf muscles and the pulses below the femoral will be absent on the affected side.

Management

This is mainly by saphenous vein bypass graft although, if the vein is unsatisfactory, endarterectomy, using a stripper (a rebore) may be done or a synthetic graft may be used as a bypass. A rebore tends to become occluded again more quickly than a bypass graft. Synthetic materials are still more thrombogenic than veins but are improving. A further possibility, especially as a limb-saving operation, is a profundoplasty, where the opening of the profunda femoris artery is widened by the insertion of a graft or vein patch.

In very extensive arterial disease affecting the popliteal artery and its main branches, long grafts have been inserted even down to the ankle. This is worth trying but is less likely to succeed than grafts higher up.

Aneurysms

An aneurysm is a dilatation of an artery. Two types have been described, saccular and fusiform. The latter is the commoner. Although in the past syphilis was an important cause of aneurysms, especially in the thoracic aorta, the main cause nowadays is atheromatous disease.

Aneurysms may occur in any artery but are found most commonly in the abdominal aorta and, in decreasing order of frequency, the popliteal, common femoral, thoracic aorta, carotid, subclavian and other arteries. The major complication is rupture; others include thrombosis, especially in popliteal aneurysms, and emboli.

Abdominal aortic aneurysm

About 90% of these aneurysms originate below the renal arteries. There may be no symptoms or the patient may be aware of pulsation in the abdomen. The aneurysm can be palpated either above the umbilicus if it is small or extending downwards and to the left if it is large. The most notable feature is expansile pulsation. Slight tenderness may be present but, if this is marked, one should suspect rupture.

On plain X-ray, calcifiction of the wall of the aneurysm may be seen. Aortography is not necessary unless one suspects that the aneurysm involves the renal or visceral arteries.

Management

As these aneurysms usually occur in the elderly and, as rupture is uncommon in those less than 6 cm in size, they may be left alone. If large, or if found in younger people, their resection and replacement by a Dacron graft should be advised.

Ruptured aortic aneurysm

This is an emergency of the gravest kind as the mortality in the elderly is very high. Abdominal pain, faintness or shock with a pulsating tender mass in the abdomen should suggest the diagnosis and indicate the need for surgery. The abdominal pain is also felt in the centre of the back and often in the left side, giving rise to the misdiagnosis of renal colic. X-rays are unnecessary.

Management

Urgent laparotomy is indicated. The aorta is clamped, the aneurysm opened and a graft inserted to establish continuity.

Thoracic aorta aneurysms

These are usually detected on a plain X-ray of the chest and can be confirmed by aortography. The risk of rupture is less than with abdominal aneurysms.

Management

Resection of an aneurysm of the ascending aorta with possible replacement of the aortic valve is a major procedure and requires cardiopulmonary bypass.

Dissecting aneurysm

This is usually caused by a splitting of the intima just distal to the aortic valve or below the origin of the left subclavian artery and is associated with mucoid degeneration in the muscle coat of the aorta.

Clinically, there is sudden, severe chest pain that radiates through to the back and possibly down to the abdomen and to the limbs. Hypertension usually precedes dissection. Depending on the extent and degree of the dissection, various branches of the aorta may be occluded.

A plain X-ray may show a widened mediastium and fluid in the left side of the chest. Confirmation is obtained by aortography.

Management

Hypertension must be brought down to normal levels. This may be all that is necessary. Severe cases require surgery. This may take the form of transection of the aorta lower down and the creation of a re-entry defect or resection of the diseased area under cardiopulmonary bypass (see p. 226).

Popliteal aneurysm

This often takes the form of a saccular aneurysm and tends to thrombose, producing severe distal ischaemia. The patient may notice a pulsating swelling behind the knee, but it often passes unnoticed until thrombosis or rupture occurs.

Aortography will outline the aneurysm and the state of the distal vessels.

Management

If asymptomatic, operation may not be necessary.

If symptomatic, the aneurysm may be resected and the artery grafted or it may be bypassed with a graft from the side of the femoral artery to the distal popliteal artery.

Vasospastic disease

Vasospasm due to increased sensitivity of the peripheral vessels to cold or temperature change results in reduced blood flow through the skin vessels with the appearance of cyanosis and a feeling of coldness and numbness or, if severe, pain.

In Raynaud's syndrome, the colour of the skin changes from white to blue and then red in response to cold. It may be related to underlying conditions such as scleroderma, rheumatoid arthritis, vibration or an auto-immune disorder. If there is no obvious underlying cause, the condition is termed 'Raynaud's disease'. Occlusion of digital vessels will produce atrophy, ulceration and even gangrene of digits. This is rare in Raynaud's disease and usually denotes a collagen disorder or vibration disease.

Management

Warm clothing, avoidance of sudden changes in temperature and vasodilator drugs should be advised. If trophic changes appear, a sympathectomy should be carried out.

Arteriovenous fistulae

Abnormal connections between arteries and veins (a–v fistulae) are either congenital or traumatic.

Congenital fistulae are usually small but are often multiple and may cause lengthening of a limb. They are also found in the brain, spinal cord and various organs.

Acquired fistulae may follow stab or bullet wounds or vascular surgery.

Typically, a thrill is present in the veins and a continuous murmur can be heard over the lesion.

Angiography will help to display the anatomy and allow planning of surgery should this be necessary.

Management

Surgery is necessary when a fistula is causing haemorrhage, expansion with aneurysm formation or a haemodynamic upset. It may be ligated, excised, repaired or embolized using beads under X-ray control.

Varicose veins

The problems arising from varicose veins have been described (p. 115–7). We are concerned here more with their management.

Management

Varicose veins are treated to prevent discomfort and to avoid complications, but most operations are carried out for cosmetic reasons on ugly veins that are causing mental anguish.

Conservative

Conservative treatment relies on compression of the veins by elastic stockings or various types of bandages. The patient should be encouraged to walk, as this helps to empty the veins by pump action of the muscles.

Surgery

Veins may be occluded by intravenous injections, ligated or excised.

With compression sclerotherapy, the object is to close the veins by stimulating endothelial reaction. This is achieved by injecting a small amount (0.5 ml) of a sclerosing agent (sodium tetradecyl sulphate) into an empty vein near an incompetent perforating vein. The veins are then kept collapsed by pressure pads, bandages and an elastic stocking. These are worn for 6 weeks, during which time the patient is encouraged to walk 3 miles (about 5 km) a day. A successful outcome is the production of a fine cord vein. Note that thrombosis is not desired and is regarded as a failure of technique. The tendency now is to use sclerotherapy for veins below the knee and surgery for those above it.

A number of surgical techniques are available including stripping and ligation. The upper end of the saphenous vein is exposed at the groin. The tributaries are ligated and the vein divided. A stripper is passed upwards from an incision in the vein just above the ankle and the whole length of the long saphenous vein is avulsed. Bleeding is reduced by tight bandaging. Multiple ligation and excision of the veins is another method. The methods may be combined.

Superficial thrombophlebitis

This is a painful complication of varicose veins when thrombosis is accompanied by pain, induration, tenderness, redness and heat along the length of the vein.

Management

Pads and bandages should be applied as in compression sclerotherapy. Tight compression of the limb does much in itself to reduce the pain and tenderness. If thrombosis spreads up to the groin, the upper end of the long saphenous vein should be ligated under local anaesthesia. It may take 6 weeks for the condition to resolve completely.

Deep vein insufficiency

This follows, and is the principal complication of, deep vein thrombosis of the iliofemoral segment. The persistent obstruction in the vein causes oedema, cellulitis with induration, dermatitis, pain on walking and ulceration.

Treatment aims at reducing the venous hypertension by compression, using bandages and heavy elastic stockings. Sitting with the legs dependent and standing will make the symptoms worse. Walking and sitting with the legs elevated will help. If an ulcer is present it will require cleaning and, if it does not disappear with pressure, may need excision and skin grafting.

Lymphatic system

Lymphoedema may be primary, when the problem is in the lymphatic vessels themselves, or secondary, when there is blockage of the lymphatic glands in a previously normal system.

Primary lymphoedema

This may be present at birth (lymphoedema praecox) but more often appears in the teens or soon after. A later stage, lymphoedema tarda, may appear in patients over the age of 35 years. The picture has already been described (p. 112).

Management

This is difficult, as one cannot replace lymphatics.

Conservative treatment

This consists of compression to empty the leg, either continuously with heavy elastic stockings or intermittently using various air compression devices.

Surgical treatment

This is only required for gross oedema that is unresponsive to conservative therapy. A number of complex operations have been devised with varying degrees of success. The commonest is to excise the subcutaneous tissue and replace the skin over the muscles so that drainage may occur via the muscle lymphatics.

VASCULAR COMPLICATIONS OF SYSTEMIC DISEASE

The vascular complications of systemic disease are numerous and may occur:

- because of changes in the blood passing through the vessels
- in response to damage to or infiltration of the vessel walls

Several factors may be operating simultaneously.

Conditions altering properties of blood passing through vessels

Many factors cause an increased tendency for blood to clot in vessels. They are mostly complex and not all are well understood.

Increased platelet stickiness

Many of the factors causing increased stickiness of the platelets are incompletely understood. In particular, mechanisms initiating their aggregation are not yet clear. There seems little doubt, however, that they do contribute to vascular occlusion in small vessels both as a result of mural thrombi and in the form of emboli.

Disseminated intravascular coagulation (DIC)

This acute form of intravascular coagulation occurs when the equilibrium between coagulation and fibrinolysis is upset. It causes a haemorrhagic diathesis due to consumption coagulopathy and microvascular obstruction. Many conditions can give rise to DIC and most are associated with the release of thromboplastic material. It is a serious condition and may complicate:

- Gram-negative septicaemia or fulminating viral infections
- oligaemic shock or incompatible blood transfusion
- certain leukaemias and carcinomas
- abruptio placentae, eclampsia or a retained dead fetus

Disorders of the haemopoietic system

Polycythaemia vera and thrombocythaemia may produce an increased clotting tendency of the blood and thus occlude medium and smaller vessels. The contraceptive pill may cause venous or arterial thrombosis.

Conditions where there is damage to vessel walls

Such damage may be due to infection or to inflammation from disorders of immunity.

Infection

Infection in vessel walls may be caused by an infected embolus or a generalized septicaemia. It may result in the formation of a localized abscess or an aneurysm (mycotic aneurysm) in arteries or to acute phlebitis with clot formation in veins.

Syphilis may involve the vessels. It is essentially a disease of the lymphatics accompanying small vessels. The basic lesion is a periarteritis; it affects the small vessels nourishing the outer and middle coats of medium and larger arteries and can thus give rise to aneurysm of the aorta, characteristically some 5–10 cm above the aortic valve. Similarly, it affects the

cerebral vessels. Tuberculosis may also involve arteries. Fortunately, both of these conditions are now rare in Britain.

Non-infective vasculitis

The immune disorders such as disseminated lupus erythematosus, polyarteritis nodosa, giant cell or temporal arteritis and rheumatoid arthritis are examples of conditions causing severe damage to vessel walls.

Disseminated lupus erythematosus

This is most common in younger people and is seen more often in females than males. It affects the small vessels of many organs, e.g. kidney, nervous tissue, skin and heart.

Polyarteritis nodosa

This affects medium and smaller vessels throughout the body and can cause a severe generalized illness with fever, leukocytosis, renal failure and hypertension.

Giant cel or temporal arteritis

This affects older patients who often present with headache or visual upset and aches and pains in the proximal joints of the limbs, especially the arms.

Systemic sclerosis

Raynaud's phenomenon and vasculitis, particularly affecting the fingers, are common forms of presentation.

Rheumatoid arthritis

In this condition, a form of vasculitis often affects small digital and other peripheral vessels as well as the small vessels supplying peripheral nerves; the latter results in a neuropathy.

Thrombophlebitis (thrombophlebitis migrans)

This is of a non-infective type and is often recurrent. It may be associated with an underlying bronchial or other neoplasm. The mechanism is not understood.

Infiltration of the vessel wall

While there is argument concerning the initiating factors in arteriosclerosis and the presence of atheroma, there is no doubt that several conditions appear to result in acceleration of the process. Such conditions are diabetes mellitus and hyperlipoproteinaemia.

Diabetes mellitus

Diabetes affects the small vessels of the kidney, retina, skin, vasaorum, coronary, cerebral and limb vessels. In the smaller vessels there may well be a specific microangiopathy. In medium-sized vessels there is an acceleration of the atheromatous process. In either case, the closest associations are with hyperglycaemia and duration of the illness. Good control and shorter duration imply less vascular damage, but it may well be an oversimplification to attribute these vascular complications to elevated blood sugar and elevated triglyceridaemia alone. The metabolic disturbance is profound and may involve other factors. It is fair to say, however, that the prognosis of a patient with diabetes is related to the degree of vascular involvement.

Hyperlipoproteinaemias

These form a large group of disorders with elevation of one or more of the elements of the blood fats. In many, there is increased deposition of cholesterol in the vessel walls, leading in the long run to vascular occlusion.

SECTION V

Principles of General Management and Treatment

GENERAL PRINCIPLES

Many patients with striking physical signs of cardiovascular disease have no disability, even on sustained exertion. As a rule it is important to treat symptoms rather than signs and, for this reason, rational therapy depends in many cases not only upon accurate diagnosis but also upon a careful assessment of functional capacity. If this is always kept in mind, much unnecessary and inappropriate treatment will be avoided.

There are, of course, exceptions to this rule, particularly in those born with malformations in whom palliative or corrective operations are often carried out to prevent deterioration in later life rather than to alleviate symptoms in childhood.

Although surgery has revolutionized many aspects of treatment, it is seldom curative, except in some congenital lesions, and in many conditions it still has little or nothing to offer. Remember too, that even where it is not possible to remove their cause, symptoms can very often be alleviated by modifying factors that aggravate them. Of these, obesity is of prime importance. Every pound of surplus weight gives the heart extra work to do.

Heart disease or the fear of it raise special doubts and worries in patients' minds. They should be encouraged to adopt an optimistic attitude to their health. A balance must be struck between regulating exertion and providing adequate rest. Patients must be taught to live within their capacity, always remembering that unnecessary restrictions are likely to be counterproductive and may lead to needless chronic invalidism. In this regard, a great deal of harm can be done with the best possible intentions. They should be encouraged to do whatever they feel able to, short of sudden and obvious overexertion.

Nowadays, with such pressure on beds and so many powerful drugs to choose from, one tends to forget that the heart has quite remarkable powers of recuperation, if it is given a chance. For patients with heart failure, bed rest and sleep, with relief of symptoms that disturbed them, used to work wonders. The regime of early to bed and late to rise with a rest in the afternoon and most of Sunday, will often 'recharge the batteries' of those with diminished cardiac reserve for many years of useful and enjoyable life.

When drugs are required, it is better to use potent remedies with which you are familiar, than to be constantly trying the latest products. Haphazard and indiscriminate prescribing is always to be deprecated. 'One thing at a time' is a golden rule that is all too

often forgotten: only in this way can its efficacy and the need for additional therapy be determined.

PRINCIPLES OF DRUG THERAPY

Objectives of treatment

If possible, the diagnosis should be firmly established before treatment is commenced. Thereafter, treatment should be kept under constant review in the light of subsequent developments and the patient's response to it.

Overprescribing is commonplace and occurs not only when unnecessary drugs are prescribed but also when necessary drugs are given in excessive doses or for too long. It often results from the desire to make certain that everything possible is being done. Underprescribing, on the other hand, or the failure to prescribe necessary drugs appropriately, is equally to be avoided.

Many beneficial drugs also have the potential to cause serious harm. It is, therefore, essential to choose those with a high therapeutic index, i.e. ones whose beneficial effects far outweigh their possible disadvantages.

No drug should be used without a clearly defined indication and, whenever possible, a familiar and well tried remedy should be used. The duration of therapy should be decided before it is started and it is important to know what response to expect or, failing this, what response to accept.

Before prescribing any drug, it is essential to find out what, if any, drugs the patient is already taking or has recently been taking. This is especially important when more than one doctor is contributing to the patient's management.

Modes of action

The mode of action of each drug used must be understood because this will enable the prescriber to predict its likely effects. This is essential when drugs acting through different mechanisms are given at the same time. There is, for example, no point in using two drugs with the same action because nothing will be obtained that could not be obtained using either drug alone. Therapy, however, can often be enhanced by prescribing simultaneously two drugs with different modes of action. Adverse effects and clinically important drug interactions can often be predicted from a knowledge of the modes of action of the drugs being used.

A knowledge of the dose–response curve for each drug being used is helpful, not only to determine the dose that should be given or changes in the dose necessitated by an inadequate response, but also to determine the likely incidence and severity of adverse effects. The dose–response curves for effects other than the desired effect should also be appreciated. They are often asynchronous with the therapeutic dose–response curve and, because of this, the potential benefit of many drugs is curtailed.

Assessment of effect

This may be subjective or objective and both assessments are important. A subjective assessment of the effect of a drug on the patient's symptoms or signs can be made either by the patient or by the doctor. The patient's own assessment is particularly important in terms of continuing compliance with the recommended therapy. Objective assessment is also important because it allows quantitation of the effects produced in response to alterations in the size and frequency of the dose and the cumulative effects of the drug.

Apparent resistance of the disease to therapy may be caused by poor compliance, failure to comprehend the instructions or interactions with other therapy.

Age and hepatic or renal disease may alter the metabolism or excretion of drugs so that smaller than usual doses may be required to produce the desired effect.

Adverse effects and interactions

Adverse effects of drugs often seriously restrict the possible benefits of therapy. Interactions with other drugs may enhance or diminish the desired therapeutic effect. It is particularly important to recognize allergy and idiosyncrasy as causes of adverse drug reactions and patients should always be asked about a past history of such reactions. With familiar drugs, the prescriber should be aware of the spectrum of known adverse effects, their incidence and severity. Adverse effects should be watched for with special care when a new drug is being used or when any drug is given for a long time.

The mechanisms underlying adverse effects and interactions must be understood, as this often determines the means of overcoming or avoiding them. Some unwanted effects can be explained on the basis of the known pharmacological effects of the drug and these need to be distinguished from true side-effects and toxicity reactions.

Not all drug interactions are clinically significant. Remember that those that are significant may occur not only with drugs that have been prescribed, but also with drugs that the patient has purchased or with 'social drugs' such as alcohol.

Finally, it is helpful to keep a detailed chronological record of all apparent adverse effects and interactions that occur during the course of therapy. Otherwise, unexpected adverse effects may not always be recognized as such and may be wrongly attributed to the underlying disease. For example, acute coronary insufficiency may follow abrupt withdrawal of β-blockade in a patient with angina pectoris or a hypertensive crisis may follow reduced dosage or withdrawal of clonidine in a patient with hypertension.

CARDIAC GLYCOSIDES, DIGOXIN

Objectives of treatment

These are primarily to control:

- cardiac failure
- atrial tachycardias, especially atrial fibrillation

Cardiac failure

Digoxin produces several beneficial effects in patients in heart failure, namely:

- an increase in cardiac output
- a decrease in heart size
- a decrease in venous pressure and blood volume
- a diuresis
- relief of oedema

In normal individuals, however, digoxin produces no significant haemodynamic change.

Atrial tachycardias

In atrial fibrillation and atrial flutter, digoxin controls

the heart by slowing conduction through the AV junctional tissues and reducing the rate of ventricular response. It may convert flutter to fibrillation.

In paroxysmal supraventricular tachycardia, it commonly restores sinus rhythm.

Direct current cardioversion is often used nowadays instead of digoxin in the management of tachycardias, but in fully digitalized patients, this procedure carries the hazard of producing ventricular dysrhythmias.

Modes of action

Cardiac failure

The main pharmacodynamic property of digoxin is its ability to increase the force of myocardial contraction by inhibiting the membrane enzyme Na/K ATPase. The resulting positive inotropic action is due to accumulation and increased availability of Ca within the cells. It is beneficial in heart failure, especially when it is accompanied by atrial fibrillation. In patients with sinus rhythm, it is less effective and may be discontinued once an adequate diuretic regime has been established.

Atrial tachycardias

In atrial fibrillation, the atrial 'input' to the atrioventricular conducting system is irregular and very rapid. Most of the atrial impulses either fail to enter the AV node or are extinguished by decremental conduction within it. The ventricular rate is also rapid and irregular; rapid because of the high frequency of atrial impulses reaching the AV node and irregular because many of the impulses that do not reach the ventricles leave the AV junctional tissues refractory to the passage of subsequent impulses. The ventricles not only contract irregularly but they often do so very early in diastole so that little or no systolic ejection occurs and no pulse is felt at the periphery, hence the 'pulse deficit'.

The action of digoxin on the AV node is complex. It prolongs the apparent or functional refractory period of the AV junctional tissues, in part by:

- increasing parasympathetic (vagal) and decreasing sympathetic activity
- direct action upon the AV node
- antagonizing adrenergic influences on the node

Digoxin, by improving the cardiac output, will also slightly reduce the heart rate in patients with heart failure who are in sinus rhythm. This change in rate is not a primary therapeutic effect, but is secondary to the improvement of the circulation. The distinction is important, because digoxin should not be used in an attempt to reduce the heart rate when sinus tachycardia is present without evidence of heart failure.

Assessment of effect

Cardiac failure

The beneficial effects should be reflected in a diuresis accompanied by a reduction in weight, oedema, hepatomegaly, venous pressure and heart size.

Atrial tachycardias

The beneficial effects are shown by a decrease in the ventricular rate in fibrillation or flutter and by return to sinus rhythm in a paroxysm of supraventricular tachycardia.

Adverse effects and interactions

Digoxin is one of the most commonly prescribed drugs, but it also has one of the lowest margins of safety. The effects of digoxin toxicity on the heart can be lethal. Recognition of the signs of toxicity that call for the cessation of therapy must therefore be known by all doctors. Digoxin toxicity is usually due to one of the following:

- cumulative effect of maintenance doses taken over a long period
- administration of excessive doses together with diuretics
- failure to adjust the dose carefully on an individual basis, e.g. in the elderly or in renal failure

Gastrointestinal adverse effects

These include:

- anorexia, nausea, vomiting
- diarrhoea
- abdominal discomfort or pain

The total dose of digoxin given before nausea and vomiting occur varies greatly from one patient to another. Gastrointestinal symptoms disappear within a few days after stopping the drug.

Cardiac adverse effects

The alterations in heart rate and rhythm that occur in digoxin poisoning may simulate almost every type of dysrhythmia encountered in clinical practice (Table 25).

TABLE 25

Dysrhythmia	Significance
Ectopic beats	
Atrial	If coupled, are called pulsus bige-
Ventricular	minus and warn of toxicity
AV block	
Partial or complete	Suspect digoxin toxicity, especially if the heart rate falls
Others	
Atrial tachycardia	Often occurs with AV block, especially in the elderly
Ventricular tachycardia	This is a prelude to ventricular fibrillation if the digoxin is not stopped
Ventricular fibrillation	This is the most common cause of death from digoxin poisoning

Before deciding whether the observed cardiac disturbances stem from digoxin toxicity or from the disease itself, it is important to consider the cardiac status before digoxin was given, the dose used and the patient's response during the period of digitalization.

Other adverse effects

These are much less common, but occur especially in the elderly and include:

- headache
- confusional states

Interactions with digoxin

The following have significant clinical application:

- digoxin potentiates the effects of β-adrenoreceptor blocking drugs on the heart rate
- the concurrent administration of antacids inhibits the absorption of digoxin
- the concurrent administration of the bile-acid sequestering resin cholestyramine, used in the management of hypercholesterolaemia, inhibits the absorption of digoxin
- quinidine potentiates the action of digoxin, largely by interfering with its renal excretion

Special precautions

Hypokalaemia

This may result from the concurrent administration of potassium-losing diuretics such as bendrofluazide, frusemide or bumetanide. It increases the risk of digoxin toxicity. A potassium-sparing diuretic, such as amiloride, spironolactone or triamterene may be the best way of avoiding or correcting such hypokalaemia.

Renal impairment

As the main route of digoxin excretion is via the kidney, patients with impaired renal function are particularly susceptible to digoxin toxicity. Nomograms for dosage guidance are available.

Advancing age

The increased sensitivity to digoxin observed in geriatric practice is related to the deterioration in renal function that occurs with advancing years. This results in a prolongation of the half-life of the digoxin in the plasma and elevation of the plasma concentration.

Myocardial infarction

Some suspect that, following acute myocardial infarction, digoxin may increase myocardial oxygen demand and the tendency to ventricular dysrhythmias. On the other hand, it may benefit the ischaemic myocardium by improving coronary perfusion. Careful supervision of therapy is necessary.

Digoxin toxicity

Sensitive, specific methods for the estimation of the plasma digoxin concentration are now used routinely in many hospitals, usually quite unnecessarily. Therapeutic plasma concentrations of digoxin (1.2–3.2 nmol/l) are usually not associated with digoxin toxicity. Thus, the plasma concentration of the drug, estimated 4 hours after the last dose, can indicate whether or not the patient has recently received digoxin and whether the plasma concentration is within an unquestionably toxic range. However, it must be remembered that the therapeutic and toxic ranges overlap considerably and vary from one patient to another. Careful clinical appraisal is still the best way of diagnosing digoxin toxicity and assay should be reserved for cases where it is difficult to believe that the patient has been taking a stated dose.

When severe digoxin toxicity is diagnosed, the digoxin should be stopped and the patient's heart rhythm monitored continuously by an ECG. Hypokalaemia should be corrected and, if necessary, intravenous phenytoin or a β-blocker given to correct serious tachycardia. Bradycardia should respond to the administration of atropine, but pacing may occasionally be required as a temporary measure. Direct current cardioversion should be avoided.

Dosage

A loading dose of 0.5–1.0 mg of digoxin is followed by 0.25 mg b.d. until the desired effect is achieved. The maintenance dose required is best decided by the clinical response: usually 0.25 mg once or twice a day, but often less in old people. If there is no urgency, the loading dose may be omitted.

In children the dose is based on body weight: 0.05 mg/kg to digitalize and 0.01 mg/kg as the daily maintenance dose.

Intravenous digoxin is seldom required except in acute left ventricular failure or when a rapid ventricular rate must be swiftly controlled. In these circumstances 0.5–1.0 mg can be given slowly, preferably under ECG control.

DIURETICS

Objectives of treatment

In heart failure, glomerular filtration is reduced, sodium reabsorption from the renal tubules is increased and aldosterone production is increased with resulting fluid retention.

Diuretics are used to decrease the amount of sodium in the body. This leads to a decrease in the amount of water associated with sodium and thus to a loss of extracellular fluids such as oedema, ascites and pleural effusions.

Diuretics are also used in patients without oedema or other forms of overt fluid retention. This is in part because they reduce plasma volume. For example, they are beneficial in the treatment of:

- hypertension
- diabetes insipidus
- hypercalciuria

The ability of diuretics to increase the excretion of water along with sodium is the basis of their use in:

- some cases of poisoning
- the syndrome of inappropriate antidiuretic hormone (ADH) secretion
- the presumed prevention or treatment of acute renal failure

Occasionally, certain diuretics are used to stimulate excretion of other substances such as calcium (in hypercalcaemia) or potassium.

Mode of action

Diuretics act on the kidneys and increase the excretion of sodium from the blood plasma. They do not mobilize accumulations of extracellular fluid and transport these to the kidneys for excretion. The reduction in sodium leads to a corresponding loss of water and a decrease in plasma volume. This reduction in the saline component of the plasma decreases the hydrostatic pressure and increases the oncotic pressure in the capillary bed with the result that excess extracellular and interstitial fluid moves into the plasma.

The pharmacological characteristics of a diuretic are determined by the localization of its action to particular parts of the nephron. The rational therapeutic selection of a diuretic depends, therefore, on an understanding of its mechanism and site of action. Combined use of diuretics that act on different parts of the nephron or by antagonizing aldosterone are often effective in resistant heart failure.

From the practical point of view, diuretics can be classified into three groups on the basis of their potency to increase the urinary excretion of salt and water.

High potency diuretics

These are often called 'loop' diuretics because their chief action is on the ascending limb of the loop of Henle. They are the most powerful diuretics available and may lead to the urinary excretion of more than 20% of the NaCl filtered by the glomeruli. They have a rapid onset and a short duration of action, e.g. frusemide starts to act immediately when given intravenously and within half an hour when given orally. Its action is complete within 4–6 hours. All diuretics in this group (frusemide, bumetanide and ethacrynic acid) are expensive.

Medium potency diuretics

These are the largest group and comprise the thiazide or benzothiadiazine family together with a few other chemically dissimilar diuretics whose pharmacological action is similar to that of the thiazides, e.g. chlorthalidone. All the thiazides have an identical mode of renal action. Their effect is exerted mainly on the proximal renal tubule but also to a lesser extent on the ascending limb (cortical diluting segment) of the loop of Henle. One important practical difference between the drugs in this group is their duration of action, e.g.:

- bendrofluazide acts for 10–12 h
- chlorthalidone acts for 48–72 h

A longer duration of action may have merit in the treatment of hypertension, but is sometimes associated with disturbing nocturia. Patients who fail to respond to one medium potency diuretic usually fail to respond to the others.

Bendrofluazide is the drug of choice in mild to moderate heart failure when severe pulmonary oedema is not a problem. It is also the standard diuretic used in the treatment of hypertension.

Low potency diuretics

Members of this mixed group of agents include:

- spironolactone
  This blocks the action of aldosterone, thereby promoting the exchange of sodium for potassium and potentiating the action of thiazide or loop diuretics. Its full effect takes 4–5 days to develop
- amiloride and triamterene
  These promote the exchange of sodium for potassium in the distal nephron. They do not compete for aldosterone binding sites. Both act within 2–3 h

They tend to be used in combination with the medium or high potency diuretics to restrict the tendency to develop hypokalaemia. Spironolactone may be indicated when there is evidence of hyperaldosteronism. All three drugs exert their effects on the distal nephron. Serum potassium levels require to be regularly checked and their use should be avoided in renal failure because of the risk of inducing fatal hyperkalaemia.

Newer compounds

Xipamide resembles chlorthalidone but is more potent than other thiazides in controlling oedema and reducing blood pressure. Indapamide, in low doses, lowers blood pressure without causing a diuresis.

Assessment of effect

Measurement of weight loss is a useful clinical means of quantitating the loss of sodium and water. Provided the serum sodium concentration remains normal, 1 kg of water loss corresponds to 140–150 mmol of associated sodium loss. Another useful approach is to measure the 24 h excretion of sodium in the urine. If this is below 10–20 mmol/day, the diuretic therapy is inadequate. If it is relatively high (> 100 mmol/day) and weight is not decreasing, sodium excretion is satisfactory but intake is excessive and should be reduced. In those at risk of developing saline depletion, the dose can be adjusted to allow a trace of ankle oedema in the evening that will clear during the night in bed.

Adverse effects and interactions

Complications

The following can occur:

- excessively rapid clearance of oedema causing malaise
- long term intensive therapy causing extracellular fluid depletion with decreased plasma volume, decreased cardiac output, prerenal uraemia and, especially in the elderly, circulatory collapse
- chronic dilutional hyponatraemia caused by the inappropriate secretion of ADH
- alkalosis caused by a relatively excessive loss of chloride (hypochloraemic alkalosis)
- hypokalaemia with increased risk of digitalis toxicity or of encephalopathy in those with liver failure
- hyperkalaemia may follow the injudicious use of the 'potassium-sparing' diuretics
- hyperuricaemia and occasionally gout (reversible)
- glucose intolerance (rare, but reversible)
- acute retention of urine in those with prostatism

- ototoxicity with tinnitus and deafness may be precipitated by high doses of frusemide or ethacrynic acid in those with renal failure
- gynaecomastia and gastrointestinal disturbances may be caused by spironolactone
- skin rashes
- myalgia may be caused by bumetanide
- thrombocytopenia is occasionally caused by thiazides and when used late in pregnancy they may cause thrombocytopenia in the baby

Interactions

Ethnacrynic acid may:

- increase the anticoagulant effect of warfarin

Frusemide may:

- have an enhanced diuretic effect in patients taking clofibrate
- cause sweating, hot flushes, variable blood pressure changes and tachycardia in patients taking chloral hydrate
- enhance the nephrotoxic effects of certain antibiotics, e.g. gentamicin

Anti-inflammatory analgesics such as indomethacin, the antipeptic ulcer drug carbenoxolone, steroids and oestrogens all cause salt retention and antagonize the action of diuretics.

Diuretics and potassium

Hypokalaemia (serum potassium < 3.5 mmol/l) occurs in some patients treated continuously for long periods with 'loop' diuretics or, especially, thiazides. However, the plasma potassium represents only 2% of the total body potassium and therefore absolute deficiency of potassium cannot reliably be detected without the use of a whole body counter. Moreover, the clinical symptoms of potassium depletion are vague and non-specific, consisting mainly of lassitude and muscle weakness.

Young ambulant patients with hypertension being treated with a thiazide diuretic usually do not develop potassium depletion and, even when mild depletion occurs, it is well tolerated. Routine potassium supplementation or the use of potassium-sparing diuretics is therefore unnecessary in such patients.

Ambulant patients after recovery from heart failure usually do not develop potassium depletion on long term treatment with a thiazide diuretic so, again, routine potassium supplements are not required. The 5–10% of such patients who develop potassium depletion do so despite the administration of potassium supplements and a potassium-sparing diuretic may then be indicated.

Prevention of potassium depletion may be particularly important in patients taking digoxin or any other cardiac glycoside because hypokalaemia enhances digitalis toxicity. Patients on high doses of long-acting diuretics, such as chlorthalidone or polythiazide, tend to develop hypokalaemia when these drugs are used for long periods. This is probably a reflection of their very prolonged duration of action compared with the thiazide or 'loop' types of diuretics. In the absence of concurrent digoxin therapy, the significance of this hypokalaemia is uncertain, but hazardous ventricular dysrhythmia may be facilitated if acute myocardial infarction occurs.

Correction of hypokalaemia has been advocated by means of dietary measures or potassium supplements. Increasing the dietary intake of potassium is expensive and tedious and has little, if any, beneficial effect.

Potassium chloride supplements are widely prescribed in inadequate amounts and, in any case, are often not taken by the patients. Slow-release preparations are less likely to cause intestinal mucosal ulceration. The amount of potassium in fixed combination diuretic-potassium tablets is trivial and most of it appears in the urine during the diuresis. If potassium is really needed, it is best given after the diuresis has occurred. The addition of a potassium-sparing diuretic, e.g. amiloride, triamterene or spironolactone, to the diuretic regime is preferable on the few occasions when hypokalaemia needs to be avoided in patients on long term diuretic therapy.

Potassium supplements must not be prescribed concurrently with potassium-sparing diuretics because of the risk of dangerous hyperkalaemia.

Dosage

Thiazides:
   Bendrofluazide (Neo Naclex):
      2.5–10 mg/day in heart failure
      5 mg/day in hypertension
   Chlorthalidone (Hygroton):
      25–100 mg/day in heart failure
      25 mg/day in hypertension

Loop:
   Bumetanide (Burinex):
      0.5–2.0 mg once or twice a day

Ethnacrinic acid (Edicrin):
    0.5–2.0 mg once or twice a day
Frusemide (Lasix):
    20–80 mg once or twice a day (up to 2 g/day in oliguria)
    20–40 mg by i.m. or slow i.v. injection

Potassium sparing:
    Amiloride (Midamor):
        5–20 mg/day
    Spironolactone (Aldactone):
        100–200 mg/day
    Triamterene (Dytac):
        100–200 mg/day

VASODILATORS

Objectives of treatment

Vasodilators are used in the treatment of hypertension to reduce peripheral vascular resistance and lower the blood pressure. They are also used in angina pectoris to decrease venous return by dilating the veins and possibly dilating the coronary arteries with the object of reducing the work load of the heart and improving its blood supply. In resistant heart failure, they may improve cardiac performance to an extent comparable with that achieved by the most potent inotropic drugs such as digoxin.

Mode of action

In hypertension

The drugs in common use are:

- hydralazine
- prazosin
- minoxidil
- sodium nitroprusside

Hydralazine acts mainly by a direct relaxation of vascular smooth muscle, the arterioles being more affected than the veins.

Prazosin acts in two ways to cause peripheral arteriolar vasodilatation; (1) direct relaxation of vascular smooth muscle and (2) interference with peripheral sympathetic function by α-adrenoreceptor blockade.

Minodoxil acts in a way that is not yet clear but peripheral vasodilatation through a direct action on

arterial smooth muscle seems most likely on present evidence.

Sodium nitroprusside acts directly on both resistance and capacitance vessels.

In angina pectoris

The drugs in common use are:

- nitrates:
    glyceryl trinitrate (trinitrin, percutol ointment, nitrolingual spray)
    isosorbide dinitrate
- calcium blockers:
    verapamil hydrochloride
    nifedipine
    perhexilene maleate

Nitrates: all the major effects are produced by the nitrite ion and by organic nitrate esters. The organic nitrates may release nitrite ions intracellularly. A direct effect producing smooth muscle relaxation seems certain. These drugs do not appreciably dilate diseased coronary arteries. They reduce venous return and, as a result, ventricular stroke volume, systolic pressure and ventricular work fall. It is likely that the recently available isosorbide mononitrate will replace the dinitrate, as this new form is not metabolized by the liver and can therefore give a more predictable clinical effect.

Calcium blockers: Verapamil acts chiefly by interfering with slow inward currents that are mainly carried by calcium ions thereby inhibiting excitation–contraction coupling. It also increases coronary blood flow by reducing coronary and peripheral vascular resistance. Cardiac contractility and myocardial oxygen requirements are both reduced.

Nifedipine exhibits potent Ca^{2+} ion current antagonism and acts mainly as a vasodilator of peripheral vessels, though also to a lesser extent on coronary vessels. It is more potent than verapamil.

Perhexilene, likewise, is thought to act through ion mechanisms. It reduces exercise-induced tachycardia, but unlike β-adrenoreceptor blocking drugs has no effect on resting heart rate and does not cause airways obstruction or precipitate heart failure.

In heart failure

Vasodilators act in heart failure by one of two mechanisms:

- arteriolar dilatation that reduces peripheral vascular resistance (reduced 'afterload') and left ventricular systolic pressure with consequent improvement in cardiac output

- venous dilatation that increases venous pooling and decreases venous return to the heart (reduced 'preload'), which in turn leads to a fall in left ventricular end-diastolic pressure

Of the drugs in increasingly common use:

- nitrates predominantly cause venous dilatation
- hydralazine predominantly causes arteriolar dilatation
- prazosin, sodium nitroprusside and phentolamine cause both venous and arteriolar dilatation

More recently, the angiotensin converting enzyme inhibitor captopril has been shown to produce significant short term haemodynamic improvement in patients with refractory heart failure and there is evidence, too, of long term symptomatic improvement. These benefits appear to result from the actions of the drug in reducing both 'preload' and 'afterload'.

Assessment of effects

In hypertension

A fall in blood pressure between pre- and post-treatment periods, both in the erect and supine positions, is the only indicator.

In angina

The assessment of antianginal drugs is difficult, especially as the symptoms may either remit or exacerbate spontaneously during the period of assessment. A placebo response also occurs commonly in patients with angina and this may even be associated with an increase in exercise tolerance. Most studies, therefore, now include a standardized exercise test using either a treadmill or a bicycle ergometer. Relief of symptoms during exercise stress testing, however, does not always correlate with ECG or haemodynamic changes nor with the level of drug in the serum.

In heart failure

Haemodynamic monitoring provides accurate assessment of vasodilator therapy. Standard clinical criteria are also of value.

Adverse effects and interactions

Hydralazine

Side-effects are very common: headache, palpitation, dizziness due to postural hypotension, sweating, anorexia, nausea and vomiting are especially troublesome. Angina may be provoked in those with coronary artery disease because of reflex sympathetic stimulation and tachycardia in response to the fall in blood pressure. Chronic therapy with doses in excess of 200 mg/day can produce an acute rheumatoid state or, less commonly, drug-induced SLE. The symptoms usually regress after drug withdrawal. Long term use may also cause fluid retention. Many of the side-effects, particularly palpitation, headache and dizziness can be minimized by the concurrent use of a β-blocker.

Prazosin

Postural hypertension may occur very soon after the drug is first given, but tolerance to this effect develops quickly. Tachycardia is less troublesome than with hydralazine. A positive antinuclear factor test may be noted after prolonged usage. Drowsiness and weakness may be troublesome. A lower dose is required in renal failure.

Minoxidil

Angina caused by tachycardia and oedema caused by salt and water retention may cause trouble if the drug is prescribed without a β-blocker and a diuretic. Darkening of the skin, hypertrichosis and coarsening of facial features are particularly distressing to women. Pericardial effusion, ECG changes, gastrointestinal upset and breast tenderness may occur, but are reversible on drug withdrawal.

Sodium nitroprusside

Most side-effects are secondary to an excessive or too rapid reduction in blood pressure: nausea, vomiting, sweating, restlessness etc. Hypothyroidism and methaemoglobinaemia are risks of other than very short term therapy.

Phentolamine

Marked tachycardia and postural hypotension are the main side-effects. Flushing may also be troublesome.

Nitrates

Headache, flushing, dizziness, weakness and postural

hypotension, especially accentuated by alcohol, are common. These drugs also raise intraocular pressure so that caution is required in patients with glaucoma.

Verapamil

This is contraindicated in heart failure, partial AV block, left bundle branch block, severe bradycardia and hypotension, because of its negative inotropic effect and action on AV conduction. It is contraindicated with, or soon after, the use of a β-blocker because of synergistic adverse effects on myocardial contraction and AV conduction.

Nifedipine

Flushing and headache due to vasodilatation and gastrointestinal intolerance are the most common side-effects. Some patients may develop acute coronary insufficiency or even myocardial infarction when the drug is suddenly withdrawn. Other hypotensive drugs are potentiated and diabetic control may be upset. The drug may have a beneficial synergistic effect when combined with a β-blocker.

Perhexilene maleate

Side-effects are common and include headaches, dizziness, flushing, nausea, vomiting and impotence. Cardiac failure and obstructive airways disease are not aggravated. Liver enzymes may be raised and peripheral neuropathy may occur with high doses. Postural hypotension may be a feature of autonomic neuropathy. Hypoglycaemia may be precipitated in diabetics. The drug is contraindicated in those with severe liver or renal disease. Marked weight loss may occur. Raised intracranial pressure has been recorded.

Captopril

Skin rashes occur in about 10% of patients. Altered taste and gastrointestinal upset are also relatively common. Serious adverse effects such as proteinuria and bone marrow depression are rare. Drowsiness, sedation and depression have not been the problem they have been with many other currently used antihypertensive drugs.

Dosage

Dosages are:

Hydralazine (Apresoline):
50–100 mg b.d., by mouth. Higher doses possible in fast acetylators of the drug

Minoxidil (Loniten):
up to 50 mg/day, by mouth in divided doses
Prazosin (Hypovase):
up to 20 mg/day, in divided dosage, by mouth
Sodium nitroprusside (Nipride):
1 μg/kg per minute i.v. initially, usual maintenance range is 200–400 μg per minute
Phentolamine (Rogitine):
5–10 mg i.v., repeated as necessary
Captopril (Capoten):
12–15 mg t.i.d., by mouth
Nitrates:
Glyceryl trinitrate:
0.5–1.0 mg sublingually, repeated as necessary
Isosorbide dinitrate (Sorbitrate):
20 mg b.d., by mouth
Calcium antagonists:
Nifedipine (Adalat):
10–20 mg t.i.d.–q.i.d., by mouth
Perhexilene (Pexid):
100–200 mg b.d., by mouth
Verapamil (Cordilox):
40–80 mg t.i.d., by mouth (also available for i.v. use – dose varies)

α-ADRENORECEPTOR BLOCKERS

These include:

- phenoxybenzamine
- phentolamine
- prazosin
- indoramin
- labetalol

Objectives of treatment

α-Blockers were not used routinely in the treatment of hypertension because they cause troublesome tachycardia and orthostatic hypotension. They were mainly used in the preoperative and operative treatment of pheochromocytoma to control paroxysmal hypertension and in the long term control of inoperable cases. Intravenous phentolamine has also proved useful in controlling severe 'rebound' hypertension associated with abrupt clonidine withdrawal and in the severe hypertensive crises associated with reaction to foods containing pressor amines in patients taking monoamineoxidase inhibitors for depressive illness.

More recently, prazosin, indoramin and labetalol have become part of the accepted treatment of hypertension.

Mode of action

α-Blockers antagonize the effects of circulatory catecholamines upon α-adrenoreceptors and act as competitive inhibitors at the alpha receptor sites in arteriolar muscle. Phenoxybenzamine produces stable covalent bonding at α-receptor sites and so antagonizes adrenergic nerve activity. It also antagonizes the transport of catecholamines into adrenergic neurons (uptake-1) or extraneuronal tissue (uptake-2). Phentolamine, on the other hand, is more effective against circulating noradrenaline than against adrenergic nerve activity. It also lowers peripheral vascular resistance by a direct action on arteriolar muscle.

Prazosin is a selective antagonist of α-adrenoreceptors. It acts on both the arterial and venous sides of the circulation. Indoramin also demonstrates selective antagonism of α-adrenoreceptors as well as other pharmacological effects. Labetalol, on the other hand, is chiefly a non-selective β-blocker like propranolol with, in addition, mild α_1 and therefore vasodilating properties.

Assessment of effect

This is made by assessing (1) the response of the blood pressure to the drug and (2) the control of other manifestations of excess circulating catecholamines.

Postural hypotension, reflex tachycardia and flushing are the main adverse effects.

Dosage

Dosage is:

Phenoxybenzamine (Dibenyline):
  40–100 mg b.d. orally
Phentolamine (Rogitine):
  5–10 mg i.v. as necessary.
Prazosin (Hypovase):
  3–20 mg daily in divided doses
Indoramin (Baratol):
  25–50 mg b.d.
Labetalol (Trandate):
  100–400 mg t.i.d.

β-ADRENORECEPTOR BLOCKERS

β-Blockers are a rapidly expanding group of drugs that includes:

- oxprenolol ⎫
- pindolol ⎬ non-cardioselective. Oxprenolol and pindolol also have intrinsic sympathomimetic activity (ISA)
- propranolol ⎭
- acebutolol ⎫
- atenolol ⎬ cardioselective
- metoprolol ⎭

Objectives of treatment

β-Blockers are widely used in:

- supraventricular dysrhythmias to slow the heart rate during attacks and to prevent the recurrence of ectopic rhythms

- angina pectoris to prevent attacks of pain during stress or exercise. They slow the heart rate and decrease myocardial contractility by blocking the sympathetic drive, thereby reducing cardiac work and oxygen demand

- hypertension of all kinds either alone or in combination with diuretics and other antihypertensive drugs: their main advantage being a once daily dose and relative freedom from side-effects

- thyrotoxicosis to control the manifestations of sympathetic overactivity and in preoperative preparation

Their role in the treatment of acute myocardial infarction to restrict infarct size and prevent serious dysrhythmias is controversial and under investigation, but recent studies have confirmed their efficacy in secondary prevention of myocardial infarction. A significant reduction in reinfarction and cardiac death rates over the next few years has been reported.

Mode of action

The β-blockers are competitive inhibitors of the natural sympathetic transmitter at receptor sites and they are capable of virtually abolishing reflex cardiac stimulation during stress or exercise. Their action in hypertension is not fully understood but possible mechanisms include:

- blockade of central beta receptors involved in blood pressure control and sympathetic outflow

- inhibition of renin production by the kidney, associated with decreased angiotensin formation and aldosterone secretion, which is partly mediated by β-adrenergic activity

Additional factors in their antihypertensive effect seem likely to include a decrease in cardiac output and an effect on baroreceptor activity.

Secondary properties of β-blockers

Partial agonist activity

The close chemical relationship between the β-blockers and the catecholamines allows some degree of direct receptor stimulation at the same time as they block the action of the normal neural and humeral transmitter. The clinical relevance of this partial agonist activity (PAA) or intrinsic sympathomimetic activity (ISA) is uncertain, but it may be of some importance in those with previous heart failure, symptomatic bradycardia, peripheral vasospasm or airways obstruction. Pinidol and, to a lesser extent, oxprenolol and acebutolol have significant partial agonist activity.

Cardioselectivity

Selective blockers for β_1-receptors, e.g. atenolol, metoprolol and acebutolol, have been developed. These permit the desired therapeutic effect on the heart or blood pressure to be obtained without producing troublesome bronchoconstriction. In this respect, cardioselectivity is more important than intrinsic sympathomimetic activity. It is important to note, however, that cardioselectivity is a relative phenomenon and that large doses of a 'cardioselective' drug will affect the β_2-receptors so that the selectivity is lost. The absence of peripheral vascular effects with cardioselective drugs may be important in those who suffer from cold hands and feet whilst taking a non-selective β-blocker.

Lipid solubility

Less lipid-soluble β-blockers such as atenolol penetrate the central nervous system poorly and are generally, though not always, associated with fewer 'central' side-effects, e.g. depression, sleep disturbance and vivid dreams.

Assessment of effect

The degree of β-blockade is generally assessed by the fall in the resting heart rate, but the response of the heart rate during a standardized exercise test is more reliable. Adequate β-blockade has been achieved when the resting heart rate falls to 55–60/min or when the rate is kept below 120/min during a standardized exercise test.

Adverse effects and interactions

Most adverse effects result from the pharmacological action or excessive dosage.

Withdrawal of cardiac sympathetic drive

Care is needed when the sympathetic drive is withdrawn from the heart in the elderly and where there is a risk of heart failure, e.g. following a recent myocardial infarction. In addition to this central effect, β-blockers may also produce cold extremities and exacerbate Raynaud's phenomenon due to a fall in cardiac output and unopposed α-receptor vasoconstriction in the skin.

Heart block

β-Blockers should be avoided in patients with heart block as they decrease conduction through the AV junctional tissues.

Central effects

Central effects may be troublesome, particularly when large doses are used. They include sleep disturbance, nightmares, hallucinations, vivid and bizarre dreams, drowsiness, lassitude and depression. High concentrations of the drug in the brain or cerebrospinal fluid are thought to be responsible.

Airways obstruction

Adverse effects on airways obstruction are troublesome, even when high doses of the so-called 'cardioselective' β-blockers are used. The concurrent use of the bronchoselective β-adrenergic agonist salbutamol is helpful in ameliorating this effect, but is only effective when a cardioselective drug such as atenolol or metoprolol has been used.

Hypoglycaemia

The hypoglycaemic action of insulin and the sulphonylurea antidiabetic drugs may be potentiated by β-blockers and there are good theoretical grounds for choosing one that is cardioselective for such patients.

Effects on skin

Skin rashes are relatively common, but the oculomucocutaneous syndrome, which caused practolol to be withdrawn from use, does not appear to be a problem with any of the other β-blockers currently in common use.

Interactions

A β-blocker should not be given to a patient already taking verapamil because this may lead to profound bradycardia, severe hypotension or asystolic cardiac arrest. β-Blockers also offset the cardiotoxic effect of digoxin.

Dosage

Hypertension – once-daily administration:
    Acebutolol (Sectral):
        400–800 mg
    Atenolol (Tenormin):
        50–200 mg
    Metoprolol (Betaloc):
        200–400 mg
    Oxprenolol (Trasicor):
        up to 320 mg
    Pindolol (Visken):
        up to 45 mg
    Propranolol (Inderal):
        up to 320 mg.

Angina – multiple doses or sustained release preparations.

In resistant cases, larger doses than normally used in hypertension may be given.

COMBINED α- AND β-BLOCKADE

The drug labetalol (Trandate) combines some α- with its β-receptor blocking activity and is a more effective antihypertensive agent than some β-blockers or an α-blocker alone. Its α-blocking activity may restrict the bronchoconstrictor effect of its β-blocking action, but postural hypotension resulting from α-blockade in the peripheral arteries severely limits its usefulness. It may be of value in hypertensive patients with angina and i.v. in hypertension resistant to other therapy.

Dosage

Dosage is:
    100–200 mg t.i.d. by mouth.
    2 mg/min to a maximum of 200 mg i.v.

ANTIHYPERTENSIVES

Objectives of treatment

Hypotensive treatment for patients with persistent hypertension or accelerated (malignant) hypertension is well established and mandatory. A reduction in the increased risk of stroke, heart failure and renal failure by sustained control of severe hypertension improves life expectancy. Even partial control is beneficial. Evidence that treatment reduces the incidence of myocardial infarction is less convincing.

Recent evidence suggests that treatment of mild hypertension is also beneficial and associated with a worthwhile improvement in prognosis. Mild hypertension is so common in Western communities, however, that the task of treating all such patients would be very considerable. The decision to treat or not to treat a patient with mild hypertension should take account of all vascular risk factors including blood lipid levels and cigarette smoking habits.

If it is decided to reduce the blood pressure, a target should be set, the aim being to prevent or reverse end-organ damage. In practice, it may not always be reached because of the disturbing side-effects of treatment, impaired autoregulation of the cerebral circulation or poor compliance with therapy.

In accelerated (malignant) hypertension the aim is to avert the risk of cerebral or myocardial damage by reducing the blood pressure to an acceptable level at which it can thereafter be maintained.

Mode of action

There are five classes of antihypertensive drugs in common use:
- thiazide diuretics
- β-adrenoreceptor blockers
- vasodilators
- centrally acting drugs
- adrenergic neuron blockers

A sixth class, calcium antagonists, e.g. nifedipine, verapamil, are gaining in popularity as antihypertensive agents, but experience with these drugs remains limited. Similarly, minoxidil and captopril are increasingly used in resistant hypertension.

Thiazide diuretics

The mechanism of action of their antihypertensive effect is uncertain. Plasma volume is certainly reduced by the excretion of sodium and water, at least during the initial weeks of therapy. Their selective depletion of sodium from the arteriolar walls may also reduce the reaction of the smooth muscle to catecholamines and angiotensin-II, thereby lowering the peripheral vascular resistance.

β-Adrenoreceptor blockers

Their mechanism of action in hypertension is complex and not fully understood. Blocking of central sympathetic outflow and of renin formation by the kidneys are both important.

Vasodilators

Drugs such as hydralazine, prazosin and minoxidil directly relax vascular smooth muscle, thereby reducing peripheral vascular resistance. Prazosin also inhibits peripheral sympathetic function, but unlike hydralazine, does not cause tachycardia. Sodium nitroprusside can be used intravenously to control severe hypertensive crises.

Centrally acting drugs

Both methyldopa and clonidine affect the sympathetic outflow from the brainstem. Clonidine probably acts as an α-adrenergic agonist upon brainstem neurons that inhibit sympathetic activity originating in the vasomotor centre. The hypotensive effect that accompanies chronic dosage may involve a different mechanism. Clonidine reduces both supine and erect blood pressure. Methyldopa, on the other hand, may enter the noradrenaline synthetic pathway and form α-methylnoradrenaline. This then stimulates presynaptic central α-adrenoreceptors in vasopressor neuron systems or postsynaptic receptors in vasodepressor neuron systems. It is usually prescribed together with a diuretic.

Adrenergic neuron blockers

Drugs such as bethanidine, debrisoquine and guanethidine inhibit the release of noradrenaline from postganglionic adrenergic neurons. This action derives from the fact that these drugs act as substrates for the membrane amine pump usually responsible for the reuptake of noradrenaline after its release by stimulation of the neuron. Guanethidine also depletes the nerve endings of noradrenaline. The pump is non-specific and so permits the neuron blockers to accumulate in the nerve terminal. This blockade leads to a reduction in the tone of the vascular smooth muscle, especially under conditions that normally result in vasoconstriction. The action of these drugs is potentiated by diuretics, but their value is often limited by their failure to control supine blood pressure without causing unacceptably severe postural hypotension.

Calcium antagonists

Drugs that specifically reduce the influx of calcium into the cell through the cell membrane and from bound sites within the cell have a vasodilator, antihypertensive action. This is substantially greater in patients with essential hypertension than in normal individuals.

Minoxidil is a new potent arterial vasodilator but has many side-effects. Captopril is a competitive antagonist of angiotensin converting enzyme and thus acts mainly by lowering arteriolar resistance.

Weight reduction

In those who are overweight, significant and sustained weight loss will lower blood pressure and may modify or obviate the need for drug therapy.

Salt intake reduction

Reduction of sodium intake permits drug treatment to be substantially reduced without loss of blood pressure control.

Combined therapy

If more than one drug is used to control blood pressure, each should be selected from a group with a different mode of action e.g. a thiazide diuretic plus a β-blocker. It is illogical to combine drugs with a similar mode of action, e.g. methyldopa plus clonidine.

Assessment of effect

This is easily determined by measuring the blood pressure, preferably at a standard time of day. When the patient is taking an adrenergic neuron blocker, it is essential to measure the standing and post-exercise pressures as well as those recorded with the patient sitting or supine.

Adverse effects and interactions

Diuretics

The side-effects of the low doses used in hypertension are infrequent and include:

- electrolyte imbalance with hypovolaemia
- a slight rise in blood urea
- skin rashes
- thrombocytopenia (rare)
- metabolic changes:
  hyperuricaemia
  hypercalcaemia
  raised blood lipids
  glucose intolerance
- a possible increased incidence of acute pancreatitis

The potassium-sparing diuretic spironolactone may cause impotence, amenorrhoea and gynaecomastia.

In the elderly, excessive use of diuretics may cause hypovolaemia and collapse.

β-Adrenoreceptor blockers

See above, p. 248.

Vasodilators

See above, p. 245.

Centrally acting drugs

Clonidine

Initially, clonidine therapy is commonly associated with a dry mouth and sedation. Impotence and failure of ejaculation have been reported. Raynaud's phenomenon may occur. In larger doses, salt and water retention occur, necessitating the use of a diuretic. Clonidine may cause or aggravate depression. Marked hyperinstability and rebound hypertension with agitation and insomnia may accompany abrupt withdrawal of the drug, especially if a β-adrenoreceptor blocking drug has been taken concurrently.

Methyldopa

Methyldopa therapy has such a high incidence of side-effects that the drug is no longer widely prescribed for new patients. Weight gain, drowsiness, nasal congestion and dizziness are common and about 20% of patients are unable to tolerate the drug. Many feel much better after the drug is withdrawn. Other fairly common side-effects include diarrhoea, depression, decreased mental acuity and drug fever. A positive Coombs test is also common, especially in those taking high doses for a long time, but the development of overt haemolytic anaemia is rare. Hepatitis or a systemic lupus erythematosus-like syndrome may occur. Severe hypotension may occur during anaesthesia.

Reserpine

This drug is now seldom used because it causes an unacceptably high incidence of severe depression.

Adrenergic neuron blockers

Postural hypotension is liable to be especially troublesome:

- early in the morning
- during micturition
- after a hot bath
- on getting out of bed during the night
- in hot weather
- after a heavy meal
- during exercise or fever

Other side-effects include failure of ejaculation and, less commonly, impotence. Diarrhoea is a common side-effect of guanethidine but less so with the other members of the group. Guanethidine may also cause parotid pain. All three drugs in this group may cause dizziness, syncope and nasal stuffiness.

Abrupt cessation causes a less severe clinical syndrome similar to the clonidine withdrawal syndrome.

Interactions

Patients taking sympathomimetics (e.g. in cold cures, as nasal decongestants or as appetite suppressants) often fail to respond to adrenergic neuron blockers. Tricyclic antidepressants block catecholamine uptake by the neurons and so also antagonize the action of the adrenergic blockers. In patients with renal failure, this group of drugs may further impair renal function by decreasing renal blood flow and drug accumulation resulting in excessive hypotension is a hazard.

Dosage

Diuretics:
> Bendrofluazide (Neo Naclex):
> 5 mg/day or equivalent dose of other diuretic

β-blockers:
> Atenolol (Tenormin):
> 100–200 mg/day
> Propranolol (Inderal):
> up to 320 mg/day or equivalent dose of other β-blocker

Vasodilators:
> Hydralazine (Apresoline):
> 50–200 mg/day
> Prazosin (Hypovase):
> up to 20 mg/day

Centrally acting drugs:
> Clonidine (Catapres):
> up to 1.2 mg/day
> Methyldopa (Aldomet):
> up to 2 g/day

Adrenergic neuron blockers:
> Bethanidine (Esbatal):
> 10–70 mg t.i.d.
> Debrisoquine (Declinax):
> 10–60 mg b.d.
> Guanethidine (Ismelin):
> 10–15 mg/day.

ANTIDYSRHYTHMIC DRUGS

Objectives of treatment

The drug treatment of dysrhythmias may be necessary for the following reasons:

- to terminate or prevent paroxysms of tachycardia that are causing troublesome or serious symptoms
- to improve cardiac output in patients with heart failure
- to suppress ectopic rhythms that may initiate a life-threatening dysrhythmia

In normal individuals, 24 h ECG tape monitoring has demonstrated a high incidence of many types of abnormal rhythm. Drug therapy is therefore not always necessary when an abnormal rhythm is detected. If treatment is necessary, a clear understanding of the underlying mechanism and the mode of action of the drugs available is required to ensure success.

Correction of electrolyte and acid-base imbalance and hypoxia may sometimes obviate the need for drug therapy.

Some tachycardias are resistant to all forms of drug therapy, and DC cardioversion, cardiac pacing or, rarely, surgery is required to terminate them. Electroversion rather than drugs should be used to terminate rapid dysrhythmias causing serious haemodynamic upset and inadequate tissue perfusion as these may directly threaten life.

Modes of action

Drugs used to treat tachycardias are usually classified according to their effect on the cardiac action potential but it is helpful to link this to their clinical roles (Table 26).

TABLE 26

Type of tachycardia	Mechanism of action	Drug(s) used
Atrial	Prolongation of the cardiac action potential (CAP) by reducing Na^+ influx	Disopyramide phosphate Procainamide Quinidine
	Increased refractoriness of the AV node	Digoxin β-Blockers Verapamil
AV junctional (nodal)	Increased vagal tone Reduced sympathetic tone Reduced influx of Ca^{2+} ions	Digoxin β-Blockers Verapamil
Ventricular	CAP upstroke delayed	Lignocaine Mexiletine
	CAP upstroke delayed, CAP duration prolonged and cardiac muscle membrane suppressed	Disopyramide Procainamide Quinidine
	Cardiac muscle membrane suppressed	β-blockers

Therapeutic approach

Atrial tachycardias

Apart from atrial premature beats, paroxysmal atrial tachycardia, atrial flutter and atrial fibrillation are common. Vagal stimulation under ECG control, (unilateral carotid sinus massage, gagging or the Valsalva manoeuvre) should be tried before drug therapy is given.

Sinus tachycardia

No treatment is required other than that of the underlying cause.

Supraventricular ectopic beats

These rarely require treatment.

Paroxysmal supraventricular tachycardia

Paroxysms can often be terminated by vagal stimulation. If this fails, and the patient is not distressed, routine digitalization can be initiated. Prolonged paroxysms associated with patient distress can be managed with either intravenous digoxin or verapamil, but verapamil should be avoided if digoxin toxicity is a possible cause because of the risk of asystole. If verapamil is used, a β-blocker is best avoided because of their combined negative inotropic effects. Direct current cardioversion is seldom necessary.

If the paroxysms are troublesome and recur frequently, then digoxin, either alone or in combination with a β-blocker, can be used to interfere with AV node re-entry by prolonging its refractoriness. If this combination is ineffective, quinidine can be tried, but although it suppresses the ectopic beats that initiate the paroxysms of tachycardia, it has little effect on AV nodal conduction. Alternative drugs to consider are disopyramide or amiodarone. In resistant cases a combination of drugs may be required. If drugs fail to control the paroxysms, a pacemaker may be tried or, rarely, surgical section of the His bundle.

Paroxysmal atrial tachycardia

When the ventricular rate is slow and the rhythm disturbance is causing no symptoms, no treatment may be required. If the ventricular rate is more rapid or the patient has symptoms, drug treatment is necessary. When the dysrhythmia is due to digitalis toxicity, the drug should be withdrawn and the rate controlled by a β-blocker.

Paroxysms may be terminated by disopyramide phosphate, procainamide or quinidine. Commonly these drugs merely slow the atrial rate and this, paradoxically, may lead to a faster ventricular response because reduced fatigue of the AV node permits more of the atrial beats to be conducted to the ventricles. For this reason, when atrial tachycardia is not associated with AV block, it must be pretreated with digoxin, a β-blocker or verapamil to slow conduction through the AV junctional tissues and consequently, the ventricular rate. A DC shock should be considered if there has been serious haemodynamic deterioration.

Atrial flutter and atrial fibrillation

Established chronic atrial tachycardias are notoriously difficult to convert to sinus rhythm but no treatment may be required if the ventricular rate is slow. Atrial flutter and atrial fibrillation are best treated by drugs that prolong the refractoriness of the AV node. Digoxin is usually given first to slow the ventricular rate and a β-blocker added, if necessary, especially in thyrotoxicosis. In those already taking verapamil, great care is necessary because severe bradycardia or asystole is a risk if digoxin is added. Urgent control of the ventricular rate can be achieved by the intravenous use of a β-blocker, but DC cardioversion should be considered if the dysrhythmia persists, is established or is causing haemodynamic deterioration. In lone atrial fibrillation, drugs seldom help to restore or to maintain sinus rhythm and are therefore best avoided. In the Wolff–Parkinson–White syndrome, digoxin is probably best avoided and a β-blocker, verapamil or amiodarone used if it is necessary to control paroxysms.

AV junctional nodal ectopic beats and tachycardias

All three classes of drugs that affect the AV junctional tissues (see Table 26) protect the ventricles from excessive stimulation by depressing the conduction of impulses through them and by delaying their recovery time. The balance between conduction delay and recovery time is crucial to the initiation and continuation of AV junctional (nodal) rhythms because most are re-entrant in type. Drug treatment aims at prolonging the recovery time so that it exceeds the circuit time of the tachycardia. The advancing depolarization front then meets tissue that has not yet recovered its excitability, is unable to conduct the impulse and the tachycardia stops.

Junctional ectopic beats

Treatment is not usually required unless palpitations are troublesome, when a β-blocker, disopyramide or quinidine can be tried.

Junctional tachycardia

In the absence of digoxin toxicity, treatment is usually not required. If it is desired to restore sinus rhythm, atropine or isoprenaline can be given to accelerate the sinoatrial (SA) node preferentially or the atrium can be paced. Alternatively, the drugs shown in Table 26 can be used to control the ventricular rate.

In the Wolff–Parkinson–White syndrome, drug therapy aims to delay the recovery of tissue excitability either in the AV tissues or in the accessory pathway.

Accelerated idioventricular rhythm

Atropine may be used to increase the sinus rate, but usually no treatment is necessary.

Digoxin toxicity

AV junctional (nodal) tachycardias are often a manifestation of digoxin toxicity. If digoxin toxicity is suspected, the drug should be discontinued and abnormally low levels of serum potassium and magnesium, which enhance the effects of digoxin, should be corrected. When severe rapid rhythms occur, e.g. paroxysmal atrial tachycardia with block or ventricular tachycardia, intravenous phenytoin or a β-blocker may be given. The use of a β-blocker may increase atrioventricular block and necessitate the use of atropine or a temporary pacemaker. Direct current shock should be avoided.

Ventricular ectopic beats and ventricular tachycardias

Ventricular ectopic beats (of the R-on-T type) and ventricular tachycardias should be treated only if they are associated with coronary or other severe heart disease or are causing symptoms. For the purpose of treatment, the definition of ventricular tachycardia must be arbitrarily determined. It may be defined as runs of more than nine consecutive ventricular extrasystoles occurring at a rate greater than 100 beats per minute.

Electroversion rather than drug therapy is indicated where there is profound hypotension, circulatory failure or loss of consciousness.

Drug treatment and prophylaxis of abnormal ventricular rhythms aim to suppress the premature beats and to make recovery of excitability in the ventricular myocardium more uniform. If a drug from one group fails to achieve its desired effect, one from another group should be tried. Intravenous lignocaine or oral mexiletine or disopyramide may be used. For recurrent ventricular tachycardia, procainamide or a β-blocker can be tried either alone or in combination.

Amiodarone, a new drug that prolongs the duration of the cardiac action potential, has proved highly effective where currently-used drugs have failed to control a tachycardia, especially when this has been associated with the Wolff–Parkinson–White syndrome.

Assessment of effect

In established rhythms the effect of treatment can be monitored by continuous observation of the ECG. In paroxysmal rhythms, it can be assessed either symptomatically, e.g. decreased frequency or abolition of palpitations, or by ambulatory ECG tape recording, which has assisted greatly in rationalizing drug therapy.

Adverse effects and interactions of drugs used in treatment of disorders of rhythm

With an increasing number of powerful drugs available for treatment, their adverse effects and interactions have become a matter of considerable importance because some of them are serious and may be life-threatening. Those in common use are shown in Table 27.

Dosage

Dosages are:
  Amiodarone (Cordarone X):
    200 mg t.i.d. for 1–4 weeks (depending on individual response), thereafter reducing to a maintenance dose of at least 200 mg/day.
  β-Blockers:
    see p. 250.
  Digoxin:
    see p. 242.
  Disopyramide (Dirythmin SA):
    150–300 mg 12-hourly by mouth; 2 mg/kg to maximum of 150 mg by slow i.v. injection or 400 μg/kg per hour by i.v. infusion
  Lignocaine (Xylocard):
    50–100 mg i.v. bolus, repeated after 5 min if necessary, followed by 2 mg/min by i.v. infusion

TABLE 27

Drug	Adverse effects	Interactions and contraindications
Digoxin	See p. 242. Therapeutic range 1.2–3.2 μmol/l	
β-Blockers	See p. 250.	
Verapamil	Nausea, dizziness (due to its vasodilator action), cardiac failure (due to its myocardial depressant action)	Asystole is a risk within 8 h of taking a β-blocker or, to a lesser extent, in those taking digoxin. Contraindicated in sick sinus syndrome unless paced
Disopyramide phosphate	Anticholinergic effects cause a dry mouth, blurred vision, urinary retention and gastrointestinal upset	Contraindicated, therefore, in those with glaucoma, prostatism or intestinal obstruction. Also contraindicated in second and third degree AV block
Procainamide	Anorexia, nausea, vomiting and diarrhoea; flushing, skin rashes and pruritis; occasionally vertigo, hallucinations, depression and acute psychotic episodes; shivering, fever, joint and muscle pain, and weakness; lupus syndrome during long term therapy (courses should therefore not exceed 6 weeks)	
Quinidine	Hearing disturbances, blurred vision, headache, dizziness and vomiting result from the central effects of high blood levels Nausea, vomiting and diarrhoea result from local gut irritation Hypersensitivity reactions, e.g. urticaria, pyrexia and thrombocytopenia, may occur Death may result from impaired ventricular conduction Acceleration in ventricular rate Risk of ventricular tachycardia or ventricular fibrillation (risk proportional to dose). Warning signs are prolonged QRS or QT intervals on ECG	Absolutely contraindicated in complete AV block with nodal or idioventricular pacemaker as it may cause ventricular arrest. Also contraindicated in second and third degree AV block Hypoprothrombinaemic haemorrhage in those receiving warfarin
Lignocaine	Convulsions, confusion, hypotension	History of thrombocytopenia during previous use
Mexiletine	Nausea and vomiting CNS upsets: drowsiness, confusion, dysarthria, tremor and hallucinations, hypotension and sinus bradycardia	Contraindicated in second and third degree AV block
Amiodarone	Corneal microdeposits, peripheral neuropathy, tremor, photosensitization and rarely skin discoloration, hyper- and hypothyroidism	Potentiates digoxin – maintenance doses of digoxin need to be halved

Mexiletine (Mexitil):
  200–300 mg t.i.d. by mouth
Quinidine (Kinidin):
  200–400 mg t.–q.i.d. by mouth (500–1250 mg b.d., if long acting)
Procainamide (Pronestyl):
  250–500 mg 4-hourly by mouth (1.0–1.5 g t.d., if long acting)
Verapamil (Cordilox):
  40–80 mg t.d. by mouth; 5–10 mg/h by i.v. infusion up to maximum of 100 mg in 24 h.

SALICYLATES

Objectives of treatment

In acute rheumatic fever salicylates are given to relieve joint pain, to reduce the fever and because of their anti-inflammatory properties.

They are used in patients with cerebral atherosclerosis who are experiencing recurrent transient cerebral ischaemic attacks because of their antiplatelet-aggregating effects.

Mode of action

Salicylates are weak inhibitors of the prostaglandin synthetase enzyme system. This is now believed to be the mechanism behind not only their anti-inflammatory properties, but also their central anti-pyretic effect and their peripheral action on pain perception.

Salicylates are also potent inhibitors of platelet aggregation by suppressing thromboxane formation and preventing the synthesis of prostacyclin in the arterial wall.

Assessment of effect

In acute rheumatic fever, salicylates have no effect on the disease process or its eventual outcome, but they do relieve joint pain and the pain of erythema nodosum, should this be present. They also lower or eliminate the fever and improve the patient's general condition. On the debit side, they may occasionally precipitate heart failure and so are best avoided if heart failure or cardiac deterioration occurs in those with carditis.

In patients with transient cerebral ischaemic attacks, the finding of impaired platelet aggregation can be used to demonstrate the beneficial effect of salicylate therapy. Some early evidence suggests that the continued use of low dose salicylate therapy in this disorder may reduce the number of ischaemic attacks, cerebral or retinal damage and the death rate, although the benefits seem more obvious in men.

Adverse effects and interactions

In adults, salicylate blood levels of 20–30 mg/100 ml are effective in suppressing the symptoms of acute rheumatic fever, whereas in children a blood level of 30–35 mg/100 ml is often required. These values are achieved by giving 65 mg/kg per 24 h to children and 130 mg/kg per 24 h to adults in six divided oral doses.

Because hepatic metabolism and renal excretion of aspirin at high dose is limited, small adjustments in dose may be sufficient to eliminate toxic symptoms and yet maintain therapeutic blood levels. Monitoring blood levels is unnecessary, because when toxic doses are reached auditory side-effects such as tinnitus and, occasionally, deafness occur. Nausea, gastrointestinal irritation and even haematemesis and melaena may ensue.

All patients taking salicylates lose a small quantity of blood in their stool as a result of the erosive effects of aspirin on the gastric mucosa, but the amount of bleeding is not paralleled by the dyspepsia. Profuse bleeding is rare.

The drug is usually taken with food to minimize gastric irritation, either as simple aspirin or as soluble aspirin, but variants such as buffered or micro-encapsulated aspirin or the enteric coated form may be tried, if gastric irritation is troublesome. Antacids merely cause more rapid elimination of the drug and hence less effective blood levels.

Drowsiness, with hyperventilation and respiratory alkalosis, may be precipitated in dehydrated children with fever, if the dose is too high. Asthma and urticaria are rare sensitivity reactions.

Salicylates inhibit the uricosuric effect of probenecid or sulphinpyrazone when these drugs are given to counteract hyperuricaemia and gout.

They may theoretically potentiate the effect of the oral anticoagulants by inhibiting the synthesis of clotting factors. In practice, salicylates appear to exert no clinically important effect on anticoagulant control. Nevertheless, they should still be avoided in patients receiving anticoagulant therapy because they increase the risk of bleeding by affecting platelet function.

Large doses of aspirin may increase the hypoglycaemic effect on the oral sulphonylureas.

STEROIDS

Objectives of treatment

Corticosteroids are used to suppress the inflammatory response in the arterial wall in a variety of disorders, including giant cell or temporal arteritis, polyarteritis nodosa, rheumatoid disease, systemic lupus erythematosus and Takayasu's disease. They are used to suppress inflammation in the persisting pericarditis that may be associated with several of these arteritides and also in idiopathic pericarditis and the pericarditis that occurs in the postmyocardial infarction syndrome.

In acute rheumatic fever, corticosteroids are used to suppress the inflammatory response and prevent decompensation in the myocardium when there is evidence of severe carditis and pericarditis. Steroids, such as methylprednisolone, may also be used in acute myocardial infarction, especially when it is associated with cardiogenic shock, in an attempt to preserve some of the acutely ischaemic myocardium. No long term benefit has been proved in either of these conditions.

Steroids, such as dexamethasone or betamethasone, are also used to minimize cerebral oedema after cerebral hypoxia has occurred during a period of cardiac arrest.

Mode of action

The anti-inflammatory actions of the corticosteroids are complex. They decrease the infiltration of inflammatory cells and stabilize the phagocytic vacuoles in infiltration polymorphs, thereby decreasing their heterolytic activity. In addition, they stabilize cell membranes and intracellular lysosomes, thereby decreasing autolysis. They also reduce the increased capillary permeability that is characteristic of acute inflammation. Tissue oedema is consequently reduced and collateral blood flow to ischaemic areas is enhanced. Prostaglandin-mediated components of inflammation may also be suppressed.

Assessment of effects

In arteritis, symptoms are suppressed by corticosteroids (prednisone up to 60 mg/day in divided doses), but they are most effective when given early in the disease and least beneficial in those with renal involvement.

In giant cell arteritis, steroids usually suppress symptoms dramatically. The aim of corticosteroid therapy is to control symptoms with the smallest dose possible and to bring the ESR back to normal or near normal, as this provides a good index of disease activity. If eye or cranial symptoms threaten, there is a grave risk of central retinal artery occlusion with consequent blindness. In these circumstances, the dose should be immediately increased to around 50 mg/day. Treatment should be continued for life and has been shown to improve prognosis.

In pericarditis, corticosteroid therapy suppresses the chest pain, friction, fever and ECG changes, and reduces the ESR. Intermittent corticosteroid therapy is sometimes possible but, in some patients, the steroids must be continued in low dosage in order to prevent a recurrence of symptoms. These drugs do not cure the underlying disorder and their long term

influence on the eventual outcome of the pericarditis is uncertain.

When severe carditis complicates acute rheumatic fever, corticosteroids may prevent heart failure and improve the patient's general condition. Like salicylates, they do not prevent permanent cardiac damage.

Adverse effects and interactions

There are three forms of serious adverse reactions:

- those that result from exaggeration of the normal physiological effect of steroids:
  hypertension
  sodium retention
  potassium loss
  muscle weakness
  diabetes
  osteoporosis
  mental disturbance
  peptic ulceration
  suppression of growth in children

- modification of the tissue response to infection, so that infection may become far advanced before it is recognized

- suppression of the normal adrenocrotical response to stress
  This may persist for up to 2 years after stopping the drug. Subsequent illness or surgery during this time necessitates further steroid therapy. Patients should therefore carry a card giving details of their steroid therapy for at least 2 years after it has been stopped. This is important during anaesthesia, because adrenal suppression may cause a precipitous fall in blood pressure

Corticosteroids may interact with aspirin and result in non-therapeutic blood levels of salicylate. Phenobarbitone enhances the metabolism of prednisone and dexamethasone and may reduce their efficacy.

Dosage

Dosages are:

Betamethasone (Betnesol) }:
Dexamethasone (Dexacortisyl)
    5 mg q.i.d. by i.m. injection and reducing, over only a few days in total.

Methylprednisolone (Medrone):
   up to 120 mg by injection or infusion
Prednisolone (Prednesol)
Prednisone (Deltacortone) } :
   Acutely, up to 60 mg/day, thereafter reducing gradually to the minimum possible dose required to control symptoms: preferably 7.5 mg or less each day.

ANTIBIOTICS

Objectives of treatment

Rheumatic fever

Prevention of rheumatic fever (both initial and recurrent attacks) depends upon control of Group A haemolytic streptococcal infections. Prevention of first attacks (primary prevention) can be accomplished by identification and adequate treatment of streptococcal upper respiratory tract infections. Patients who have had rheumatic fever are particularly susceptible to recurrent attacks and require continuous protection to prevent recurrences (secondary prevention).

Acute infections are best treated by an intramuscular administration of a single dose of 900 mg repository benzathine penicillin G. This is more reliable than oral therapy as it ensures treatment for an adequate length of time. If oral therapy is used, 500 mg penicillin V must be given three or four times daily for a full 10 days.

Drugs other than penicillin offer no advantage in the treatment of streptococcal infection. Their use should be limited to patients who are allergic to penicillin, e.g. erythromycin 65–110 mg/kg per day (not to exceed 1 g/day) in divided doses for 10 days. Tetracycline should not be used because of the very high prevalence of strains that are resistant to this antibiotic. Sulphonamides fail to eradicate the streptococcus when given for acute tonsillitis or pharyngitis.

Continuous antibiotic prophylaxis is recommended for patients who have a well documented history of rheumatic fever or Sydenham's chorea or those who show definite evidence of rheumatic heart disease. The risk of recurrence declines with increasing age and the interval since the most recent attack, so that lifelong antibiotic prophylaxis is sometimes relaxed. Adults with a high risk of exposure to streptococcal infection include parents of young children, school teachers, physicians, nurses and allied medical personnel and those in military service.

The disadvantaged have a high risk of recurrent infection, especially those with rheumatic heart disease and those who have had a recent attack or multiple attacks of rheumatic fever.

An injection every 4 weeks of 900 mg of the long-acting intramuscular benzathine penicillin G is the most effective method of secondary prevention. Many children do not like the injection and prefer oral prophylaxis. Some physicians elect to switch patients to oral prophylaxis when they have reached late adolescence or young adulthood and have remained free of rheumatic attacks for at least 5 years. Oral prophylaxis can be achieved with sulphadiazide (0.5 g once a day for those under 30 kg and 1.0 g once a day for those over 30 kg) or 500 mg penicillin V daily. Erythromycin 250 mg twice a day can be used in those sensitive to both penicillin and the sulphonamides.

Bacterial endocarditis

Prophylaxis

When selecting antibiotics for the prophylaxis of endocarditis, one should consider both the types of bacteria that are likely to enter the blood stream and those that are most likely to cause infection. Certain species of micro-organisms cause the majority of cases of infective endocarditis and their antimicrobial sensitivity patterns have been defined. Despite this, there has been no definite clinical documentation of the efficacy of antibiotics in preventing valvular infections in man.

Several regimens have been recommended for procedures involving the oropharynx and these are primarily directed against streptococci of the viridans type, but it now seems likely that a single oral dose of 3 g amoxycillin given 1 h before the procedure provides optimum prophylaxis.

In patients who are already taking penicillin or who are allergic to penicillin, erythromycin stearate 500 mg orally in adults (20 mg/kg in children) $1\frac{1}{2}$–2 h before the procedure and then 250 mg orally (10 mg/kg in children) four times a day for the remainder of that day and for 2 days thereafter, can be given. Vancomycin 500 mg i.v. or cephaloridine 1 g i.m. followed by erythromycin 500 mg q.i.d. for 2 days are suitable alternatives.

Prophylactic antibiotic therapy for genitourinary and lower gastrointestinal tract procedures should be primarily directed against S. faecalis. The recommended regime is to give ampicillin 1 g and gentamicin 100 mg, 30 min before the procedure. Vancomycin, cephaloridine or erythromycin can be used in those who are allergic to penicillin. Therapy may be required for longer periods to cover operative as opposed to investigative procedures.

Established bacterial endocarditis

In established bacterial endocarditis, the organism must be correctly identified and the antibiotic sensitivity accurately assessed. A bactericidal antibiotic(s) must be used and the dose and duration of therapy must be adequate. The drug(s) may be given intermittently or continuously. Side-effects of treatment must be minimized.

For streptococcal infections, penicillin plus gentamicin is the treatment of choice and relapse is most unlikely if these drugs are given for at least 4 weeks. Most physicians still prefer to initiate treatment with parenteral penicillin, but adequate blood levels can be achieved with oral therapy. Phenoxymethylpenicillin 1.0 g and probenecid 0.5 g can be given every 6 h, but even better levels can be achieved with amoxycillin, which is better absorbed when given by mouth and much less protein bound than phenoxymethylpenicillin.

Infections with other organisms are treated according to antibiotic sensitivity testing.

Cases of endocarditis with negative blood cultures should be treated with a combination of broad spectrum antibiotics.

Mode of action

All penicillins are bactericidal and act by interfering with bacterial cell wall synthesis. The aminoglycosides are also bactericidal.

Erythromycin arrests cell growth and is bacteriostatic.

The sulphonamides are bacteriostatic, stopping growth by competitive inhibition of para-aminobenzoic acid.

Assessment of effects

Rheumatic fever

The success of rheumatic fever prophylaxis can be assessed by the incidence of streptococcal tonsilitis and pharyngitis (including asymptomatic infections) and by the recurrence of rheumatic fever.

Bacterial endocarditis prophylaxis

The effectiveness of prophylaxis against bacterial endocarditis has not been clearly shown. Asymptomatic transient bacteraemia in man is exceedingly common, whereas endocarditis in susceptible persons is remarkably uncommon. It is therefore difficult to obtain proof of the efficacy of bacterial endocarditis prophylaxis.

Established bacterial endocarditis

In established bacterial endocarditis, the bactericidal capacity of the serum should be determined. If it is bactericidal at a dilution of 1:5 or more for about half the interval between doses, the therapy is almost certainly adequate. Peak and trough serum concentrations of each antibiotic should be determined by microbiological assay twice weekly and the doses adjusted appropriately. Adequate treatment coincides with corresponding improvements in the haemoglobin, white cell count, ESR and signs of embolism. Low levels of serum complement return to normal and assays of serum immune complexes may confirm the disappearance of antigen (the causal organism).

Adverse effects and interactions

Intramuscular benzathine penicillin G is painful enough to cause some patients to discontinue rheumatic fever prophylaxis or to switch to oral preparations. Allergic reactions, which occur in only a small percentage of patients, include urticaria and angioneurotic oedema. A serum sickness-like reaction, characterized by fever and joint pains, may be mistaken for rheumatic fever. As with all penicillins, anaphylaxis may occur in rare instances. A careful history of allergic reactions to penicillin should always be taken.

Reactions to sulphadiazine are infrequent and usually minor. Leukopenia has been reported, so the white count should be checked if a rash develops in association with a sore throat or fever. Prophylaxis with sulphonamides may be contraindicated in late pregnancy because of transplacental passage of the drug and competition with bilirubin for albumin sites in the neonate.

Gentamicin is toxic to the vestibular component of the 8th cranial nerve and, to a lesser extent, to the kidney. Excretion is principally via the kidney so that ototoxicity is most likely to occur in those with renal failure or the elderly in whom renal drug excretion is usually impaired. Potentially ototoxic diuretics such as frusemide should be avoided when gentamicin is being given. If renal function is impaired, the interval between doses should be increased and if necessary, the amount of each dose reduced. They are best avoided in pregnancy because they cross the placenta and could cause 8th nerve damage in the fetus.

Erythromycin estolate, if given for more than 14 d, can cause either cholestatic or hepatocellular jaundice. Other forms, e.g. stearate or ethylsuccinate compounds, can be used instead in patients with liver disease.

ANTICOAGULANTS

The anticoagulant drugs in use at the present time inhibit the action or formation of one or more clotting factors. Patients receiving them in adequate amounts are continually on the brink of a bleeding state. Anticoagulant therapy is of value when thrombus formation, or its subsequent growth, is critically dependent on the accumulation of significant amounts of fibrin, i.e. in the venous rather than the arterial side of the circulation.

Objectives of treatment

Venous thrombosis of the legs

Anticoagulants are used to prevent calf vein thrombosis progressing to iliofemoral thrombosis with consequent swelling of the leg and thigh. They may also be given prophylactically during surgery or immobilization to prevent thromboembolism and in patients with recurrent deep vein thrombosis. Well controlled therapy aims at avoiding pulmonary embolism.

Pulmonary embolism

Anticoagulants are used to prevent massive and potentially fatal emboli and also to prevent recurrent emboli.

Myocardial infarction

Short term treatment with anticoagulants, in those who have prolonged immobilization or cardiac failure following an acute myocardial infarct, aims at preventing thromboembolic complications from mural thrombus or venous thrombosis in the legs.

Transient cerebral ischaemic attacks

Anticoagulants are used in an attempt to diminish their frequency. Their benefit here is uncertain.

Cardiac valve disease

Patients with clinically significant mitral stenosis, especially those with atrial fibrillation or a previous history of embolism, receive long term anticoagulant treatment in an effort to reduce the incidence of cerebral or peripheral embolism from thrombi formed because of stasis in the enlarged left atrium.

Prosthetic heart valves

Improved valve design has reduced the incidence of thromboembolism in patients with prosthetic heart valves, but long term anticoagulant therapy is still necessary to protect patients from this hazard.

Mode of action

Heparin

The anticoagulant activity of this mucopolysaccharide is related to its sulphuric acid content and to its molecular shape and size. The drug inhibits factors involved in the conversion of prothrombin to thrombin and, unlike the oral anticoagulants, it does not block prothrombin synthesis in the liver. The anticoagulant action of heparin requires the presence of the η-globulin heparin cofactor. It inhibits the clotting of blood both *in vitro* and *in vivo*. Recent evidence suggests that coating of the venous endothelium may play a major role in achieving its clinical benefit. It neither crosses the placenta nor passes into maternal milk. Heparin is best given by intravenous infusion. An oral anticoagulant is started at the same time and the heparin withdrawn after 3 d.

Oral anticoagulants

The coumarin (e.g. warfarin) and indandione (e.g. phenindione) derivatives all have essentially only one major pharmacological effect, the inhibition of blood clotting mechanisms by interfering with the hepatic synthesis of vitamin K dependent clotting factors.

Unlike heparin, they exert their effect only *in vivo* and after a latent period of 12–24 h necessary for the disappearance of already circulating clotting factors. In addition to diminishing the plasma prothrombin (factor II) level, the oral anticoagulants depress the plasma concentrations of factors VII, IX and X.

Assessment of effect

Laboratory

Heparin

The drug prolongs the whole-blood clotting time, the thrombin time and the one-stage prothrombin time. It also makes thromboplastin generation abnormal. With therapeutic doses, the bleeding time is usually unaffected so that the patient can lead a normal life without danger of bleeding. In clinical practice, the thrombin clotting time, partial thromboplastin time or whole-blood clotting time is used to monitor its anticoagulant effect.

Low dose subcutaneous heparin is used to prevent deep vein thrombosis and pulmonary embolism without laboratory control.

Oral anticoagulants

Therapy with either warfarin or dindevan requires adequate laboratory monitoring facilities and utilizes the thrombotest or the prothrombin time, which should be prolonged to two to three times normal. These drugs antagonize the effects of vitamin K and take 36–48 h to exert their effect.

Clinical

Anticoagulant therapy is mainly of value on the venous side of the circulation. Adequately controlled long term studies have confirmed its benefits in venous thromboembolism and in mitral stenosis. In myocardial infarction early studies suggested that there is little or no reduction in the mortality or reinfarction rate with the long term use of anticoagulants, but recent work is more encouraging. In peripheral arterial disease and following coronary artery bypass grafting, there is no well-controlled evidence to support their use. In transient cerebral ischaemic attacks, the incidence of the attacks is said to be diminished by their use, but no improvement in the patient's lifespan has yet been demonstrated.

In patients with a stroke, anticoagulants may cause extension of a cerebral haemorrhage or haemorrhage into a cerebral infarct.

Adverse effects and interactions

Heparin

The main danger from heparin is bleeding, especially from an unsuspected peptic ulcer. The drug is therefore contraindicated in patients with active bleeding, a bleeding tendency, severe hypertension, suspected intracranial haemorrhage etc. The effect of heparin can readily be reversed, if necessary, by the intravenous administration of its specific antagonist protamine sulphate (1 mg/100 u heparin over 15 min with a maximum dose of 50 mg), but usually it is sufficient to withdraw therapy if bleeding occurs because heparin is rapidly excreted.

Oral anticoagulants

Changes in the availability of vitamin K alter the response to oral anticoagulants. This may result from the presence in the colon of certain antibacterial drugs that alter the normal microflora and so interfere with an important source of vitamin K. Patients with decreased hepatic function and the newborn are especially sensitive to the effects of oral anticoagulants.

Induction of hepatic microsomal enzymes that metabolize the coumarins is the most important cause of diminished therapeutic response to the oral anticoagulants. After 2 days of concurrent barbiturate administration, the reduced effect of an oral anticoagulant is already significant; after a week, a new steady state is reached, characterized by an increased requirement for the anticoagulant. If such an enzyme-inducer is withdrawn, it may take several weeks before the half-life of the anticoagulant returns to normal.

Similarly, many drugs can enhance the action of the oral anticoagulants through several possible mechanisms so that the dose requires to be adjusted, e.g.

- aspirin (see p. 257)
- phenylbutazone displaces the anticoagulant from its plasma albumin binding sites
- clofibrate inhibits the hepatic microsomal enzymes

Bleeding is the most important adverse effect of the oral anticoagulants and occurs in almost 5% of patients. It occurs from the mucous membranes, into the skin and into the gastrointestinal and urinary tracts. Minor bleeding is usually manifest by bruising, haematuria or melaena. Massive bleeding may occur into muscles, viscera or the brain. During pregnancy placental and fetal haemorrhage may occur.

Asymptomatic haematuria is the most common complication, but about 25% of all deaths from therapy are due to major gastrointestinal bleeding from unsuspected peptic ulceration or carcinoma. Cerebral haemorrhage may complicate the use of these drugs in subacute bacterial endocarditis.

Minor bleeding necessitates only the omission of a few doses of the drug. Major bleeding may require blood transfusion and phytomenadione (vitamin K_1) 10–20 mg i.v. This may take up to 12 h to act and thereafter oral anticoagulants will be ineffective for several days or longer.

Dosage

Dosages are:
  Heparin (Pularin):
    40 000 u over 24 h by i.v. infusion, 5000 u subcutaneously before surgery or bed rest and 5000 u 12-hourly till ambulant again
  Phenindione (Dindevan):
    200 mg on first day, 100 mg on second day, thereafter 50–150 mg daily
  Warfarin (Marexan):
    10 mg daily for 3 d, thereafter 3–10 mg daily.

FIBRINOLYTICS

Objectives of treatment

Fibrinolytic agents can be used to speed the lysis of thrombi in massive pulmonary embolism, acute myocardial infarction, deep vein thrombosis and a variety of other thrombotic disorders but, so far, have not had much clinical success.

Mode of action

Streptokinase and urokinase

Streptokinase is derived from the β-haemolytic streptococcus. The more expensive urokinase is derived from human urine or cultured kidney cells. They are polypeptides that stimulate the dissolution of fibrin (fibrinolysis) by activating plasminogen to form plasmin, an enzyme that degrades not only fibrin but also a number of the clotting factors. As fibrinolysis is theoretically important in the resolution of both arterial and venous thrombi, fibrinolytic agents may act as thrombolytic agents when given intravenously. Therapy is controlled by measuring the thrombin clotting time.

Assessment of effects

The results of controlled clinical trials that have been completed in pulmonary embolism, myocardial infarction and, less extensively, in deep vein thrombosis, are indicated below. Less well-controlled studies have been done in other thrombotic disorders.

Pulmonary embolism

Serial angiographic and haemodynamic changes confirm that fibrinolytic agents do speed the resolution of massive pulmonary emboli, but unfortunately this is not associated with a decrease in the mortality rate. They offer an alternative to surgical embolectomy in those with pre-existing pulmonary or cardiac insufficiency, but their value in this situation has not been critically appraised.

Myocardial infarction

No consistent beneficial effect of fibinolytic on the size of myocardial infarcts has yet been proved and they appear to have little or no effect on mortality.

Deep vein thrombosis

Angiographic and radio-labelled fibrinogen studies confirm that fibrinolytic agents lead to the more rapid resolution of venous thrombi and that subsequent valve damage and the postphlebitic syndrome are favourably affected. The incidence of pulmonary embolism, however, is unaltered. Fibrinolytic agents may best be reserved for those with persisting, and especially those with extending, deep vein thrombosis affecting the iliofemoral veins.

Acute arterial thromboembolism

Fibrinolytic therapy is of little or no value and surgical treatment is preferred.

Adverse effects and interactions

The production of a fibrinolytic state interferes with haemostasis more profoundly than does conventional anticoagulant therapy. Fibrinolytic agents are therefore contraindicated whenever there is an increased risk of bleeding, as in:

● recent surgical or biopsy procedures
● lumbar or sternal puncture

- bleeding diatheses
- active peptic ulceration
- severe hypertension or known intracranial haemorrhage
- excessive menstruation

Fibrinolytic-induced bleeding necessitates immediate cessation of the therapy, administration of fresh frozen plasma or clotting factor concentrate and the use of antifibrinolytic agents – aminocaproic acid or tranexamic acid. Heparin is contraindicated during fibrinolytic therapy, but warfarin may be used in the latter stages to avoid 'rebound' thrombosis.

Corticosteroids and antihistamines may be used concurrently to minimize sensitivity reactions. Repeat therapy carries the risk of severe anaphylaxis and, in any case, is ineffective for 4–6 months because of resistance to its effect.

Dosage

This is:

Streptokinase:
250 000 u over 30 min by i.v. infusion; thereafter 100 000 u/h for up to 1 week.

LIPID LOWERING DRUGS

Objectives of treatment

Data derived from several studies confirm that people with high plasma cholesterol levels have more and earlier coronary heart disease than those with low cholesterol levels. The 'lipid hypothesis' postulates that reduction of plasma cholesterol levels will reduce the risk of coronary heart disease. To date, there is no definite proof that drug treatment will do so. Drug intervention in hyperlipidaemia should, therefore, be highly selective and largely confined to young patients with severe hyperlipidaemia who have a bad family history of vascular disease or who already have established vascular disease. Lipid lowering therapy aims to restore levels of cholesterol and triglyceride to as near normal as possible. As a lifelong commitment for patients who will usually have no symptoms, it should ideally be readily acceptable and free of side-effects, neither of which goals is easily achieved.

Mode of action

No single drug is effective against all forms of hyperlipidaemia. It is usual to start treatment with dietary changes; occasionally this is all that is necessary. Diets are usually continued during drug therapy, though this is not necessary when bile-acid binding resins are used.

Clofibrate

This branched chain fatty acid ester has many effects on the body, including changes in the blood coagulation and fibrinolytic systems as well as in lipoprotein metabolism. It decreases the synthesis of very low density lipoprotein (VLDL) and, perhaps more importantly, enhances its catabolism. Very low density lipoprotein and intermediate low density lipoprotein (ILDL) levels usually decrease predictably. Low density lipoprotein (LDL) levels are also reduced, but usually to a lesser extent. High density lipoprotein (HDL) levels may rise or fall. The drug increases the faecal excretion of sterols derived from cholesterol.

Cholestyramine and colestipol

These are resins that are completely unabsorbed. In the small bowel they exchange ions for bile acids, thus interrupting the latter's enterohepatic circulation. This results in increased cholesterol catabolism to bile acids and lower plasma cholesterol levels. Levels of LDL fall, but their effects on VLDL are variable. HDL levels increase during therapy.

D-thyroxine

It has been assumed that, like L-thyroxine, D-thyroxine acts by enhancing the catabolism of LDL. Its effects on VLDL are variable. The faecal excretion of sterols is increased.

Neomycin

Its mechanism of action is not dependent on its antibiotic action on the intestinal flora, but seems rather to be secondary to the disruption of the micelles and formation of insoluble complexes with bile acids in the intestine, thus decreasing cholesterol and bile acid absorption. It is assumed that its hypolipidaemic action is due to an increase in LDL catabolism. HDL levels are increased.

Nicotinic acid

Its mode of action in pharmalogical doses is complex.

The drug inhibits adipose tissue lipolysis and depresses free fatty acid levels. It decreases VLDL synthesis and the production of LDL from VLDL.

Probucol

This is a new biphenol drug whose mode of action is obscure. It reduces serum cholesterol and both HDL and LDL without affecting triglycerides. It appears to have a cumulative effect over months of administration.

Chenodeoxycholic acid

This drug reduces the synthesis of VLDL and triglycerides in the liver. It has no action on serum cholesterol, LDL or HDL levels in the blood.

Assessment of effects

Clofibrate

This reduces the concentration of pre-β-lipoprotein, but sometimes β-lipoprotein levels rise. Serum triglyceride concentrations fall by 20–50% and serum cholesterol levels by 7–20%. Two trials in the UK reported that morbidity and mortality rates in patients with angina were decreased by clofibrate, but there is a general consensus that a clear demonstration of long term benefit from clofibrate therapy is still lacking. There is also a consensus that, so far as the community is concerned, the increase in non-cardiac deaths in those on long term therapy outweighs the decrease in deaths from coronary heart disease.

Cholestyramine, D-thyroxine and neomycin

Cholesterol levels may be reduced by up to 20% but long term benefit on morbidity and mortality have not yet been shown.

Nicotinic acid

Its main effect is to reduce pre-β-lipoprotein levels. It reduces serum cholesterol by 15–20% and serum triglycerides by 30–50%. In the USA Coronary Drug Project, the drug appeared to produce a modest but significant decrease in the frequency of non-fatal recurrences of coronary heart disease.

Combined drug therapy

A combination of hypolipidaemic agents that act by different mechanisms has sometimes proved to be highly efficacious in controlling raised serum lipoprotein and lipid levels, e.g. cholestyramine and nicotinic acid or clofibrate and cholestyramine.

Adverse effects and interactions

Clofibrate

Clofibrate administration is not usually associated with serious adverse effects. Nausea, diarrhoea and weight gain are infrequent and usually transient. Rare, but more serious, side-effects include myopathy with raised serum creatine kinase levels (especially in patients with renal failure), skin rash, abnormalities of liver function and frequent ventricular ectopic beats. The prevalence of gallstones is markedly increased.

Clofibrate potentiates the hypoprothrombinaemic effects of warfarin sodium, probably by displacing it from albumin binding sites, so the dosage of warfarin and related drugs should be halved initially when clofibrate is added to the treatment schedule. It may have similar effects on other protein bound drugs like diphenylhydantoin (phenytoin).

Cholestyramine and colestipol

The most frequent side-effects are gastrointestinal. Constipation is seen especially in older patients and may aggravate angina. Many patients find the taste of cholestyramine unpleasant and nausea, vomiting and abdominal distension with cramps may occur. Steatorrhoea may occur in those with pre-existing asymptomatic malabsorption. Those on large doses should be monitored annually for evidence of malabsorption of vitamins D and K.

Since cholestyramine is an ion exchange resin, it has a strong affinity for acidic compounds. It decreases the absorption of concomitantly administered digitalis glycosides, warfarin sodium, thiazides, thyroxine, folic acid, phenylbutazone and tetracycline. These drugs should be taken 2–4 h before cholestyramine, their blood concentrations or clinical effects should be monitored and their dosage adjusted appropriately. Children receiving the resin should be given a routine folic acid supplement.

D-thyroxine

This drug may produce excessive cardiovascular morbidity and mortality in those with symptoms or signs of coronary heart disease or with unstable cardiac rhythm. It has, however, been prescribed with propranolol 20 mg three times a day to minimize possible thyrocardiac effects. Other less common side-effects include glucose intolerance, abnormalities of liver function tests and neutropenia.

The drug increases the hypoprothrombinaemic effect of warfarin sodium but the mechanism of this interaction is unclear.

Neomycin

Nausea, vomiting and mild diarrhoea are fairly common side-effects. Its potential for impairing renal function and auditory acuity has inhibited its use, although absorption only occurs in those with inflammatory bowel disease or liver failure. Drug interaction is not a problem.

Nicotinic acid

Until tolerance is established, each dose of nicotinic acid is followed by severe flushing and pruritus. Nausea, vomiting and diarrhoea commonly occur, but are usually transient. Raised aminotransferase levels are frequent and a dose-related cholestatic jaundice is common. Hyperuricaemia, gout, impaired glucose tolerance and skin pigmentation may also occur.

Probucol

No serious side-effects are known, though mild nausea can occur.

Chenodeoxycholic acid

Dose-related diarrhoea is frequent and may limit the amount that can be taken. Minor changes in serum enzyme activity (As.T) and gama-glutamyl transpeptidase have been noted, but do not appear to be of clinical significance.

Dosage

Dosages are:
Cholestyramine (Questran):
12–16 g/day in divided doses in liquid
Clofibrate (Atromid):
2 g/day in divided doses after meals
Colestipol (Colestid):
10–20 g/day in divided doses in liquid
D-thyroxine (Choloxin):
1–2 mg/day increasing to a maximum of 8 mg/day

Neomycin:
0.5–2 g/day
Nicotinic acid
1–2 g t.d.
Probucol (Lurselle):
250–500 mg b.d.
Chenodeoxycholic acid (Chendol):
750 mg/day.

CARDIAC ARREST

Introduction

Although cardiac arrest occurs in death from all causes, the term is customarily used when cessation of the circulation is due to:

- coronary heart disease
- pulmonary embolism
- drowning
- electrocution
- drug overdose

This restriction is applied because, usually, resuscitation is indicated only when one of these conditions is responsible for the arrest.

Clinical features

A cardiac arrest can be distinguished from other conditions that cause sudden loss of consciousness, such as vasavagal syncope or epilepsy, by pulselessness. The diagnosis must therefore be confirmed by absence of the carotid pulse. Absence of breathing is usually also noticeable, but is an unreliable sign because the patient may continue to breathe for some seconds after the circulation stops. If the pupils are dilated, this indicates that cerebral anoxia has already developed.

Management

The management of cardiac arrest is termed 'cardiopulmonary resuscitation' and its objectives are twofold:

- to simulate circulation and respiration so that oxygenation of the brain is maintained

• to restore normal rhythm

When the facilities are immediately available, as in a coronary care unit (CCU), observe the ECG and carry out defibrillation if this is appropriate. If a defibrillator is at hand, it is justifiable to give a 200 J DC shock even in the absence of an ECG, because ventricular fibrillation is by far the most likely abnormality of rhythm.

In other circumstances, cardiopulmonary resuscitation should be carried out as follows:

• ensure the patient is lying supine on a firm surface

 The floor, or a bed with a firm wooden or metal base and no springs, may be used.

• strike the lower sternum once

 This is performed by making a clenched fist and striking the lower sternum with the medial aspect of the hand. Care should be taken to avoid striking the ribs or xiphoid process which, if fractured, may penetrate the liver and cause fatal haemorrhage. This manoeuvre occasionally restores normal heart rhythm. If it is unsuccessful, desist from further attempts.

• restore the circulation

 Lean over the patient and place the outstretched arms vertically over the chest so that the palms of the hands, one above the other, are placed over the lower sternum, avoiding the xiphoid. The arms are then pressed downwards intermittently so that the heart is compressed between the sternum and the spine. Pause when the chest is maximally compressed. The heart should be compressed about 60 times per minute. When cardiac massage is carried out in this way, a circulation of about one third of normal can be maintained, only effective in oxygenating the brain if air or oxygen can be made to reach the pulmonary capillaries by artificial respiration.

• establish a patent airway

 Remove false teeth and vomitus where necessary, then place one hand under the neck, elevate it and raise the chin. This ensures that the tongue is not blocking the pharynx. An airway should be inserted in the mouth if one is available.

 If technical aids are not to hand, adequate artificial respiration can be achieved by mouth to mouth breathing. To do this effectively, the attendant should pinch the patient's nose, exhale into the mouth and ensure that no air escapes between his mouth and the patient's mouth. Between inflations, the patient's lungs must be given time to expire passively.

 Artificial respiration can be performed more pleasantly and efficiently with a face mask and a rubber bag. It will be even more effective if an oxygen supply is attached to the bag.

 The best method of artificial respiration involves the insertion of a cuffed endotracheal tube attached to a rubber bag with a supply of oxygen. This prevents vomitus entering the lungs and enables 100% oxygen to be given. However, intubation should only be attempted by a doctor who is confident of completing the procedure in under 20 seconds. A longer delay will cause cerebral hypoxia.

 The aim should be 12–14 breaths per minute, i.e. one breath after every fifth cardiac compression, although some now say that cardiac massage and artificial ventilation can be conducted simultaneously and there is no need to pause between cardiac compressions to allow ventilation to take place.

• give i.v. sodium bicarbonate

 The dose is about 1 mmol/kg immediately, followed by the same dose every 10 min until the circulation is restored (8.4% sodium bicarbonate contains 1 mmol/ml). Correction of acidosis renders cardioversion more likely and improves cardiac output if normal circulation is restored.

An ECG should be recorded as soon as possible to identify the heart rhythm. This enables the second objective to be attempted, i.e. the restoration of normal heart rhythm. The form of management is dependent on which of the three fatal heart rhythms is encountered:

• ventricular fibrillation
• ventricular asystole
• agonal rhythm

Ventricular fibrillation (VF)

A 200 J d.c. shock should be administered and a second shock of 400 J should be given if the first does not restore sinus rhythm. If the patient is refractory to 400 J and the amplitude of fibrillary deflections on the ECG is large, a 400 J shock should be repeated after an i.v. bolus of 100 mg lignocaine. If the deflections are small, 10 ml of i.v. 1:10 000 adrenaline may make the dysrhythmia more susceptible to electrical cardioversion. Some suggest that 3–5 ml of 1:1000 is more effective.

Ventricular asystole

A dose of 10 ml of 1:10 000 adrenaline and 10 ml 10% calcium choride should be given intravenously and, in a CCU where facilities permit, a transvenous pacing catheter should be inserted into the right ventricle. If asystole persists after intravenous adrenaline, the same dose may be injected directly into the left ventricle, taking care not to inject into the wall of the heart. Drugs should not be mixed with the intravenous sodium bicarbonate; laevulose, dextrose or N saline are preferred.

Agonal rhythm

This is an idioventricular bradycardia with very broad QRS complexes. Management is the same as for ventricular asystole.

Prognosis

If cardioversion has been started promptly, and if the patient was not suffering from shock or pulmonary oedema, restoration of sinus rhythm is usual in ventricular fibrillation, rare in ventricular asystole and almost never achieved in agonal rhythm.

After cardiac arrest, the pupils dilate. This does not mean that death is inevitable. However, if dilatation persists for several minutes, despite what appears to be satisfactory resuscitation, the patient should be considered dead and attempts at resuscitation should be discontinued.

Following successful resuscitation, the heart rhythm should be monitored continuously and, if necessary, steroids should be given to reduce cerebral oedema.

SURGERY

During the past 35 years, surgical treatment has revolutionized the treatment of many types of acquired and congenital heart disease. It started with relatively simple operations, such as the relief of mitral stenosis, ligation of the persistant ductus arteriosus and resection of coarctation in the aorta. These could be carried out on the beating heart without interrupting the circulation. Now that cardiopulmonary bypass can maintain an adequate circulation while the heart is out of circuit, complex procedures are carried out on the cardioplegic open heart and, with the aid of patches, grafts, artificial valves and conduits, few purely mechanical problems remain outside the scope of surgery.

In many conditions, however, myocardial and pulmonary vascular disease play an important role in the disability, especially when this has been longstanding, and for this reason, despite much spectacular progress, many operations must still be regarded as palliative rather than curative.

When considering whether or not to recommend cardiac surgery, which is by any standards a major assault on the person, one must make a careful assessment of the benefits that might be expected and weigh them against the risks involved in attempting to achieve them. By and large, only patients with severe lesions are considered for surgical treatment and then only when they have symptoms that cannot be relieved by adequate medical therapy. Exceptions to this rule occur mostly with congenital malformations, where severe lesions are dealt with to prevent future disability.

Acquired heart disease

This is concerned mainly with attempts to improve the function of valves and to increase the supply of blood to the myocardium when it has been impaired by coronary atheroma. Aneurysms of the heart and aorta and some cases of constrictive pericarditis are also amenable to surgical treatment. The surgery of acquired heart disease is, therefore, mostly palliative surgery; the aim being to relieve symptoms and, hopefully, to prolong life, knowing that the benefits are unlikely to be permanent.

Valve disease

Valve disease that is severe enough to require surgical treatment is most commonly the result of rheumatic carditis; other causes are infection, degenerative lesions and trauma. The mitral valve and, less frequently, the aortic valve are the valves most often affected.

Surgery aims at preserving the valve whenever possible. This is especially important in the mitral area, where the valve is a complex structure involving chordae and papillary muscles. Also, the prostheses themselves are not without complications. It is not simply a question of deciding whether or not to replace a faulty valve with an artificial one and then forgetting about it: patients with prosthetic valves still require careful medical management for one or more of the following reasons: (1) some of the permanent damage that has already been done to the heart by years of faulty action is still present, (2) the underlying disease may still be active, (3) the valve may function in a less than perfect manner and is subject to wear and tear, as are the blood corpuscles passing through it, (4) the valve may become the seat of infection, sometimes fungal infection that is difficult or impossible to eradicate, and (5) blood may leak around the valve because of faulty placement or damage to surrounding tissues during placement.

In general, artificial aortic valves function more satisfactorily than artificial mitral valves. They do not project into the ventricular cavity and do not interfere with the ejection of blood from it. Also, they have left ventricular systolic pressure to open them and aortic diastolic pressure to close them, so there is no lack of motive power to keep them functioning. Mitral valves, on the other hand, have only left atrial pressure to open them. As many candidates for valve replacement are fibrillating, even atrial contraction is missing and such patients have to rely on the pressure that builds up during ventricular systole to open their mitral valves. Another reason why mitral prostheses function less satisfactorily than aortic prostheses is that not only is the anterior mitral cusp missing (an important structure in guiding blood into and out of the ventricle), but the valve itself projects into the ventricular cavity and interferes with its contractile function.

For these reasons, one has to think carefully before advising valve replacement. The patient must be considerably handicapped before such a serious step is warranted. At present, moderate disability is not an indication for valve replacement.

Mitral stenosis

Until recently this was by far the commonest lesion requiring surgical treatment. Now, with the near disappearance of acute rheumatic fever, new cases of pure mitral stenosis are uncommon in the UK.

Stenosed valves with pliable cusps that have become fused along their edges can usually be opened manually by a finger inserted through an opening in the left atrial appendage (a mitral valvotomy). Where this proves difficult or inadequate, a mechanical dilator is introduced through a stab wound near the apex of the left ventricle and guided into the valve by a finger in the left atrium.

When the cusps are thickened and contracted or are heavily calcified, the left atrium should be opened and the valve inspected using cardiopulmonary bypass. If satisfactory relief of the obstruction cannot be obtained, the valve should be replaced.

Occasionally, mitral valvotomy results in serious mitral regurgitation. Minor degrees of regurgitation present before valvotomy or resulting from valvotomy are usually of little significance.

Mitral regurgitation

The surgical treatment of mitral regurgitation requires open heart surgery. It is sometimes possible to achieve satisfactory results by cosmetic surgery on the patient's own valve but, as a rule, when regurgitation is severe enough to merit surgery, the patient ends up with a prosthetic valve.

Aortic stenosis

Acquired aortic stenosis seldom causes symptoms until late middle life, by which time the valve has nearly always become heavily calcified. In most cases, the only way to restore anything like adequate function is to remove the valve and insert a prosthesis.

Aortic regurgitation

As with the mitral valve, if regurgitation is sufficiently severe to require surgical treatment, valve replacement is usually necessary.

Artificial valves

The type of prosthesis to use when a valve has to be replaced still presents a problem. Basically, two types of valve are available: biological valves and mechanical valves.

Biological valves may be homografts, where a whole valve is used, or they may have artificial rings of one sort or another to which cusps fashioned from human or animal tissues, such as dura mater, pericardium or fascia lata, are attached. These mimic the function of the patient's own valve. They do not traumatize the blood flowing through them and seldom produce emboli. Patients with biological valves do not require anticoagulant therapy, so these valves are specially suitable for women of childbearing age. In many cases, however, they have a limited life (±10 years). Homografts are liable to calcification and artificial cusps may become contracted or detached.

Many types of mechanical prostheses have been

tried. Basically, they are either 'ball in cage' or 'lavatory seat' type valves. Over the years, their design and the materials used in their construction has improved but, though durable, they are traumatic and require long-term anticoagulant therapy. In older patients, many of whom are already on anticoagulants because of atrial fibrillation, they are probably the valves of choice. Developments are still in progress.

Coronary heart disease

The surgery of coronary heart disease is mainly concerned with attempts to revascularize myocardium that has become ischaemic because its blood supply has been reduced by atheroma in the coronary arteries. The patient's saphenous vein is used to construct new blood conduits arising from the aorta and inserted into one or more of the three main coronary arteries distal to the site of obstruction (coronary artery bypass grafts).

At present, the main indication for coronary artery surgery is anginal pain that has proved resistant to medical treatment. The operation is undoubtedly effective in relieving symptoms and improving the quality of life in a high proportion of such patients. There is some evidence that it may also improve the prognosis in certain cases, particularly when the left main coronary artery or its anterior descending branch is severely affected, but its role in preventing myocardial infarction is controversial.

Localized obstructions near the origins of the arteries are much easier to bypass than extensive disease spreading out into the peripheral vessels and no amount of vascular reconstruction will have much effect on a dilated ventricle that is no longer able to contract properly. Selection of patients suitable for surgical treatment depends, therefore, not only upon the extent of atheroma in the coronary arteries but also upon the quality of left ventricular function. This is assessed by angiocardiographic studies carried out during the course of left heart catheterization.

Following such an assessment, significant obstruction in one, two or three of the main coronary arteries can be bypassed if the peripheral arterial circulation and left ventricular function appear adequate. Unfortunately, because of severe structural damage, surgery often has least to offer those who need it most.

Surgery can also be used to improve left ventricular function when complications of coronary heart disease are causing a greatly reduced cardiac output or frank heart failure. An aneurysm at the site of myocardial infarction or a grossly akinetic segment of myocardium can be excised. A mitral valve that has been rendered grossly incompetent by papillary

muscle damage can be replaced. A defect resulting from rupture of an infarct in the ventricular septum can be closed. Whenever possible, patients with such lesions should be managed by intensive medical therapy in the acute stage of myocardial infarction because of the high risk associated with surgery during this phase of the illness. Surgical treatment should be considered only when more conservative measures are clearly inadequate.

Congenital cardiac malformations

The principles used in the selection of patients for surgical treatment and its timing are given on pp. 181–190. As most malformations are now detected at or soon after birth, the surgery of congenital cardiac malformations is becoming more and more concerned with infants and small children. Recent advances have revolutionized the prognosis, particularly for those born with the types of severe lesions that used to carry a high mortality in the first year of life. Very few conditions cannot now be at least alleviated.

Generally speaking, the operations used are either curative or palliative.

Curative operations relieve the circulatory embarrassment by removing the cause and restoring a normal circulation as, for example, when a persisting ductus arteriosus is ligated or a coarcted segment in the aorta is excised.

Many curative operations, however, require open heart surgery and although open heart surgery is clearly the answer to most serious problems arising in infancy, it demands considerable skill and resources that are not yet available in many places. For this reason, it is often best to gain time by doing a palliative operation and postponing the curative procedure until later.

Palliative procedures have stood the test of time and are still widely used by cardiovascular surgeons:

- when the facilities required for curative operations are not available
- to tide patients over until a curative operation is possible
- to prepare the heart for the haemodynamic consequences of a curative operation
- in situations where no curative operation is feasible

Though not without some risk, they are quicker and easier to do and give small patients time to grow. They improve the circulation without restoring it to normal. They may do this by tackling the lesions directly or indirectly. In critical pulmonary or aortic stenosis, the stenosed valve can be enlarged by inserting a bougie or dilating instrument through a small incision made in the wall of the heart.

More commonly, another malformation is created to counter the effects of the congenital one. In Fallot's tetralogy, for example, where very little blood can reach the lungs because of an extremely narrow right ventricular outflow tract, a communication is made between the systemic and pulmonary circuits by bringing down a subclavian artery and anastomosing it to one of the main pulmonary arteries (a Blalock–Taussig shunt). This creates an artificial ductus and decreases the central cyanosis by increasing the flow of blood through the lungs.

Where the flow of blood through the lungs is already greatly increased by a large left to right shunt through a septal defect, the pulmonary artery pressure rises. After a few years, the raised pressure causes permanent narrowing of the pulmonary arterioles, the pulmonary hypertension becomes irreversible and it is then too dangerous to attempt to close the defect. To prevent this chain of events, a band is placed around the pulmonary trunk to decrease the amount of blood flowing to the lungs. The banding reduces the pulmonary artery pressure by creating an artificial pulmonary stenosis and prevents the onset of serious pulmonary vascular disease.

For those with severe malformations that are not associated with a high mortality in the first year of life, surgical treatment can be delayed until the optimum time; most operations being done, if possible, before the patient goes to school.

Those with less severe malformations that may or may not require surgical treatment are followed in the outpatient department and surgery is carried out when and if it appears to be necessary; the general rule being not to delay once it becomes obvious that an operation is needed.

Patients with serious malformation who present later in life, often present special problems. They require detailed investigation and careful consideration before surgical treatment is recommended to improve the quality of life or to prevent it from deteriorating. Fortunately, they are a diminishing group because, sometimes, the difficult decision has to be made that it would be safer to leave things the way they are; and such a recommendation is always difficult to explain to those who are most intimately concerned.

TEST-YOURSELF QUESTIONS
Sections IV and V

1. List eight risk factors for coronary heart disease.

2. Which of the following statements is/are true of angina?
a) The usual site is over the centre of the praecordium
b) It can waken the patient from sleep
c) The pain may radiate down the right arm
d) The resting ECG is usually abnormal
e) Exercise testing may be useful diagnostically

3. Which of the following statements is/are true about the size of β-adrenoreceptor blockers?
a) The presence of heart failure is a contraindication
b) The presence of bronchial asthma is a contraindication
c) The starting dose would be small and increased progressively
d) Therapy can be discontinued suddenly
e) B2-receptors are found mainly in the heart
f) They should not be used along with calcium antagonists

4. The pulse in patients with acute myocardial infarctions gives information. For each pulse rate on the left select the most appropriate condition on the right.

a) 38/min   1) Sinus bradycardia
b) 120/min and regular 2) Atrioventricular block
c) 160/min and regular 3) Supraventricular
d) 172/min and irregular   tachycardia
                       4) Sinus tachycardia
                       5) Atrial fibrillation

5. List four complications that can follow myocardial infarction
1) immediately
2) after one or more days
3) later

6. List eight causes of secondary hypertension.

7. The five enzymes on the right are commonly measured in patients with suspected infarcts. For each of the time sequences on the left select the most appropriate enzyme on the right.

a) Level rises at 6 hours and 1) SGOT
   peaks at 18–36 hours   2) SGPT
b) Level rises at 12–24   3) Creatinine
   hours and peaks at   phosphokinase
   34–48 hours   4) Lactic acid
c) Level rises after 2–3   dehydrogenase (LDH)
   days and remains
   raised for up to one
   week

8. List five major and five minor criteria (Duckett Jones) for rheumatic fever.

9. Which of the following are typical of pericarditis in rheumatic heart disease?
a) Pain affected by respiration
b) To and fro sound of friction heard on auscultation
c) Widespread ST depression in the ECG
d) Indicates pancarditis
e) Heals with no residual damage

10. Which of the following statements is/are true about mitral stenosis?
a) The apex beat is classically tapping in nature
b) A right ventricular heave may be palpated
c) On auscultation the first sound is usually decreased
d) An 'opening snap' is heard following the first heart sound
e) In patients with atrial fibrillation the presystolic accentuation of the murmur is usually marked

11. List five complications of mitral stenosis.

12. Match the murmurs on the left with one or more features on the right.
a) Mitral incompetence 1) Radiation to the neck
b) Aortic stenosis   2) Hepatic pulsation

c) Tricuspid regurgitation

3) Mid systolic crescendo
4) Reversed splitting of the second heart sounds on inspiration
5) Pansystolic murmur conducted to axilla
6) Increased on inspiration
7) Prominent V waves in the neck

13. List the three causes of aortic stenosis.

14. Fourteen days after a cholecystectomy a 55-year-old woman complains of sudden dyspnoea and collapses.
What is the most likely diagnosis and what would you expect to find on the ECG?

15. Which of the following statements is/are true of chronic cor pulmonale?

a) An important factor in its development is pulmonary vasoconstriction caused by hypoxia
b) Peripheral vasoconstriction is typically found
c) The pulmonary component of the second heart sound is usually soft
d) Peaked P waves may be found on the ECG
e) The typical blood gas picture is that of a compensated respiratory acidosis

16. For each of the statements on the left select the most appropriate lesion on the right.

a) The commonest congenital cardiac malformation
b) The most frequent cause of heart failure in babies without cyanosis
c) The finding of clinical cyanosis, a loud systolic murmur, an ECG that shows tall R waves in V1 with a sudden change to R and S waves of approximately equal amplitude in V2
d) A continuous murmur that builds up to a crescendo in late systole and continues through the second heart sound into diastole

1) Ventricular septal deficit
2) Atrial septal deficit
3) Co-arctation of the aorta
4) The tetralogy of Fallot
5) Pulmonary stenosis
6) Persistence of the ductus arteriosus

(continued next column)

e) A systolic murmur heard over the left upper precordium propagated upwards and towards the left shoulder

17. List eight causes of pericarditis.

18. Which of the following statements is/are true of chronic constrictive pericarditis.

a) The first complaint often is of abdominal swelling
b) Peripheral oedema is usually marked
c) The heart size is usually large
d) Echocardiography is usually diagnostic
e) Patients who are incapacitated should have pericardectomy

19. With which of the features on the right are each of the names on the left associated?

a) Lutembacher
b) Leriche
c) Carey Coombs
d) Graham Steell
e) Kussmaul

1) Quiet low pitched mid-diastolic murmur
2) Pulmonary incompetence
3) Mitral stenosis accompanied by an atrial septal deficit
4) Venous pulsus paradoxus
5) Impotence, absent femoral pulses and intermittent claudication
6) Temporal arteritis

20. How do patients with SBE most commonly present?

21. For each of the rhythms on the left select the most likely response to vagal simulation on the right.

a) Sinus tachycardia
b) Paroxysmal atrial tachycardia
c) Atrial flutter
d) Atrial fibrillation
e) Paroxysmal supra-ventricular tachycardia

1) Nil or increased AV block
2) Usually nil, may slow VR
3) Slows
4) Nil or may stop

22. List seven causes of atrial fibrillation.

23. For each condition on the left note appropriate drugs on the right.

a) Ventricular tachycardia

1) No therapy

b) Supraventricular
   ectopics
c) Ventricular fibrillation
d) Paroxysmal atrial
   tachycardia
e) Junctional tachycardia
f) Atrial flutter
g) Atrial fibrillation

2) Digoxin
3) β-blocker
4) Atropine
5) D C shock
6) Lignocaine
7) Disopyramide

24. For each of the presentations on the left, select the most likely type of cardiomyopathy.

a) Increasing
   breathlessness
b) Signs of right
   ventricular failure
c) Breathlessness with
   effort syncope and
   angina

1) Constrictive
   cardiomyopathy
2) Congestive
   cardiomyopathy
3) Obstructive
   cardiomyopathy

25. List three approaches to reducing the incidence of post-operative deep vein thrombosis.

26. What is the usual presenting feature in a patient with a carotid artery transient ischaemic attack?

27. A 60-year-old patient presents with headache, visual upset and aches and pains in the arms.
What condition should you suspect?

28. Which of the following statements are true of digoxin?

a) Spironolactone given with digoxin may result in hypokalaemia
b) Antacids may inhibit the absorption of digoxin
c) Digoxin potentiates the effect of β-blockers on the heart rate
d) The half-life of digoxin in the plasma is decreased in the elderly
e) Headache is a recognised adverse effect of digoxin

29. In which of the following conditions may diuretics be indicated?

a) Oedema
b) Hypertension

c) Diabetes insipidus
d) Hypercalciuria
e) Inappropriate ADH secretion

30. Match the drugs on the left with the most appropriate side effect on the right.

a) Captopril
b) Nitrates
c) Minoxidil
d) Bumetanide
e) Spironolactone

1) Headache and flushing
2) Myalgia
3) Skin rash
4) Gynaecomastia
5) Darkening of the skin

31. What five classes of antihypertensive drugs are in common use?

32. Match the drugs on the left with the most appropriate adverse effect on the right.

a) Lignocaine
b) Mexiletine
c) Amidarone
d) Quinidine
e) Disopyramide

1) Corneal microdeposits
2) Convulsions
3) Dysarthria
4) Urine retention
5) Hearing disturbance

33. In the prophylaxis of subacute bacterial endocarditis which antibiotic would you use before.

a) tooth extraction
b) genitourinary procedure?

34. For each of the statements on the left select the most appropriate answer on the right.

a) Main danger is
   bleeding
b) Effect reversed by
   protamine sulphate
c) Effect reversed by Vit
   K1
d) Aspirin enhances its
   action
e) Takes 36–48 hours to
   exert an effect

1) Applies to heparin
2) Applies to warfarin
3) Applies to both
   heparin and warfarin
4) Applies to neither

35. List the steps in cardiopulmonary resuscitation when an ECG is not available.

ANSWERS TO TEST-YOURSELF QUESTIONS

Sections I, II and III

1. 1 – b (page 3); 2 – b (page 3); 3 – c (pages 4–5); 4–c (pages 4–5); 5 – d (page 2)
2. a – Yes (page 16); b – No (page 17); c – No (pages 17–18); d – No (page 21); e – Yes (page 22)
3. d, a, c, b (pages 17–19)
4. a The resistance to flow through a vessel varies inversely with the fourth power of its radius
   b The flow decreases sixteenfold (page 24)
5. 1 – d (page 31); 2 – b (page 31); 3 – a (page 30); 4 – e (pages 33–34); 5 – c (page 33)
6. a – Yes (page 38); b – Yes (page 39); c – No (page 39); d – No (page 39); e – No (page 39)
7. Q-wave, ST elevation, T wave inversion (page 43)
8. a – 3; b – 4; c – 1; d – 2 (page 43)
9. a – Yes (page 48); b – Yes (page 49); c – Yes (page 49); d – No (page 52)
10. a – Yes; b – Yes; c – No; d – Yes; e – No (page 47)
11. a – 1; b – 1; c – 2; d – 1; e – 2 (pages 67–68)
12. Compare your answer with the list on page 71
13. Is it regular, how fast is it, how does it start, how does it stop, how long does it last, how frequently does it occur? (page 75)
14. Compare your answer with the list on page 75
15. a – Sinus arrhythmia; b – Pulse deficit; c – Pulsus bigeminus; d – Pulsus alternans; e – Waterhammer pulse (page 82)
16. a – 5; b – 1 or 5; c – 2; d – 3; e – 4 (pages 85–88)
17. Coronary artery disease; Systemic hypertension; Valvular heart disease; Disturbance of heart rhythm; Thyroid disease (page 98)
18. Compare your answers with those on pages 100–101
19. Compare your answer with the list on page 63
20. 1 – General causes: cardiac failure, hepatic disease, renal disease. 2 – Local causes: varicose veins, venous thrombosis in leg, venous or lymphatic obstruction, arthritis, immobility or prolonged standing (pages 103–104)
21. 1 – Orthopnoea; 2 – Effort dyspnoea; 3 – Angina (page 103)
22. Compare your answer with the list on pages 104–105
23. a – 3; b – 2; c – 1; d – 2; e – 3 (page 107)
24. Compare your answer with the table on page 108
25. Compare your answer with the table 14 on page 113
26. a – Emboli from the heart following a recent myocardial infarction; b – At the bifurcation of the common femoral artery, the common iliac artery and the aorta (page 114)
27. 1 – Deep venous thrombosis; 2 – Pelvic tumours; 3 – Constipation (page 116)
28. 1 – Bed rest or immobility; 2 – The post-operative state; 3 – Oral contraceptives; 4 – Pregnancy; 5 – Obesity; 6 – Neoplastic disease (page 118)

Sections IV and V

1. 1 – Plasma lipids; 2 – Cigarette smoking; 3 – Blood pressure; 4 – Diabetes mellitus; 5 – Obesity; 6 – Lack of physical activity; 7 – Stress; 8 – Oral contraceptives (pages 126–128)
2. a – Yes (page 129); b – Yes (page 129); c – Yes (page 129); d – No (page 130); e – Yes (page 131)
3. a – Yes; b – Yes; c – Yes; d – No; e – No; f – No (pages 132–133)
4. a – 2; b – 4; c – 3; d – 5 (pages 135–136)
5. Compare your list with the list on page 140
6. Compare your answer with the list on page 147
7. a – 3; b – 1 and 2; c – 4 (page 139)
8. Compare your answers with the list on page 157
9. a – Yes; b – Yes; c – No; d – Yes; e – Yes (page 157)
10. a – Yes; b – Yes; c – No; d – No; e – No (pages 161–162)
11. Atrial fibrillation; systemic embolus; pulmonary infarction; chest infection; subacute bacterial endocarditis (page 164)
12. a – 5; b – 1, 3 and 4; c – 2, 6 and 7 (page 167)
13. Congenital; Rheumatic; Sclerotic (page 168)
14. A massive pulmonary embolism.
    The ECG may be normal or show signs of right heart strain (see tracing on page 176)
15. a – Yes; b – No; c – No; d – Yes; e – Yes (pages 178–180)
16. a – 1; b – 3; c – 4; d – 6; e – 5 (pages 182–185)
17. Compare your list with the list on page 190
18. a – Yes; b – No; c – No; d – No; e – Yes (page 192)
19. a – 3 (page 159); b – 5 (page 115); c – 1 (page 157); d – 2 (page 162); e – 4 (page 191)
20. Patients with endocarditis usually present with vague malaise and other 'flu'-like symptoms. The condition must be suspected in the absence of florid clinical signs (page 193)
21. a – 3; b – 1; c – 1; d – 2; e – 4 (page 197)
22. Compare your answer with the list on page 199

23 a – 3, 5, 6, 7 (page 203); b – 1, 3, 7 (page 205); c – 5 (page 203); d – 1, 2, 3, 5 (page 198); e – 1, 4 (page 199); f – 2, 3, 5 (page 199); g – 1, 2, 3, 5 (page 200); h – 1, 4 (page 209)

24 a – 2; b – 1; c – 3 (pages 213–214

25 1 – Early ambulation exercises; 2 – Heparinization; 3 – Dextran (page 223)

26 Contralateral hemiparesis often with sensory and speech loss lasting usually 5–30 minutes (page 229)

27 Temporal arteritis (page 234)

28 a – No; b – Yes; c – Yes; d – No; e – Yes (page 241)

29 a – Yes; b – Yes; c – Yes; d – Yes; e – Yes (page 242)

30 a – 3 (page 247); b – 1 (page 246); c – 5 (page 246); d – 2 (page 242); e – 4 (page 242)

31 Thiazide diuretics; β-blockers; Vasodilators; Centrally acting drugs; Adrenergic neuron blockers (page 250)

32 a – 2; b – 3; c – 1; d – 5; e – 4 (page 256)

33 a – Amoxycillin is first choice. In patients already taking penicillin or sensitive to penicillin use erythromycin, or vancomycin or cephaloridine followed by erythromycin; b – Ampicillin and gentamycin. In patients allergic to penicillin, vancomycin, cephaloridine or erythromycin can be used (pages 259–260)

34 a – 3; b – 1; c – 2; d – 2; e – 2 (page 262)

35 1 – Lie the patient on firm surface; 2 – Strike the lower sternum once; 3 – Restore the circulation; 4 – Establish a potent airway; 5 – Give IV sodium bicarbonate (page 267)

INDEX

Japan 2
pathology 228
Chagas' disease 31
and heart 211, 220
Charcot–Bouchard aneurysms 153
chest examination 90–2
children and heart disease
infections 216
reassurance 96, 217
rhythm disturbances 217
tropics 216, 217
chlorthalidone 243
dose 244
cholesterol
blood levels 146
coronary heart disease 126
chordae tendinae rupture 165
chromaffin cells 22
circulation 16, 17
blood distribution 16, 17
pressures 28
pulmonary, blood content 17
response in heart failure 67
systemic 16
claudication
arm muscles 230, 231
estimates of distance 93, 115
see also intermittent claudication
clofibrate and cholesterol levels 126, 265
clonidine 251, 252
coarctation of the aorta
angiocardiography 64
congenital
features and surgery 185
incidence 182
features and management 150
hypertension 150
palpation 80
pulse 81
congenital cardiac malformations 8, 168, 173, 181–90, 217
causes 181, 182
cyanosis 107
detection and age 186, 187
diagnosis and investigations 187, 188
finger clubbing 107
frequency and types 182–5
incidence 181
management and degree 188, 189
mortality 186
multiple 185
murmurs 186
prophylactic measures 189, 190
risks and counselling 189
surgery 270, 271
see also individual malformations
congenital heart disease 165
causes 30
hospital stay 4
moartality, age and sex 3
connective tissue disorders, heart
involvement 212, 213
Conn's syndrome and hypertension 151, 154
aldosterone 151
conus ligament 12
coronary arteriography
angina pectoris 131, 132
indications 131, 132
techniques 64, 65, 131
coronary artery disease 128
coronary bypass surgery 133, 270
coronary care units, mobile 139

coronary heart disease 124–46
angina pectoris 128–33
clinical patterns 31, 32
community studies 124
falling mortality 124
hospital stay 4
international comparison 3, 4
mortality, age and sex 2
myocardial infarction 134–45
prognosis 132
risk factors 126–8
surgery 270
UK variation 3, 4, 124
see also myocardial infarction
coronary insufficiency, acute 134
coronary spasm 133, 134
cor pulmonale 73, 176–81
acute 176–8
diagnosis 176
electrocardiogram 176, 177
fatal 177
features 176
management and seriousness 177, 178
chronic 178–81
causes and pathology 178, 179
clinical features 179
electrocardiogram 179, 180
failure signs 179
management 180, 181
precautions 181
tropical 220
X-ray 180
Corrigan's sign 81
cough 179
cardiac disease 102
cardiovascular and respiratory disease 73, 102
features and sounds 73
creatinine phosphokinase
cardiac isoenzyme 137
features in myocardial infarction 137, 138
Cushing's disease 150
Cushing's syndrome and hypertension
causes 150
features 150, 151
management 151
cyanosis
blood pigments 107
causes and features 78, 79, 106, 107
central 107
neonatal 186, 187
oxygen use 180
peripheral 106, 107
right-to-left shunt 107
cyclimorph 139

DC cardioversion 200, 203, 240
DC shock 198, 199, 202, 267
deep venous thrombosis 221–4
causes 221
clinical features 222
fate of thrombus 221, 222
insufficiency 234
investigations 222, 223
management of established 223, 224, 262, 263
predisposition 222
prophylaxis 223
surgery 224
depolarization 35, 36; see also
electrocardiogram
dextran 223

diabetes mellitus
atherosclerosis 127
hypertension 150
vasculitis 236
diagnosis and presentation 98–119
diazepam 139
diazoxide 154, 155
diet and lipids 146
digitalis 164
electrocardiogram 46
toxicity dysrhythmias 210
digoxin
doses 242
drug interactions 241
mode of action 240
plasma levels and toxicity 241, 242, 256
management 255
poisoning 241
uses and effects 239, 240
disopyramide 253–6
disseminated intravascular coagulation 235
diuretics
adverse effects 243, 244
assessment 243
doses 247, 253
hypertension 251, 252
interactions 244
mode of action and potency 242, 243
potassium effects 244, 245
uses 242
driving after myocardial infarction 145
drugs
anticoagulant 178
antihypertensive 250–3
assessment 239
diuretic 155
modes of action 238, 239
principles of treatment 238
respiratory stimulation 181
thrombolytic 177
see also individual drugs, groups and
adverse reactions
ductus arteriosus
changes at birth 8
fetal circulation 8
persistent
features and management 184
incidence 182
murmurs 88
dyspnoea 169, 171
causes 100, 101
examination 101
features and occurrence 72, 100
grading 100, 160
mechanism 100
mitral stenosis 160
paroxysmal nocturnal 72, 100
patient history 101
dysrhythmias
focal automaticity 142
importance 141, 142
incidence after myocardial infarction 141, 142
management 142, 256
prognostic value 142
types 142, 143

Ebstein's anomaly 173
echocardiography
aortic valve 58, 60
cross sectional 59–61
left ventricle 56